Dup copy

Handbook of
Black American Health

Library of Congress Cataloging-in-Publication Data

Handbook of Black American health : the mosaic of conditions, issues,
   policies, and prospects / edited by Ivor Lensworth Livingston.
       p.   cm.
     Includes index.
     ISBN 0–313–28640–X (alk. paper)
     1. Afro-Americans—Health and hygiene.   2. Afro-Americans—Medical
   care.   I. Livingston, Ivor Lensworth.
   RA448.5.N4H364   1994
   362.1′089′96073—dc20   93–4852

British Library Cataloguing in Publication Data is available.

Library of Congress Catalog Card Number: 93–4852
ISBN: 0–313–28640–X

First published in 1994

Greenwood Press, 88 Post Road West, Westport, CT 06881
An imprint of Greenwood Publishing Group, Inc.

Printed in the United States of America

The paper used in this book complies with the
Permanent Paper Standard issued by the National
Information Standards Organization (Z39.48–1984).

10 9 8 7 6 5 4 3 2 1

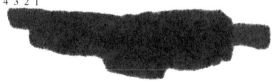

Handbook of
Black American Health

THE MOSAIC OF CONDITIONS, ISSUES, POLICIES, AND PROSPECTS

Edited by
Ivor Lensworth Livingston

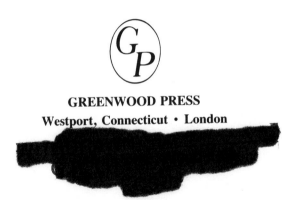

GREENWOOD PRESS
Westport, Connecticut • London

To my wife, "Toy," daughter, Litonya Selima, and son, Stefan Lensworth.

&

To the millions of African Americans and other minority people of color who are today suffering the effects of an unequal society, but who will, indeed, have a healthier "2000" tomorrow.

Contents

Illustrations

FIGURES

Foreword

The year 1993 is both a difficult and an opportune time for a book on the health of Black Americans. It is difficult because it has now been eight years since the Secretary's Task Force Report on the health of Blacks and other minorities. This report related, among other things, that there were 60,000 excess deaths per year among Blacks when compared with Whites with appropriate adjustment for age and sex. From those who monitor life and death statistics, we know that things have not improved and may, in fact, be worse, with a significant increase in the number of excess deaths per year. Thus, one might be tempted to look askance at a book about the health of Black Americans in 1993.

On the other hand, 1993 is a most opportune time to examine in depth the health status of Blacks because significant changes in health care and health professions education are on the horizon. A majority of Americans of all races and social classes are demanding such changes. Major national councils, commissions and organizations are documenting the need for such changes. Further, we have recently elected a new administration in Washington that is clearly committed to such change. In the near future, that administration will present to Congress a proposal for major health care reform in this nation. Congress will carefully examine and debate this proposal, but when deliberations are concluded, we will be moving toward major health care reform.

Because the present health care system has not been effective in bridging the gap in health status between Blacks and Whites through prevention, early diagnosis, or medical treatment, we must expect that health care reform holds hope for improving both health and health professions education for Blacks. Beyond the reform of health care and the health care system, we are also challenged to escalate our attention to, and our support for, the prevention of disease and disability.

A book that examines the health status of Blacks from a multidisciplinary perspective—clearly defining etiology, prevention strategies, enhancement of early diagnosis, and models of successful interventions—could be very timely. This is such a book. It is significant that the editor, Dr. Livingston, is trained in behavioral science, public health, and epidemiology and brings these perspectives to the book. The *Handbook of Black American Health* brings together some of the best and most committed minds on the subject of black health in a most organized and deliberate fashion. Moving from cardiovascular and general conditions through mental/behavioral-related problems and social/political conditions, the book ends with an examination of legal and social policy issues. The most recent findings and experiences with hypertension, various forms of cancer, and mental health problems are presented clearly, and questions for further examination are posited. The problem of HIV/AIDS, which was not dealt with in the Secretary's Report of 1985 but is now a leading cause of death and disability in Blacks, is thoroughly examined, including the controversy surrounding etiology and various forms of therapy. In this book, the health care system is challenged to become not only more aware, but also more representative, more culturally sensitive, and more user-friendly.

From all indications, health care reform will include incentives for both individuals and the health care system to focus more attention on prevention and health promotion. Given such a push for prevention, we will be challenged as never before to develop, implement, and evaluate the technology of prevention. Among other things, this will challenge our ability to understand and modify individual and group behavior relative to diet, exercise, stress management, sexual activity, and the avoidance of toxins. Meeting this challenge will require the most multidisciplinary health care team that we can form. Expertise in medicine, nursing, allied health, behavioral science, anthropology, ethics and economics will be brought to bear upon this effort. Most of all, it will require knowledgeable and highly motivated individuals and families.

The perspective of the broadly trained and sensitive editor, Dr. Livingston, is reflected throughout the book as these various subjects are brought together in an interdisciplinary fashion. We are reminded again of the four categories of determinants of health and illness as defined by the Surgeon General in 1979: life-style, environment, genetic/biology, and access to medical care. Although past writings have noted that life-style accounts for over 50 percent of the risk and environment and biology account for another 40 percent, leaving only 10 percent for medical care access, this book makes it clear that the interaction among these factors is a dimension that cannot be easily measured. The interaction of health factors, as seen with HIV/AIDS, is emerging as a major player. For example, when life-style and medical care cooperate, we are more likely to control hypertension, prevent cancer, and advance the immune system. Likewise, the environment where Blacks live is disproportionately burdened with toxins, including lead and carcinogens. When health care workers add their expertise and testimony to those calling for environmental changes, we can make significant progress in creating more healthful environments.

Perhaps, as never before, the *Handbook of Black American Health* makes clear why the health care work force must be interdisciplinary in function and more diverse in racial and sociocultural backgrounds. The World Health Organization was and is correct when it stated, "Health is not merely the absence of disease but the presence of complete physical, mental and social well-being." In order to protect and promote health, the health work force must be distributed equitably; however, it must also be more culturally sensitive and aware and more user-friendly and trustworthy.

Finally, we must begin to give prevention and health promotion the kind of primacy that they have not heretofore received. Such a focus not only will help to maintain and improve health, but will also help to control costs and to assure better quality. It was John Gardner who said, "Life is full of golden opportunities carefully disguised as irresolvable problems." As we move to reform our health care system, we must not miss the golden opportunity to enhance the health care and health work force role of Black Americans and other minorities. This book will be an invaluable resource as we move in that direction.

David Satcher MD., Ph.D
President
Meharry Medical College

Preface

The *Handbook of Black American Health: The Mosaic of Conditions, Issues, Policies, and Prospects,* is a 27 chapter collection of original (except for one chapter) scholarly presentations covering a variety of areas relating to the health of Blacks or African Americans. It must be noted that the terms Black and African American are used interchangeably throughout the book. Because of the varying views expressed by certain authors, the decision was made to include both terms; however, an attempt was made to have consistency within a chapter, when either term was used.

Initial thoughts about this book began approximately ten years ago, when I was pursuing postgraduate work in public health at the Harvard School of Public Health (HSPH). During this period I was responsible for coordinating a conference entitled "Selected Health Care Issues in the Black American Community," sponsored, in part, by the minority students at the HSPH. Apart from this conference, the class discussions at the HSPH and later experiences I had while pursuing postdoctoral studies in the Department of Behavioral Sciences and Health Education, at the Johns Hopkins School of Hygiene and Public Health, helped to stimulate my ideas for the book. These experiences also formulated my professional research agenda relating to my decade-long pursuit of the social epidemiology of cardiovascular and immunological diseases in Black populations in America, Africa and the Caribbean. These initial experiences, and also my subsequent research over the years in the area of Black and minority health, uncategorically suggested a void in the comprehensive illumination of "salient" health problems and issues in Black America and hence the need for this volume, its scope, and its timely importance.

As I labored over the scope and the ultimate direction the volume would take, I came to one inescapable conclusion: that, when completed, the volume must make a contribution. This need for the volume to make a contribution led in turn to the purpose of the book, which is threefold: (1) To go beyond the traditional areas covered in past publications on the health of Blacks (i.e., cardiovascular and cerebrovascular disease and cancer) and adopt a multidisciplinary focus on a variety of other conditions and issues. (2) Apart from presenting a representative selection of conditions and issues that contribute to poorer morbidity and mortality rates for Blacks, to provide practical strategies, models, and recommendations to address these conditions and issues. (3) Lastly, based on the two previous objectives, to provide an illuminating forum to provoke dialogue and debate for academicians, clinicians, researchers, and politicians alike to debate and discuss the urgency of the Black health crisis and, it is hoped, how best to intervene now and in the future to reduce racial disparities in health.

Blacks in this country have made improvements in their health; however, a multitude of racial disparities still exists. A major reason is that, although legislation (e.g., Medicaid and Medicare in 1965) may have made health care relatively more available and affordable, the fundamental and unequal structure of American society, which is primarily responsible for racial disparities in health, did not and has not changed.

The Report of the Secretary's Task Force on Black and Minority Health (1985), a landmark clarion call for change, was revealing, showing, for example, that there are 60,000 excess Black deaths annually compared with White Americans. However, since its publication much has changed for the worse and little has changed for the better. Not only do Black babies die earlier than White babies, but in recent years reports suggest that a continued reduction and leveling off in life expectancy for Blacks has occurred while there has been, in contrast, an extension for Whites.

Understanding health in general is a difficult undertaking, and understanding Black health in particular is perhaps even more difficult. The complexities associated with understanding Black health are compounded by several factors, for example, intraracial variations, socioeconomic status or poverty, racial admixture, health practices, and the compelling realities of an unequal, unjust, insensitive, and institutionally racist American society. Many changes over the last twenty-five years in the geopolitical, sociopolitical, and technological arenas, both in this country and overseas, while ushering in many new opportunities, have also brought new miseries or exacerbated old ones (such as toxic-waste dumping, chemical abuse/dependency, urban congestion, fatalistic attitudes, and unemployment), especially for minority communities.

This volume is not intended to provide an exhaustive coverage for *all* major conditions and issues affecting the health of Blacks. Instead, its 27 chapters, divided among the 5 parts of the book, provide a mosaic of salient conditions, issues, and policies related to Black American health, heretofore (to the best of my knowledge) not covered under a single volume. The multidisciplinary approach to health adopted in this volume is one of its major advantages. The forty-four contributing authors, drawn from institutions across America, are premier scholars in their respective fields. The scope and multidisciplinary nature of the volume are, in part, reflected in the areas from which these authors came: clinical medicine, epidemiology, health care administration, medical sociology, nursing, nutritional sciences, political science, psychology, public health, and social work, to mention only a few. A related advantage is the public health background of most of the authors, which lent itself not only to an illuminating presentation of epidemiologic data, where applicable, but also to the discussion of designated problems from prevention and interventionist points of view. It also supported the discussions of how best to intervene to address a problem, allowing authors to discuss prospects and suggest recommendations.

By way of a summary, two questions need to be answered about this handbook: (1) Who is the intended audience? (2) What is its significance?

Because of the multidisciplinary focus of this handbook it can be used by a variety of professionals and disciplines in the behavioral sciences, allied sciences, and clinical sciences. Whether the volume is used as a reference text, a main text, or a supplementary text from which selected readings are taken, it provides a cross-section of readers with a wealth of current information pertaining to the disproportionate incidence of morbidity and mortality in the Black American population.

This handbook is significant because of (a) its timely presentation of crucial issues pertaining to the health of Black Americans, especially now when the Clinton Administration, policy-makers, and others are debating the need and direction of health care reform; (b) its multidisciplinary and public health foci; (c) its ability to stimulate and provoke serious thought, debate, and policy decisions in a variety of forums involving crucial areas influencing the health of Blacks living in America; and (d) the variety of models and recommendations suggested by knowledgeable scholars, all within a framework for social action and change, during the remainder of this century as well as in the 21st century. While racial parity in health will not be achieved by Blacks "overnight," it is my hope that this handbook will contribute important information to early and sustained improvements in health for vast numbers of the at-risk Black American population. Therefore, as we look toward a brighter 21st century, which involves racial parity in health, it is further hoped that this handbook will help to make a brighter future out of the darkness of the past.

> The philosophies of one age have become the absurdities of the next, and the foolishness of yesterday has become the wisdom of tomorrow.
>
> Sir William Osler

Acknowledgments

The writing and completion of this volume is the outcome of the work of a collective group of persons who, although not necessarily knowing each other, were bonded by a dedication to show, yet another time, the disheartening realities and disparities regarding the health of Blacks living in America today. The individual and collective assistance I received from these persons is reflected in the quality of this completed volume.

Although the list seems endless, I would particularly like to thank certain individuals who did indeed make a difference. Thanks first of all goes to my family, who fully supported me throughout the entire period of the project. My wife's unyielding support was especially helpful, not only from a clinical sense regarding verification and clarification of information, but from a "partner's" sense, supporting me during the "aching-back" hours of the morning. In a similar manner, the unyielding support received from my relatively young children, although difficult at times for them, was particularly gratifying.

Various persons were very helpful in the early stages of the project, especially when I was crystallizing my thoughts about directions to take and areas to cover in the volume. From a clinical point of view, Drs. Charles Curry and Otelio Randall of Howard University and Dr. David Levine of Johns Hopkins University were especially helpful and generous with their time. Directions for the overall book were well received from my colleagues in the department, Drs. Ralph Gomes, Ron Manuel, G. Franklin Edwards, and James Scott. My former classmates at the Harvard School of Public Health, Drs. J. Jacques Carter, Deborah Blocker, Gerald Groves, and Omowale Amuleru-Marshall, who also contributed chapters to the volume, were helpful with ideas regarding the direction of the book.

My home institution, Howard University, and the Department of Sociology/

Anthropology provided me with sabbatical leave at the onset of the project that was most helpful in the writing and submitting of the prospectus. Dr. Florence Bonner, Chairperson of the Department, was especially supportive of my involvement with the project and gave me "full access" to all available resources of the department. I would like to thank the secretarial staff, especially Ms. Odette Davis, for the help rendered throughout the project. The checking and verification of references were ably carried out by my graduate assistants Ms. Anyasa Otado and Mr. Douglas Fuller.

Finally, I want to thank my contributing authors who worked diligently to produce outlines, drafts, and final chapters. In many cases, there were severe time and other professional constraints; yet, as professionals, they came through. Without this kind of professional dedication and commitment, this important volume on Black American health would have remained just an idea. I would be remiss if I did not express my appreciation to the publisher, Greenwood Publishing Group, Inc. First, to the staff members who were very diligent and professional in their duties, especially my assigned production editor, Julie Cullen. Second, to Dr. James Sabin, Executive Vice President, who was readily accessible and who helped provide the opportunity for publishing the ideas expressed by a variety of scholars across the country on important issues affecting the health of Blacks living in the United States.

Ivor Lensworth Livingston

Abbreviations

CHAPTER 1

AMI	Acute myocardial infarction
CHD	Coronary heart disease
HD	Hypertensive disease
HHD	Hypertensive heart disease
ICD-9	International Classification of Diseases, 9th
IDS	Ill-defined stroke
IH	Intracranial hemorrhage
NCHS	National Center for Health Statistics Revision
NHANESII	Second National Health Nutrition and Examination Survey
NHANESI	First National Health Nutrition and Examination Survey
NHDS	National Hospital Discharge Survey
NHIS	National Health Interview Survey
TES	Thromboembolic stroke

CHAPTER 2

CAD	Coronary artery disease
CHD	Coronary heart disease
HDL	High density lipoprotein
IHD	Ischemic heart disease

| LDL | Low density lipoprotein |
| MI | Myocardial infarction |

CHAPTER 3

MRFIT	Multiple risk factors intervention trial
SAH	Subarachnoid hemorrhage
TIA	Transient ischemic attacks

CHAPTER 4

CHW	Community health worker
DBP	Diastolic blood pressure
ESRD	End-stage renal disease
HBP	High blood pressure
HDFP	Hypertension Detection and Follow-up Program
NHANESII	Second National Health Nutrition Examination Survey
SHEP	Systolic Hypertension in the Elderly Program
TOHP	Trials of hypertension prevention

CHAPTER 5

ADPKD	Autosomal dominant polycystic kidney disease
CAPD	Continuous ambulatory peritoneal dialysis
ESRD	End-stage renal disease
GN	Glomerulonephritis
HCFA	Health Care Financing Administration
MRFIT	Multiple risk factors intervention trial
NIDDK	National Institute of Diabetes and Digestive Kidney Disease
NIDDM	Non-insulin dependent diabetic mellitus
SLE	Systemic lupus erythematosus
USRDS	United States Renal Data System

CHAPTER 6

ACS	American Cancer Society
CDC	Centers for Disease Control
NCHS	National Cancer for Health Statistics
NCI	National Cancer Institute
SEER	Surveillance, Epidemiology and End Results

CHAPTER 7

| BMI | Body-mass index |
| FBS | Fasting blood sugar |

GDM	Gestational diabetes mellitus
IGT	Impaired glucose tolerance
IDDM	Insulin-dependent diabetes mellitus
OGGT	Oral glucose tolerance test
NDDG	National Diabetes Data Group
NIDDM	Non-insulin-dependent diabetes mellitus

CHAPTER 8

COPD	Chronic obstructive pulmonary disease
DHHS	Department of Health and Human Services
FEV-1	Forced expiratory volume in one second
FVC	Forced vital capacity
ICD	International Classification of Disease
NCHS	National Centers for Health Statistics
NHANES	National Health and Nutrition Examination Survey
NHANES I	First National Health and Nutrition Examination Survey
NHANES III	Third National Health and Nutrition Examination Survey
NHIS	National Health Interview Survey
WHO	World Health Organization

CHAPTER 9

CIPI	Chronic Illness Problem Inventory
EPO	Erythropoietin
GHQ	General health questionnaire
Hgb-F	Fetal hemoglobin
HU	Hydroxyurea
SCA	Sickle cell anemia
SCD	Sickle cell disease
SFS	Social functioning schedule

CHAPTER 10

CSME	Clinically significant macular edema
DRS	Diabetic retinopathy study
ETDRS	Early treatment diabetic retinopathy study
IRMA	Intra-retinal microvascular abnormalities
NVD	Neovascularization of the optic disc
NVE	Neovascularization elsewhere

| PDR | Proliferative diabetic retinopathy |
| PSR | Proliferative diabetic retinopathy |

CHAPTER 11

CDC	Centers for Disease Control
HIV	Human immunodeficiency virus
IDU	Injection drug use
SIV	Simian immunodeficiency virus

CHAPTER 12

| ECA | Epidemiologic catchment area |

CHAPTER 13

| FARS | Fatal accident reporting system |

CHAPTER 14

AA	Alcoholics Anonymous
AOD	Alcohol and other drug use
ECA	Epidemiologic Catchment Area
FDA	Food and Drug Administration
IVDU	Intravenous drug users
LAAM	Levo-alpha acetylmenthadol
NA	Narcotics Anonymous
NHSDA	National Household Survey on Drug Abuse

CHAPTER 15

GAO	General Accounting Office
IGUR	Intrauterine growth retardation
IMR	Infant mortality rate
IOM	Institute of Medicine
LBW	Low birth weight
MLBW	Moderately low birth weight
NAPARE	The National Association of Perinatal Addiction Research and Education
NMR	Neonatal mortality rate
PMR	Postneonatal mortality rate
SES	Socioeconomic status
VLBW	Very low birth weight

CHAPTER 16

| ACTH | Adrenocorticotropic hormone |
| GAS | General Adaptation Syndrome |

| SES | Socioeconomic status |
| SPPM | Sociopsychophysiological model |

CHAPTER 17

DIS	Diagnostic Interview Schedule
ECA	Epidemiologic Catchment Area
PTSD	Post-traumatic stress disorder

CHAPTER 18

ARIC	Atherosclerosis risk in communities
CARDIA	Coronary artery risk development in young adults
HDLC	High density lipoprotein cholesterol
HTN	Hypertension
LDLC	Low density lipoprotein cholesterol
NHANES II	Second National Health and Nutrition Examination Survey
NHIS	National Health Interview Survey
PUFAS	Polyunsaturated fatty acids

CHAPTER 19

| HCHP | Health Care for the Homeless Program |
| NACHC | National Association of Community Health Centers |

CHAPTER 20

ICPSR	Inter-university Consortium for Political and Social Research
NCHS	National Center for Health Statistics
NHANES	National Health Nutrition Examination Survey
NHIS	National Health Interview Survey
SOA	Supplement on Aging

CHAPTER 21

FFIEC	Federal Financial Institution Examination Council
LULU	Locally unwanted land use
NIMBY	Not in my backyard

CHAPTER 22

AFDC	Aid to Families with Dependent Children
AIDS	Acquired Immunodeficiency Syndrome
LD	Learning disabilities
MCH	Maternal child health

NBCDI	National Black Child Development Institute
WIC	Women, Infants and Children

CHAPTER 23

AAMC	Association of Educational Progress
GMENAC	Graduate Medical Examination National Advisory Committee
HBCUS	Historically Black colleges and universities
MARC	Minority access to research careers
MBRS	Minority Biomedical Research Support
NAEP	National assessment of educational progress
NIGMS	National Institute of General Medical Sciences

CHAPTER 24

HMO	Health maintenance organization
IPA	Independent practice association
PPO	Preferred provider organization
OMP	Office of Minority Programs

CHAPTER 27

E-I-O	Environment, Individual, Organization
HFC	Health Field Concept

Introduction

Ivor Lensworth Livingston

For many persons concerned with the public's health, the year 2000 and beyond hold a special importance. The year 2000 will bring to its conclusion a tumultuous century, which was characterized by wars, famines, scientific achievements, rapid population growth, and increased life expectancy for Americans as a whole. For the federal government the year 2000 and beyond are particularly important, because its *Healthy People 2000* initiative aims to significantly improve the nation's health in the twenty-first century.

For some skeptics who look beyond the posturing of program bureaucrats and technocrats and other like-minded persons, the belief is that the needed ''seeds'' have not been adequately sown to reap the intended harvest, especially as it relates to improvements in the health conditions of Blacks living in the United States. The *Handbook of Black American Health: The Mosaic of Conditions, Issues, Policies, and Prospects* provides authoritative, factual, and insightful information and guidelines about how the ''seeds'' can, and should, be sown to reap the intended harvest of eventual racial parity in health now and into the 21st century.

This 27 chapter volume shows the complexity and scope of conditions and issues that contribute to racial disparities in health. In the book's comprehensive view, these conditions and issues include, but are not limited to, the leading causes of morbidity and mortality (e.g., cardiovascular disease, cerebrovascular disease and stroke). Some rarely addressed areas (i.e., as contributors to the morbidity and mortality of Blacks) are included: ophthalmology (especially the problem of glaucoma), the politics of health and health care, unintentional injuries (e.g., drownings), homelessness, and the relatively new area of toxic pollution in the context of environmental racism.

The plight of Blacks is particularly devastating and urgent because, as a group, they experience a disproportionate burden of poverty, sickness, and death. By way of summary statistics, one-third of Blacks live in poverty, a rate three times that of the White population. Over half live in central cities, areas characterized by poverty, urban congestion, poor schools, a pervasive drug culture, unemployment, and stress. However, the best cumulative statistic that underscores the racial disparities in health is life expectancy, in which Black males (64.8) and females (73.5) trail behind their White male (72.7) and female (79.2) counterparts.

This volume is not intended to examine exhaustively all critical areas affecting the health of Blacks. However, as a call for action, its 27 chapters represent a variety of conditions and issues, all of which need serious examination in any attempt to achieve racial parity in health.

The handbook is organized into 5 parts, within which chapters are grouped according to one or more commonalities.

In Part I, "Cardiovascular and Related Chronic Conditions," there are five chapters. This section holds priority status, because cardiovascular diseases are the number-one killer of all Americans. Chapter 1, by Richard Gillum, introduces the area with an overview of cardiovascular diseases. Chapter 2, by Charles Curry, looks specifically at coronary heart disease, its clinical manifestations and risk factors. Chapter 3, by Gary Friday, examines cerebrovascular disease in Blacks, the number-three killer of all Americans. He looks at the various types of stroke and their treatment and risk factors. In Chapter 4, Lee Bone and colleagues discuss hypertension in Blacks. They highlight its epidemiology and the value of health education to intervene to control hypertension in community populations of at-risk Blacks. A case study of an East Baltimore community is presented to buttress their views. In Chapter 5, Camille Jones and Lawrence Agodoa examine the issue of end-stage renal disease in both children and adults, discussing its causes, distribution, and treatment in the general population.

In Part II, "General Chronic Conditions," comprising five chapters, a selected number of general (or noncardiovascular) chronic diseases are grouped. As with Part I, the diseases discussed in this part, or their sequelae, substantially contribute to the disproportionate incidence of morbidity and mortality among Blacks. In Chapter 6, Ki Moon Bang looks at cancer among Blacks, examining epidemiological studies and risk factors. In Chapter 7, Eugene Tull, Mohammed Makame, and Jeffrey Roseman look at diabetes mellitus in the African-American population, considering the different types of diabetes, the etiology of diabetes, and its risk factors and treatment modalities. In Chapter 8, Ki Moon Bang looks at chronic obstructive pulmonary disease (COPD) and discusses its etiology, distribution, risk factors, and treatment modalities. In Chapter 9, Kermit Nash and Joseph Telfair look at sickle cell anemia and use a biopsychosocial model to suggest better ways to understand the disease and to intervene when it becomes necessary. In Chapter 10, Steven McLeod and Maurice Rabb look at ophthalmology in Blacks, with an emphasis on selected entities. Some of these entities, which present differently and are sometimes disproportionately seen in Blacks, include cataract, glaucoma, and diabetic retinopathy. The distribution of these entities are discussed, as are their risk factors and treatment.

Part III, "Mental and Behavior-Related Conditions," comprises eight chapters, making it the largest section. Several conditions that have a mental and/or behavioral component are included. In Chapter 11, Wayne Greaves looks at the epidemiology of HIV infection, AIDS, and sexually transmitted diseases. He discusses the subgroups who are at risk and the various treatment modalities that are available. In Chapter 12, Darnell Hawkins, Alexander Crosby, and Marcella Hammett examine the epidemiology of intentional injuries, emphasizing homicide, suicide, and assaultive violence. In Chapter 13, Christine Branche-Dorsey, Julie Russell, Arlene Greenspan, and Terence Chorba discuss the epidemiology of unintentional injuries, focusing on motor-vehicle injuries, fire and burn injuries, drowning, unintentional firearm injuries, and occupational injuries. In Chapter 14, Gerald Groves and Omowale Amuleru-Marshall look at the epidemiology of chemical use and dependency, using national data sets to make their claims regarding etiology, treatment, prognosis, and distribution. They focus on alcohol consumption, tobacco use, illicit drug use, and co-morbidities associated with using/abusing these substances.

Feroz Ahmed, in Chapter 15, looks at the epidemiology of infant mortality in the District of Columbia as well as over the entire U.S. population. He discusses risk factors and related issues associated with infant mortality among Blacks. In Chapter 16, Ivor Lensworth Livingston examines the role stress plays in the health of Blacks, especially those who are at risk because of their low socioeconomic status. He uses a sociopsychophysiological model (SPPM) of the stress process to illustrate his claims. In Chapter 17, David Williams and Brenda Fenton examine the epidemiology of mental health among African Americans. Their discussion focuses, in part, on the Epidemiologic Catchment Area Study (ECA) to derive population-based estimates of mental disorders among Blacks. Their discussion also includes risk factors, treatment, and emergent issues. Chapter 18, by Deborah Blocker, looks at nutrition concerns of Blacks. The diet-related diseases and problems she examines include coronary heart disease, hypertension, diabetes mellitus, obesity, and selected cancers. She suggests several recommendations to reduce dietary-related diseases and other problems among Blacks.

In Part IV, "Sociopolitical Conditions and Related Issues," five chapters deal with areas that are not directly disease-oriented. However, these conditions and issues are important contributors to the morbidity and mortality of Blacks. The concerns grouped in this section have become issues for the health of Blacks, and they have arisen because of deficiencies or inaction associated with the social and political realms of society. Chapter 19, by Gregg Barak, deals with the expanding problem of homelessness in America. Looking at the epidemiology of homelessness, he discusses its emergence, existence, and eradication in the context of a class-driven and materialist economy. He suggests several strategies for its ultimate eradication. In Chapter 20, Ron Manuel looks at the physical, psychological, and social health of the Black elderly in America. Using national data sets, he examines trends, vulnerability and health of the Black elderly compared with their White counterparts.

In Chapter 21, which was originally published in the Urban League's *State of Black America 1992*, Robert Bullard discusses the urban infrastructure, focusing on the social, environmental, and health risks to Blacks. He emphasizes the problems associated with urban congestion and, very important, toxic pollution/dumping in minority communities. He studies various major cities to buttress his points about the realities associated with acts of environmental racism. In Chapter 22, Dionne Jones and Veronica Roberts discuss crucial problems and issues relating to the growth, development, and health of Black children. In Chapter 23, John Ukawuilulu and Ivor Lensworth Livingston look at issues relating to the underrepresentation of Black health care professionals and related personnel. The authors discuss why the problem exists and offer a variety of solutions.

In Part V, "Legal and Social Policy Issues" 4 chapters deal with and/or are affected by legal and/or social policy considerations. In Chapter 24, Stephanie Kong, B. Waine Kong, and Singleton McAllister examine the correlation of politics and health in an American society that is both multiracial and multicultural in composition. They argue for policies that reflect these realities and offer a variety of recommendations to augment their positions. In Chapter 25, Woodrow Jones, Jr., and Antonio Rene discuss problems and solutions related to barriers to health services. A review of the literature, along with national data, augments their claims that Blacks experience barriers when they use health care services. In Chapter 26, Collins Airhihenbuwa and Agatha Lowe discuss how empowerment as health education-intervention can improve the health of African Americans. In Chapter 27, the concluding chapter of the volume, Ivor Lensworth Livingston and J. Jacques Carter discuss ways of improving the health of the Black community, now and as we approach the 21st century. An Environment-Individual-Organization Model (E-I-O) is presented and discussed as a framework for social action. Various improvement strategies are also discussed for action, within the context of the E-I-O model.

A CALL FOR ACTION

This volume identifies a variety of conditions, issues, and policies that both directly and indirectly influence the health of Blacks living in the United States. It also offers information on prospects now as we approach the 21st century and beyond. Consistent with the theme of the book, most of the chapters not only discuss the respective conditions, issues, and policies that are detrimental to the health of Blacks, but they also offer information, guidelines, and/or recommendations to remedy the problem. In many cases (e.g., Chapters 9, 16 and 27) original models are introduced as frameworks for action. Sixty-thousand excess deaths a year for Blacks is an excessive price to pay, especially when, as a nation, we have the ''tools'' to prevent this problem. It is hoped that the array of information presented in this volume will serve to further inform and reawaken the need to use these ''tools'' to achieve parity in health for Blacks living in the United States.

I

Cardiovascular and Related Chronic Conditions

1

The Epidemiology of Cardiovascular Diseases: An American Overview

Richard F. Gillum

Major cardiovascular diseases were the cause of 931,838 deaths in the United States in 1989 (Advance Report, 1991). Heart disease was the leading cause of death, and cerebrovascular disease was the third leading cause of death (Advance Report, 1991). Of the 2,150,466 total deaths, heart disease accounted for 733,867 (34.1%) and cerebrovascular disease for 145,551 (6.8%). The patterns of mortality and morbidity from these and other cardiovascular diseases generally display strong associations with race, age, and gender. Using data from the National Center for Health Statistics (NCHS), this chapter will highlight selected aspects of these patterns, focusing particular attention on disparities adversely affecting Black Americans.

DISEASES OF THE HEART

In 1989 age-adjusted death rates for all causes were 60 percent higher in Black men than in White men, and 56 percent higher in Black women than in White women (Advance Report, 1991). Heart disease accounted for the following percentages (number of deaths) of total deaths by sex and race: White male (WM) 34.2 (325,397), White female (WF) 35.8 (323,469), Black male (BM) 26.2 (38,321), and black female (BF) 32.3 (39,110) (Advance Report, 1991). Table 1.1 shows age-adjusted death rates for diseases of the heart for selected years from 1950 through 1989 (National Center for Health Statistics [NCHS], 1992). This category is defined since 1979 by the following codes of the International Classification of Diseases, Ninth Revision (ICD-9), for the underlying cause of death: 390–398, 402, 404–429. In 1989, age-adjusted rates were 87 percent higher in males than in females and 43 percent higher in Blacks than in

Table 1.1
Age-adjusted Death Rates for Diseases of the Heart by Race and Sex: United States, 1950–1989

Year	White Male	White Female	Black Male	Black Female	Race Ratio Male	Race Ratio Female
1950	381.1	223.6	415.5	349.5	1.09	1.56
1960	375.4	197.1	381.2	292.6	1.02	1.48
1970	347.6	167.8	375.9	251.7	1.08	1.50
1980	277.5	134.6	327.3	201.1	1.18	1.49
1983	257.8	126.7	308.2	191.5	1.20	1.51
1984	249.5	124.0	300.1	186.6	1.20	1.50
1985	244.5	121.7	301.0	186.8	1.23	1.53
1986	234.8	119.0	294.3	185.1	1.25	1.56
1987	225.9	116.3	287.1	180.8	1.27	1.55
1988	220.5	114.2	286.2	181.1	1.30	1.59
1989	205.9	106.6	272.6	172.9	1.32	1.62

Source: Data from *Health United States, 1991,* National Center for Health Statistics (1992).

Whites. The ratio of rates in Blacks to those in Whites was much higher for younger persons than for older persons.

Data from the 1989 National Hospital Discharge Survey (NHDS) indicate an estimated 3.0 million discharges among Whites, 381 thousand among non-Whites, and 357 thousand among persons of unknown race with a first-listed diagnosis of heart disease (ICD-9 Clinical Modification 391–392.0, 393–398, 402, 404, 410–416, 420–429) (Graves, 1992). It should be noted that NHDS samples discharges, not individual patients. Because of the relatively large number of surveyed cases with race not recorded on the face sheet of the medical record, race-specific analyses are hindered and must be interpreted with caution. Pending resolution of this problem, a few studies have used various analytic techniques to make racial comparisons for specific diseases using NHDS data. The results of some of these studies follow.

Coronary Heart Disease

Mortality

Over half the deaths due to heart disease in 1989 were attributed to coronary heart disease (CHD) (ICD-9 410–414), the percentage being lower for Blacks than Whites: WM 72.0 percent (234,365), WF 67.2 percent (217,443), BM 52.8 percent (20,243), and BF 54.0 percent (21,133). Table 1.2 shows death rates for CHD by age, sex, and race (NCHS, 1989). Also shown are rates for two CHD subgroups, acute myocardial infarction (AMI) (ICD-9 410) and chronic IHD (ICD-9 412, 414). At younger ages, rates were higher in Black than White men. At all ages below 75, rates were higher in Black than White women. Black-White ratios were higher for chronic CHD than for acute myocardial infarction (AMI). Recent analyses of data from 40 states revealed that CHD death was more likely to occur out of hospital or in emergency rooms in Blacks than in Whites, in men than in women, and in younger than in older persons (Gillum, 1989b). In 1968–75 CHD death rates declined faster in Blacks than Whites, while in 1976–85 rates in White males declined faster than in Blacks or in White women (Sempos, Cooper, Kovar & McMillen, 1988).

Morbidity

In the United States in 1989, 571,000 Whites, 55,000 non-Whites, and 69,000 patients with race not stated were discharged with a first-listed diagnosis of AMI (Graves, 1992). Additional discharges with other CHD diagnoses were coronary atherosclerosis: 351,000 Whites, 25,000 non-Whites, and 31,000 with race not stated; other ischemic heart disease: 727,000 Whites, 82,000 non-Whites, and 84,000 with race not stated. Using imputation of missing data for race or case-control techniques, several analyses of NHDS data indicated that AMI discharge rates were lower and in-hospital AMI mortality rates were higher for Blacks than for Whites in the United States in the 1980s (Roig et al., 1987; Gillum, 1987c). In 1973–1984, AMI case fatality rates were 11 percent in Whites and 16 percent in non-Whites aged 55–59 (Roig et al., 1987). Further, coronary artery bypass surgery rates were lower among Blacks than Whites (Ford, Cooper, Castaner, Simmons & Mar, 1989; Gillum, 1987d). In 1981, age-adjusted rates per 100,000 for coronary artery bypass surgery for persons aged 35–74 years were 51.9 for Blacks and 186.1 for Whites; age-adjusted rates for coronary angiography were 109.3 for Blacks and 236.4 for Whites (Gillum, 1987d).

The prevalence of coronary heart disease was estimated in the Health Examination Survey of 1960–62 using all available clinical data (NCHS, 1965; Gillum, 1982). At ages 55–64, percentages with definite CHD were WM 10.3, BM 5.7, WF 4.7, and BF 5.5. Percentages with definite or suspect CHD were WM 14.4, BM 13.4, WF 10.0, and BF 9.8. However, more recent estimates have been based on self-reported history of diagnosis or on symptom questionnaires (Ries, 1990; Collins, 1988; Havlik et al., 1987; LaCroix, Haynes, Savage

Table 1.2
Death Rates for Ischemic Heart Disease by Age, Sex, and Race: United States, 1989

Age (years)	Men White	Men Black	Women White	Women Black	Ratio* Men	Ratio* Women
			Rate per 100,000			
			Ischemic Heart Disease			
35-44	28.3	44.6	5.6	15.9	1.6	2.8
45-54	125.9	177.7	30.3	68.0	1.4	2.2
55-64	386.0	421.9	129.6	236.8	1.1	1.8
65-74	917.9	835.4	418.0	578.2	0.9	1.4
75-84	2239.4	1785.6	1370.2	1411.2	0.8	1.0
0-85+**	148.2	142.9	71.0	90.9	1.0	1.3
			Acute Myocardial Infarction			
35-44	16.7	23.7	3.4	8.6	1.4	2.5
45-54	76.9	95.1	18.5	39.8	1.2	2.2
55-64	227.4	231.3	77.8	134.4	1.0	1.7
65-74	507.0	454.6	237.8	316.0	0.9	1.3
75-84	1129.5	892.1	681.9	705.0	0.8	1.0
0-85+**	80.0	75.4	36.7	48.1	0.9	1.3

Table 1.2—Continued

Age (years)	Men		Women		Ratio*	
	White	Black	White	Black	Men	Women

Chronic Ischemic Heart Disease

Age (years)	White	Black	White	Black	Men	Women
35–44	11.2	20.6	2.1	7.0	1.8	3.3
45–54	47.3	79.0	11.4	26.4	1.7	2.3
55–64	154.1	182.9	50.5	98.2	1.2	1.9
65–74	403.0	368.9	176.7	254.3	0.9	1.4
75–84	1094.7	865.8	678.0	689.7	0.8	1.0
0–85+**	66.8	65.3	33.6	41.5	1.0	1.2

Source: Unpublished data from the National Vital Statistics System, National Center for Health Statistics.

*Black/White.

**Age-adjusted by the direct method, standard: 1940 U.S. population.

& Havlik, 1989). Data from the National Health Interview Survey (NHIS) yielded average annual self-reported prevalence rates per 1,000 of reported CHD at ages 55–64 in 1982–84: WM 141.7, BM 59.7, WF 59.7, and BF 38.0 (Havlik et al., 1987). At ages 45–64 in 1985–87, reported prevalence did not vary among Blacks with family incomes less than $20,000 compared to those with incomes of $20,000 or more (Ries, 1990). However, prevalence was inversely related to family income in Whites, resulting in greater Black-White differences in lower than in higher income persons.

The NHIS estimated that 286,000 Blacks suffered from CHD in the United States (Ries, 1990). Despite pooling three years of data, estimates for Blacks had relative standard errors of 30 percent or greater. Further, substantial underreporting among Blacks is possible in this survey. The London School of Hygiene Chest Pain Questionnaire was administered in the Second National Health and Nutrition Examination Survey (NHANESII), yielding age-adjusted prevalence rates of angina pectoris at ages 25–74 of BM 6.2 percent (1.1), BF 6.8 percent (1.1), WM 3.9 percent (0.4), and WF 6.3 percent (0.5) (LaCroix et al., 1989). Thus no firm conclusions were possible about racial differences in CHD prevalence for the United States, because of varying results of surveys, which depended on the methods used and the years covered (Gillum, 1982).

The NHANESI Epidemiologic Follow-up Study (NHEFS) provided estimates of CHD incidence. However, because of the limited numbers of Blacks in the cohort, the precision of estimates for Blacks was limited. After 10 years of follow-up, the incidence of CHD events (percent of group) by baseline ages was as follows: 55–64, WM 17.4, WF 8.0, BM 11.6, BF 10.1; 65–74, WM 28.1, WF 22.7, BM 23.4, BF 21.7 (Leaverton, Havlik, Ingster-Moore, LaCroix & Cornoni-Huntley, 1990). Case ascertainment was based on death certificate and hospital discharge diagnoses, with data limitations as described elsewhere (Madans, Kleinman et al., 1986; Madans, Cox et al., 1986). Systolic blood pressure in men and diabetes in women were significant predictors of CHD in Blacks (Leaverton et al., 1990). However, follow-up of larger cohorts of Blacks would be desirable to attain the statistical power needed to assess all risk factors of interest. Two recent analyses suggested that elevated pulse rate and relatively low serum albumin concentration may be cardiovascular risk factors in Blacks (Gillum, Makuc & Feldman, 1991; Gillum & Makuc, 1992). Useful analyses of total mortality have appeared for both Blacks and Whites (Madans, Cox et al., 1986; Cornoni-Huntley, LaCroix & Havlik, 1989). Adjusting for six major cardiovascular risk factors (smoking, systolic blood pressure, cholesterol level, body mass index, alcohol intake, and diabetes) decreased the excess total mortality in Blacks compared to Whites in the NHEFS cohort by 31 percent; a further 38 percent was accounted for by family income, leaving 31 percent unexplained (Otten, Teutsch, Williamson & Marks, 1990).

Epidemiologic patterns and trends in coronary heart disease risk factors in Blacks have been extensively reviewed elsewhere (Gillum & Grant, 1982; Eaker, Packard & Thom, 1989). National levels and trends in the major risk factors, elevated blood pressure, cigarette smoking, and elevated serum cholesterol are published regularly (NCHS, 1992). The higher prevalence of cigarette smoking as well as hypertension are continuing causes of concern for Blacks. For example, in 1988 the prevalence of current cigarette smoking among persons aged 45–64 was BM 43.2 percent, WM 30.0 percent, BF 29.5 percent, and WF 27.7 percent (NCHS, 1992). Further, knowledge about cardiovascular disease risk factors was lower in Blacks than Whites, even after controlling age and education, in the United States in 1985 (Ford & Jones, 1991). The need persists for longitudinal studies to establish the relative importance of coronary risk factors in Blacks, especially in Black women.

Other Heart Diseases

Nearly half the deaths from diseases of the heart were attributed to causes other than coronary heart disease among Blacks. Data from NCHS have been used to examine epidemiologic patterns of several other heart diseases. In 1982, age-adjusted death rates for acute rheumatic fever and rheumatic heart disease combined (ICD-9 390–398) were higher in women than in men and slightly lower in Blacks than Whites (Gillum, 1986a). Death rates for congestive heart failure (ICD-9 428) were higher in older than younger, male than female, and Black than White persons in 1981 (Gillum, 1987a). A similar pattern was seen for hospital discharge rates. Cardiomyopathy (ICD-9 425) death rates were higher in older than younger, male than female, and non-White or Black than White persons (Gillum, 1986b; Gillum, 1989a). Blacks had age-adjusted hospital discharge rates 2.2 times higher than Whites aged 35–74. Pulmonary embolism (ICD-9 415) death and hospital discharge rates were also higher in Blacks than Whites (Gillum, 1987b).

Summary

Heart disease was the leading cause of death for Blacks and Whites in the United States in 1989. The majority of these deaths were attributed to coronary heart disease. The apparent distribution of CHD manifestations was different in Blacks compared to Whites. Death rates for CHD were higher in Blacks than Whites for women and for younger persons. A greater percentage of deaths occurred out of hospital in Blacks than in Whites. The incomplete morbidity data suggest angina pectoris and chronic CHD excesses in Blacks with AMI excesses in Whites. However, AMI case fatality may have been higher in Blacks. Further studies are needed to determine whether these patterns can be validated and whether a combination of adverse risk factor profiles (especially in Black women), poorer access to preventive care, pre-hospital AMI care, and surgical care for angina combined to produce preventable coronary mortality in Blacks.

STROKE

Mortality

In 1989, cerebrovascular diseases (ICD-9 430–438) was the third leading cause of death in BF and WF and the fourth leading cause in BM and WM (Advance Report, 1991). Cerebrovascular diseases accounted for the following percentages (number of deaths) of total deaths by sex and race: WM 5.1 (48,563), WF 8.5 (76,953), BM 5.3 (7,739), and BF 8.4 (10,240). Table 1.3 shows age-adjusted death rates for selected years from 1950 through 1989 by sex and race (NCHS, 1992). In 1989, age-adjusted death rates were 89 percent higher in Blacks than in Whites. The relative excess mortality among Blacks rose sharply with decreasing age. Stroke mortality rates among Blacks were much higher in the Southeast than in other U.S. regions in 1980 (Rocella & Lenfant, 1989).

The long-term decline in stroke mortality rates accelerated after 1973 for each race and sex group (Klag, Whelton & Seidler, 1989; Gillum, 1988). Between 1980 and 1989, age-adjusted death rates declined for each major sex and race group (Table 1.3). A recent report indicated that the rate of decline was less

Table 1.3
**Age-adjusted Death Rates for Cerebrovascular Disease by Sex and Race: United
States, 1950–1989**

Year	White Male	White Female	Black Male	Black Female	Race Ratio Male	Race Ratio Female
1950	87.0	79.7	146.2	155.6	1.68	1.95
1960	80.3	68.7	141.2	139.5	1.76	2.03
1970	68.8	56.2	124.2	107.9	1.81	1.92
1980	41.9	35.2	77.5	61.7	1.85	1.75
1983	35.2	29.6	64.2	53.8	1.82	1.82
1984	33.9	28.9	62.8	51.8	1.85	1.79
1985	32.8	27.9	60.8	50.3	1.85	1.80
1986	31.1	27.1	58.9	47.6	1.89	1.76
1987	30.3	26.3	57.1	46.7	1.88	1.78
1988	30.0	25.5	57.8	46.6	1.93	1.83
1989	28.0	24.1	54.1	44.9	1.93	1.86

Source: Data from *Health United States, 1991,* National Center for Health Statistics (1992).

from 1979 through 1986 than from 1973 through 1978 (Cooper, Sempos, Hsieh
& Kovar, 1990). These and other epidemiologic patterns of stroke mortality
were recently reviewed (Gillum, 1988).

Since the late 1970s improved diagnostic accuracy of death certificate diagnoses may have made more valid the examination of death rates for stroke
subgroups (Iso, Jacobs, Wentworth, Neaton & Cohen, 1989). Therefore data on
three subgroups were examined for 1979–1988 (Table 1.4). At ages 65–74,
ratios of rates in Blacks to those in Whites were similar for thromboembolic
stroke (TES) (ICD-9 433–434) and for intracranial hemorrhage (IH) (ICD-9 431–
432). However, race ratios were much higher for ill-defined stroke (IDS) (ICD-
9 436.0-437.1). This suggests that access to diagnostic services such as CT
scanning was poorer for Blacks and did not improve over the decade. Sex ratios
in 1988 were similar for the subgroups in Blacks (male/female about 1.3 for IH,
1.2 for TES and IDS) and in Whites (IH 1.3, TES 1.4, IDS 1.4). Between 1979
and 1988, the relative decline in rates was greater for TES than for IH or IDS
in both Blacks and Whites. The percentage differences between 1979 and 1988

Table 1.4
**Death Rates for Cerebrovascular Disease by Race and Sex among Persons Aged
65–74 Years: United States, 1979–1985**

Year	White Male	White Female	Black Male	Black Female	Race Ratio Male	Race Ratio Female

Intracranial Hemorrhage*						
1979	39.46	30.57	66.66	57.18	1.69	1.87
1980	34.94	27.36	64.16	47.53	1.84	1.74
1981	33.36	27.00	50.88	40.35	1.53	1.49
1982	33.51	25.89	54.83	40.85	1.64	1.58
1983	30.15	25.01	51.66	41.87	1.71	1.67
1984	31.78	26.02	51.96	47.43	1.63	1.82
1985	32.44	25.17	54.33	35.98	1.67	1.43
1986	30.75	26.25	47.86	38.34	1.56	1.46
1987	29.25	25.31	49.31	36.62	1.69	1.45
1988	31.10	24.40	55.59	41.99	1.79	1.72

Thromboembolic Stroke**						
1979	58.64	38.87	91.84	68.92	1.57	1.77
1980	52.88	36.05	89.19	68.78	1.69	1.91
1981	49.43	33.26	78.52	62.05	1.59	1.87
1982	43.24	28.67	69.24	49.24	1.60	1.72
1983	38.57	25.95	63.60	46.73	1.65	1.80
1984	36.32	24.46	59.86	47.07	1.65	1.92
1985	34.67	24.38	55.78	43.91	1.61	1.80
1986	31.81	22.86	55.60	43.01	1.75	1.88
1987	28.81	20.72	52.40	37.88	1.82	1.83
1988	27.30	18.95	44.38	35.78	1.63	1.89

Table 1.4—Continued

Year	White Male	White Female	Black Male	Black Female	Race Ratio Male	Female
			Ill-defined Stroke***			
1979	132.51	91.64	278.19	220.36	2.10	2.40
1980	132.97	90.88	282.57	214.48	2.13	2.36
1981	123.48	86.17	270.77	210.77	2.19	2.45
1982	116.95	82.53	270.83	184.34	2.32	2.23
1983	110.30	77.63	245.35	186.21	2.22	2.40
1984	103.84	73.59	236.16	181.45	2.27	2.47
1985	100.24	72.02	216.22	170.81	2.16	2.37
1986	92.92	71.55	203.00	157.70	2.18	2.20
1987	90.82	66.79	189.54	155.90	2.09	2.33
1988	89.29	66.03	194.52	156.69	2.18	2.37

Source: Unpublished data from the National Vital Statistics System, National Center for Health Statistics.

*ICD-9 431-432

**ICD-9 433-434

***ICD-9 436.0-437.1

rates were TES WM -53.4, WF -51.3, BM -51.7, BF -48.1; IH WM -21.2, WF -20.2, BM -16.6, BF -26.6; IDS WM -32.6, WF -27.9, BM -30.1, BF -28.9. While tending to decline, IH rates for BF showed considerable year-to-year variation. Further studies of the validity of death certificate diagnoses of stroke subgroups are needed from all regions of the United States for Blacks and Whites to confirm these findings. Studies of access to care, especially CT scanning by race and income, would also be valuable.

Morbidity

Epidemiologic patterns treated in a recent article and review included stroke prevalence, incidence, hospitalization, and risk factors, all generally higher in Blacks than Whites (Gillum, 1988; Gillum, 1986c). In the 1982–84 National Health Interview Surveys, the average rates for stroke prevalence by history per

1,000 persons aged 65 and over were WM 62.9, BM 108.0, WF 50.4, BF 75.8 (Havlik et al., 1987). These rates were for the civilian noninstitutionalized population. In 1985–87 there were an estimated annual average 305,000 Black survivors of stroke in the U.S civilian, noninstitutionalized population (Ries, 1990).

National estimates of stroke incidence by sex and race were produced from the NHANESI Epidemiologic Follow-up Study; however, the small size of the Black cohort limited the precision of these estimates (White, Losonczy & Wolf, 1990). A subsequent analysis examined the Black-White difference in stroke incidence in detail (Kittner, White, Losonczy, Wolf & Hebel, 1990). At ages 65–74, ten-year incidence rates per 100 were as follows: Black men 14.6, White men 12.6, Black women 12.1, and White women 9.2. In persons aged 35–74, the age-adjusted relative risk for Blacks versus Whites was 1.3 in men and 1.8 in women. Only a portion (50% in women) of the excess risk in Blacks could be explained by adjusting for systolic blood pressure and diabetes in addition to age.

Age-adjusted hospital discharge rates in the NHDS for first-listed cerebrovascular disease were 30 percent higher in Blacks than in Whites at ages 35–74 years in 1981 (Gillum, 1986c). Limited published data suggest poorer survivorship after acute stroke in Blacks than Whites (Gillum, 1988); data are needed on short- and long-term prognosis after acute stroke in Blacks.

Data from large longitudinal or well-designed case-control studies of Blacks are needed to assess many putative risk factors in Blacks including cigarette smoking, diabetes, serum total cholesterol and lipoproteins, and alcohol intake (Gillum, 1988). In a national cohort (NHEFS), systolic blood pressure and diabetes had similar relations to risk of stroke in Blacks and in Whites (Kittner et al., 1990). For example, the relative risks associated with diabetes were BM 2.5, WM 2.5, BF 2.4, and WF 2.5.

Summary

Cerebrovascular diseases was the third leading cause of death in Blacks and Whites in 1989, with age-adjusted death rates 89 percent higher in Blacks. Between 1979 and 1988 death rates declined more for TES and IDS than for IH. Prevalence, incidence, and hospitalization rates for stroke were higher in Blacks than in Whites in recent surveys. Further studies are needed on mortality, incidence, survivorship, access to care, trends, and risk factors for stroke and stroke subgroups in Blacks.

HYPERTENSIVE DISEASE

Hypertension acting in concert with other risk factors determines many patterns of cardiovascular mortality and morbidity. In addition to considering its contribution to mortality and morbidity from cerebrovascular diseases and diseases of the heart, it is useful to examine deaths and illness attributed to hypertensive disease (ICD-9 401–405) and hypertensive heart disease (ICD-9 402, 404). Surveys of the NCHS also provide extensive data on the prevalence of hypertension and elevated blood pressure as well as hypertension awareness, treatment, and control in the United States.

Mortality

Vital statistics data from NCHS provided information on patterns and trends of death rates from hypertensive disease (HD) and hypertensive heart disease (HHD) in the United States from 1979 through 1988. In 1988 the numbers of deaths with the underlying cause coded as HD were as follows: WM 9,550, WF 13,555, BM 3,631, and BF 4,579. Numbers of HHD deaths were as follows: WM 6,801, WF 9,871, BM 2,884, and BF 3,400. That the data on underlying cause of death underestimate the impact of hypertension is illustrated by the following: Essential hypertension not specified as malignant or benign (ICD-9 401.9) was listed as the underlying cause of death 3,581 times but as a secondary cause 74,026 times. Similarly HHD not specified as malignant or benign (ICD-9 402.9) was listed as the underlying cause 20,850 times and as a secondary cause 19,150 times. Analyses of multiple causes of death have attempted to assess the broader impact of hypertension on mortality of Blacks and Whites in the United States (Wing & Manton, 1983; Tu, 1987).

Rates of HD and HHD death increase with age, with higher rates in males than females below age 75. In 1988 age-adjusted death rates per 100,000 for HD were as follows: WM 6.1, WF 4.7, BM 27.7, and BF 22.9. Age-adjusted death rates for HHD were as follows: WM 4.5, WF 3.5, BM 21.8, and BF 17.1.

Age-adjusted rates by sex and race for 1979–1988 declined for HD and HHD in each sex and race group, e.g., for BM HD −13.3 percent, HHD −14.3 percent; BF HD −10.6 percent, HHD −17.4 percent. The ratio of rates in non-Whites to those in Whites was reported to have decreased between 1968 and 1978, reflecting greater declines in rates among non-Whites than among Whites (Persky, Pan, Stamler, Dyer & Levy, 1986). However there were no consistent trends in sex-specific ratios between 1979 and 1985 reflecting similar relative declines for non-Whites and Whites. However the percentage declines in comparisons between 1979 and 1988 figures tended to be slightly greater for Whites than for Blacks: WM HD −21.8, HHD −23.7; WF HD −23.0, HHD −25.5.

Death rates for HD and HHD varied considerably among states for each sex and race group. For HD in 1979–1988 combined, rates for Black men aged 55–64 were generally highest in south Atlantic states, and also relatively high in other southern states as well as Illinois, Missouri, and California. For example, the death rate per 100,000 was 141 in the District of Columbia, 129 in California, 128 in Maryland, and 125 in Florida compared to only 63 in New York and 50 in Pennsylvania. A similar pattern was seen for Black women. For HHD in 1979–1988 combined, the pattern was largely the same, since HHD deaths made up the majority of HD deaths. The great variation among states, resulting in a nearly three-fold variation in rates, points to major variations in hypertension prevalence, treatment, control, and possibly other factors, including death certification for sequelae of hypertension.

Morbidity

A number of NCHS publications and reports based on NCHS data document epidemiologic patterns and trends in hypertension and blood pressure distributions in the United States (Ries, 1990; Collins, 1988; Persky et al., 1986; Drizd, Dannenberg & Engel, 1986; Roberts & Maurer, 1977; Dannenberg, Drizd, Horan, Haynes & Leaverton, 1987). Possible explanations for the well-documented higher prevalence and incidence of hypertension in Blacks than Whites have been reviewed (Gillum, 1979). Comparison of data from NCHS surveys conducted in 1960–62, 1971–74, and 1976–80 revealed decreases in mean systolic blood pressure (SBP), the proportion with SBP greater than or equal to 140 mm Hg, and increases in the proportions of hypertensives who where treated and controlled among all race and sex groups (Dannenberg et al., 1987). However, among men only 20 percent of Blacks and 25 percent of Whites who had definite hypertension had their blood pressure controlled to less than 160/95 mm Hg in 1976–80 (Drizd et al., 1986). Data from NHEFS indicated that frequency of medication use among hypertensive Blacks was higher in 1982–1984 compared to 1976–80 (Havlik, LaCroix, Kleinman, Ingram, Harris & Cornoni-Huntley, 1989). Among BF, rates of uncontrolled hypertension and severe blood pressure elevations were higher in the Southeast than in other regions, corresponding to higher stroke mortality rates (Rocella & Lenfant, 1989). Higher rates of severe hypertension in BM in the Southeast were also consistent with higher stroke, HD, and HHD mortality.

Data from the National Health Interview Survey were examined for the years 1983–1987 combined in a preliminary analysis to assess variation in prevalence of self-reported high blood pressure and heart disease by region and urbanization. Even combining five years of data, too few Blacks were included in the sample to examine rates at each urbanization level for each region. Data were most adequate for the South and the total United States, with only partial data for other regions. The highest prevalence of heart disease and high blood pressure was in the nonmetropolitan South; so few Blacks lived in nonmetropolitan areas outside the South that U.S. nonmetropolitan rates are essentially identical with those in the South. In the United States and the South, rates in metropolitan areas outside central cities ("suburbs") were the lowest. Although these two patterns are generally consistent with those observed for mortality, these data must be interpreted with great caution because of large sampling errors due to the small samples of Blacks and possible bias in self-reported diagnoses.

National data on the prevalence of HHD are more limited. In the Health Examination Survey of 1960–1962, the prevalence of HHD was derived from physical examination, electrocardiogram, and chest X-ray of a national sample aged 18–79 years (Gordon & Devine, 1966). Among men aged 55–64, rates were 33.1 percent in Blacks and 11.7 percent in Whites. Among women of the same age, rates were 46.4 percent in Blacks and 19.5 percent in Whites. Recent analyses of data from the NHANESI Epidemiologic Follow-Up Study demonstrated higher prevalences of left ventricular hypertrophy by several electrocardiographic criteria in Blacks than Whites (Rautaharju et al., 1988). For example, 30.1 percent of Black men compared to only 6.3 percent of White men had left ventricular hypertrophy by Sokolow-Lyon criteria.

Incidence rates of hypertension over an average follow-up of 9.5 years were estimated from NHEFS data. Incidence in Whites increased from about 5 percent at ages 25–34 to over 20 percent at age 65–74. Incidence rates were about twice as great in Blacks as in Whites (Havlik et al., 1989). Body mass index was positively related to the incidence of hypertension in each sex and race group. Another analysis of NHEFS data showed risk factors for incidence of hypertension in Blacks to include elevated body mass index, advanced age, and possibly lower educational attainment (Ford & Cooper, 1991). Findings were similar for Whites. Associations of a number of other physiologic, behavioral, and dietary factors with hypertension incidence could not be confirmed in Blacks or Whites in multivariate analyses.

Summary

Aside from its effects on mortality from ischemic heart disease and cerebrovascular disease, hypertension produces substantial numbers of deaths attributed to HD including HHD, a disproportionate number occurring in Blacks. This indicates that despite the improvements in hypertension control of the past two decades, vigorous efforts still need to be directed to Blacks, particularly in the south Atlantic states.

PERIPHERAL ARTERIAL OCCLUSIVE DISEASE

Few epidemiologic data are available on peripheral arterial disease in Blacks. Chronic peripheral arterial disease of the extremities (ICD9-CM 440.2, 443.9, or 447.1) was listed as the underlying cause for fewer than 4,000 deaths in 1985 (Gillum, 1990). For 1979–85, average annual age-adjusted death rates per 100,000 were 1.3 in non-White males, 0.8 in White males, 0.9 in non-White females, and 0.5 in White females. Rates were higher in non-Whites than in Whites at each age. Rates at age 75–84 were NWM 20.1, WM 15.8, NWF 17.2, and WF 9.0.

In 1985–1987 an average of 332 thousand Whites and 44 thousand Blacks were discharged from U.S. hospitals with any such diagnosis among up to seven diagnoses coded per discharge. Average annual diagnosis rates at ages 65 and over were 891 per 100,000 for Whites and 1,192 for Blacks. About 3 million days of care for Whites and 605 thousand for Blacks were associated with a mention of these diagnoses. However, a peripheral arterial disease was the first-listed diagnosis (or principal diagnosis) in only about 99 thousand discharges for all ages and races combined (Gillum, 1990). Further these estimates must be viewed with caution because about 23 thousand discharges with any diagnosis had unknown race, and a single patient might have multiple diagnoses and discharges and hence be counted more than once. Despite these severe limitations, the data suggest peripheral vascular disease is a significant problem among Blacks.

GOALS FOR THE YEAR 2000

National health promotion and disease prevention objectives have been published for the year 2000, with Blacks identified as a high-risk population needing special attention (NCHS, 1992; *Healthy People 2000,* 1991). One of three overarching goals is to reduce health disparities among Americans. Cardiovascular diseases account for a major portion of the excess mortality of Blacks. In order to attain the health status objectives of reducing coronary heart disease deaths in Blacks from 163 per 100,000 in 1987 to 155 in 2000 (nearly 30% for ICD-9 410–414, 402, 429.2), reducing stroke deaths from 51.2 per 100,000 in 1987 to 27 in 2000 (nearly 50%), and reversing the increase in end-stage renal disease incidence, risk reduction objectives were specified (Table 1.5). These include increasing the proportion of people with high blood pressure whose blood pressure is under control; reducing the mean blood cholesterol among adults and reducing the prevalence of elevated blood cholesterol (levels of 240 mg/dL or greater); reducing the prevalence of overweight; increasing regular physical activity; and reducing the prevalence of cigarette smoking. In addition health services and protection objectives were set forth: increasing to at least 90 percent the proportion of adults who know whether their blood pressure was normal or high in the preceding two years (baseline 61% in 1985), increasing to 75 percent the proportion of adults having had their blood cholesterol measured within the preceding 5 years (baseline 52–59% in 1988), increasing to 75 percent the proportion of primary-care providers who initiate appropriate therapy for elevated blood cholesterol, increasing to 50 percent the proportion of worksites with 50 or more employees with high blood pressure and/or cholesterol education and control activities (baseline 17% in 1985), and increasing to 90 percent the percentage of clinical laboratories meeting standards for accuracy for cholesterol measurement (baseline 53% in 1985). Personnel needs, surveillance and data needs for tracking progress, and research needs were also listed. Achieving these objectives will require the efforts of providers and policy makers, of the public and private sectors. It is hoped that the present volume will contribute to this effort.

Table 1.5

Heart Disease and Stroke: National Health Promotion and Disease Prevention Objectives for the Year 2000 for Blacks

Health Status and Risk Reduction Objectives

- Reduce coronary heart disease deaths to no more than 115 per 100,000 (baseline: 163 per 100,000 in 1987 for ICD-9 410-414, 402, 429.2).

- Reduce stroke deaths to no more than 27 per 100,000 (baseline: 51.2 per 100,000 in 1987).

- Reverse the increase in end-stage renal disease to attain an incidence of no more than 30 per 100,000 (baseline: 32.4 per 100,000 in 1987).

- Increase to at least 50% the proportion of persons with high blood pressure whose blood pressure is under control (baseline: 24% in 1982-84).

- Increase to at least 90% the proportion of persons with high blood pressure who are taking action to control their blood pressure (baseline: 79%--63% of black hypertensive men aged 18-34--in 1985).

- Reduce cigarette smoking to a prevalence of no more than 18% among people aged 20 and older (baseline: 34% in 1987).

- Reduce the mean serum cholesterol level among adults to no more than 200 mg/dL (baseline 213 mg/dL in 1976-80).

- Reduce the prevalence of blood cholesterol levels of 240 mg/dL or greater to no more than 20% among adults (baseline: 27% in 1976-80).

- Increase to at least 60% the proportion of adults with high blood cholesterol who are aware and taking action to reduce their cholesterollevels (baseline: 11% in 1988).

Table 1.5—Continued

• Reduce dietary fat intake to an average of 30% of calories or less
and average saturated fate intake to less than 10% of calories
among people aged 2 and over (baseline: 36% from total fat and 13%
from saturated fat for ages 20-74 in 1976-80).

• Reduce overweight to no more than 20% of black men and 30% of black
women aged 20 and older and no more than 15% among persons aged 12-19
(baseline: 26% for all persons and 44% for black women aged 20-74 in
1976-80).

• Increase to at least 30% the proportion of people aged 6 and older
who engage regularly in light to moderate physical activity for at least
30 minutes per day (baseline: 22% in 1985).

Source: Healthy People 2000 (1991).

CONCLUSIONS

In 1989 heart disease was the leading cause of death and cerebrovascular disease the third leading cause of death for both Blacks and Whites in the United States. Despite improvements in hypertension control and declines in mortality rates for all groups, Blacks continue to experience excess mortality compared to Whites from all heart disease, from coronary heart disease in younger men and in women, from stroke, and from hypertensive disease. Data are needed on peripheral arterial disease in Blacks. Epidemiologic monitoring of several indicators of disease over time can assist in guiding research and prevention efforts. Longitudinal studies including sizable numbers of Blacks are needed to enhance understanding of factors influencing cardiovascular risk. Ambitious yet achievable goals for cardiovascular prevention and health promotion have been set forth for the year 2000 to guide the efforts of health care providers and policy makers.

NOTE

Address correspondence and reprint requests to R. F. Gillum, M.D., Office of Analysis and Epidemiology, National Center for Health Statistics, 6525 Belcrest Road, Hyattsville, MD 20782.

REFERENCES

Advance Report of Final Mortality Statistics, 1989. (1991). National Center for Health Statistics. *Monthly Vital Statistics Report, 40* (Supp. 8), 1–52.

Collins, J. G. (1988). Prevalence of selected chronic conditions, United States, 1983–85. *Advance Data from Vital and Health Statistics.* (No. 155. DHHS Publication No. PHS 88-1250). Hyattsville, MD: Public Health Service.

Cooper, R., Sempos, C., Hsieh, S. C., & Kovar, M. G. (1990). The slowdown in the decline of stroke mortality in the United States, 1978–1986. *Stroke, 21,* 1274–9.

Cooper, R. S., & Ford, E. (1990). Coronary heart disease among blacks and whites in the NHANES-I Epidemiologic Follow-up Study: Incidence of new events and risk factor prediction. *Circulation, 81,* 723.

Cornoni-Huntley, J., LaCroix, A. Z., & Havlik, R. J. (1989). Race and sex differentials in the impact of hypertension in the United States. National Health and Nutrition Examination Survey I Epidemiologic Follow-up Study. *Archives of Internal Medicine, 149,* 780–8.

Dannenberg, A. L., Drizd, T., Horan, M. J., Haynes, S. G., & Leaverton, P. E. (1987). Progress in the battle against hypertension. Changes in blood pressure levels in the United States from 1960 to 1980. *Hypertension, 10,* 226–33.

Drizd, T., Dannenberg, A. L., & Engel, A. (1986). Blood pressure levels in persons 18–74 years of age in 1976–80, and trends in blood pressure from 1960 to 1980 in the United States. *Vital Health Statistics, 11* (234), 1–68.

Eaker, E. D., Packard, B., & Thom, T. J. (1989). Epidemiology and risk factors for coronary heart disease in women. *Cardiovascular Clinics, 19,* 129–145.

Ford, E., Cooper, R., Castaner, A., Simmons, B., & Mar, M. (1989). Coronary arteriography and coronary bypass survey among whites and other racial groups relative to hospital-based incidence rates for coronary artery disease: Findings from NHDS. *American Journal of Public Health, 79,* 437–440.

Ford, E. S., & Cooper, R. S. (1991). Risk factors for hypertension in a national cohort study. *Hypertension, 18,* 598–606.

Ford, E. S., & Jones, D. H. (1991). Cardiovascular health knowledge in the United States: Findings from the National Health Interview Study, 1985. *Preventive Medicine, 20,* 725–736.

Gillum, R. F. (1979). Pathophysiology of hypertension in blacks and whites. A review of the basis of racial blood pressure differences. *Hypertension, 1,* 468–475.

Gillum, R. F. (1982). Coronary heart disease in black populations. I. Mortality and morbidity. *American Heart Journal, 104,* 839–851.

Gillum, R. F., & Grant, C. T. (1982). Coronary heart disease in black populations. II. Risk factors. *American Heart Journal, 104,* 852–864.

Gillum, R. F. (1986a). Trends in acute rheumatic fever and chronic rheumatic heart disease: A national perspective. *American Heart Journal 111,* 430–432.

Gillum, R. F. (1986b). Idiopathic cardiomyopathy in the United States, 1970–1982. *American Heart Journal, 111,* 752–755.

Gillum, R. F. (1986c). Cerebrovascular disease morbidity in the United States, 1970–1983. Age, sex, region, and vascular surgery. *Stroke, 17,* 656–661.

Gillum, R. F. (1987a). Heart failure in the United States 1970–1985. *American Heart Journal, 113,* 1043–1045.

Gillum, R. F. (1987b). Pulmonary embolism and thrombophlebitis in the United States, 1970–1983. *American Heart Journal, 114,* 1262–1264.

Gillum, R. F. (1987c). Acute myocardial infarction in the United States, 1970–1983. *American Heart Journal, 113,* 804–811.

Gillum, R. F. (1987d). Coronary artery bypass surgery and coronary angiography in the United States, 1979–1983. *American Heart Journal, 113,* 1255–1260.

Gillum, R. F. (1988). Stroke in blacks. *Stroke 19,* 1–9.

Gillum, R. F. (1989a). The epidemiology of cardiomyopathy in the United States. *Progress in Cardiology, 2,* 11–21.

Gillum, R. F. (1989b). Sudden coronary death in the United States: 1980–1985. *Circulation, 79,* 756–765.

Gillum, R. F. (1990). Peripheral arterial occlusive disease of the extremities in the United States: Hospitalization and mortality. *American Heart Journal, 120,* 1414–1418.

Gillum, R. F., Makuc, D. M., & Feldman, J. J. (1991). Pulse rate, coronary heart disease, and death: The NHANESI Epidemiologic Follow-up Study. *American Heart Journal, 121,* 172–177.

Gillum, R. F., & Makuc, D. M. (1992). Serum albumin, coronary heart disease, and death. *American Heart Journal, 123,* 507–513.

Gordon, T., & Garst, C. C. (1965). Coronary heart disease in adults, United States, 1960–62. *Vital and Health Statistics.* (Series 11, No. 10, PHS Publication No. 1000). Washington, DC: U.S. Government Printing Office.

Gordon, T., & Devine, B. (1966). Hypertension and hypertensive heart disease in adults, United States, 1960–62. *Vital and Health Statistics.* (Series 11, No. 13. PHS Publication No. 1000). Washington, DC: U.S. Government Printing Office.

Graves, E. J. (1992). National Hospital Discharge Survey: Annual summary, 1989. National Center for Health Statistics. *Vital Health Statistics, 13* (109), 1–51.

Havlik, R. J., Liu, B. M., Kovar, M. G., Suzman, R., Feldman, J. J., Harris, T., & Van Nostrand, J. (1987). Health Statistics on Older Persons, United States, 1986. *Vital and Health Statistics.* (Series 3, No. 25 DHHS Publication No. PHS 87-1409). Washington, DC: U.S. Government Printing Office.

Havlik, R. J., LaCroix, A. Z., Kleinman, J. C., Ingram, D. D., Harris, T., & Cornoni-Huntley, J. (1989). Antihypertensive drug therapy and survival by treatment status in a national survey. *Hypertension 13* (Supp. 1), I28–I32.

Healthy People 2000. (1991). National health promotion and disease prevention objectives. DHHS Publication No. (PHS) 91-50212. Washington, DC: Government Printing Office.

Iso, H., Jacobs, D. R., Wentworth, D., Neaton, J. D., & Cohen, J. D. (1989). Serum cholesterol levels and six-year mortality from stroke in 350,977 men screened for the Multiple Risk Factor Intervention Trial. *New England Journal of Medicine, 320,* 904–910.

Kittner, S. J., White, L. R., Losonczy, K. G., Wolf, P. A., & Hebel, R. (1990). Black-white differences in stroke incidence in a national sample: The contribution of hypertension and diabetes mellitus. *Journal of the American Medical Association, 264,* 1267–1270.

Klag, M. J., Whelton, P. K., & Seidler, A. J. (1989). Decline in U.S. stroke mortality: Demographic trends and antihypertensive treatment. *Stroke, 20,* 14–21.

LaCroix, A. Z., Haynes, S. G., Savage, D. D., & Havlik, R. J. (1989). Rose Questionnaire angina among United States black, white, and Mexican-American women and men. Prevalence and correlates from the Second National and Hispanic Health and Nutrition Examination Surveys. *American Journal of Epidemiology, 129,* 669–686.

Leaverton, P. E., Havlik, R. J., Ingster-Moore, L. M., LaCroix, A. Z., & Cornoni-Huntley, J. C. (1990). Coronary heart disease and hypertension. In J. C. Cornoni-Huntley, R. R. Huntley, & J. J. Feldman (Eds.), *Health status and well-being of the elderly* (pp. 53–70). New York: Oxford University.

Madans, J. H., Kleinman, J. C., & Cox, C. S., Barbano, H., Feldman, J. J., Cohen, B., Finucane, F., & Cornoni-Huntley, J. (1986). Ten years after NHANES I: Report of initial follow-up, 1982–84. *Public Health Report, 101,* 465–473.

Madans, J. H., Cox, C. S., Kleinman, J. C., Makuc, D., Feldman, J. J., Barbano, H., & Cornoni-Huntley, J. (1986). Ten years after NHANES I: Mortality experience at initial follow-up, 1982–84. *Public Health Report, 101,* 474–481.

National Center for Health Statistics. (1992). *Health, United States, 1991.* DHHS Publication No. (PHS) 92-1232. Washington, DC: Government Printing Office.

National Center for Health Statistics. (1989). *Vital statistics of the United States, 1986, Vol. II. Mortality, Part A.* DHHS Publication No. (PHS) 89-1101. Washington, DC: Government Printing Office.

Otten, M. W., Teutsch, S. M., Williamson, D. F., & Marks, J. S. (1990). The effect of known risk factors on the excess mortality of black adults in the United States. *Journal of the American Medical Association, 263,* 845–850.

Persky, V., Pan, W. H., Stamler, J., Dyer, A., & Levy, P. (1986). Time trends in the U.S. racial difference in hypertension. *American Journal of Epidemiology, 124,* 724–737.

Rautaharju, P. M., LaCroix, A. Z., Savage, D. D., Haynes, S. G., Madans, J. H., Wolf, H. K., Hadden, W., Keller, J., & Cornoni-Huntley, J. (1988). Electro-cardiographic estimate of left ventricular mass versus radiographic cardiac size and the risk of cardiovascular disease mortality in the epidemiologic follow-up study of the First National Health and Nutrition Examination Survey. *American Journal of Cardiology, 62,* 59–66.

Ries, P. (1990). Health of black and white Americans, 1985–1987. *Vital and Health Statistics.* Series 10, No. 171, DHHS Publication No. PHS 90-1599. Washington, DC: Government Printing Office.

Roberts, J., & Maurer, K. (1977). Blood pressure levels of persons 6–74 years, United States, 1971–74. *Vital and Health Statistics.* Series 11, No. 203. DHEW Publication No. HRA 78-1648. Washington, DC: Government Printing Office.

Rocella, E. F., & Lenfant, C. (1989). Regional and racial differences among stroke victims in the United States. *Clinical Cardiology, 12,* 18–22.

Roig, E., Castaner, A., Simmons, B., Patel, R., Ford, E., & Cooper, R. (1987). In-hospital mortality rates from acute myocardial infarction by race in U.S. hospitals: Findings from the National Hospital Discharge Survey. *Circulation, 76,* 280–288.

Sempos, C., Cooper, R., Kovar, M. G., & McMillen, M. (1988). Divergence of the recent trends in coronary mortality for the four major race-sex groups in the United States. *American Journal of Public Health, 78,* 1422–1427.

Tu, E. J. (1987). Multiple cause-of-death analysis of hypertension-related mortality in New York state. *Public Health Reports, 102,* 329–335.

White, L. R., Losonczy, K. G., & Wolf, P. A. (1990). Cerebrovascular disease. In J. C. Cornoni-Huntley, R. R. Huntley, & J. J. Feldman (Eds.), *Health status and well-being of the elderly* (pp. 115–135). New York: Oxford University Press.

Wing, S., & Manton, K. G. (1983). The contribution of hypertension to mortality in the U.S.: 1968, 1977. *American Journal of Public Health, 73,* 140–144.

2

Coronary Artery Disease in Blacks

Charles Curry

Atherosclerosis is a condition marked by loss of elasticity and thickening of the intima of blood vessels. This condition may progress until the lumen of the affected blood vessel is partially occluded, leading to diminished blood flow through the affected vessel.

The development of this process in the coronary arteries is called coronary artery disease. When there is cardiac malfunction as a result of the ischemia induced by atherosclerosis, the process is called coronary atherosclerotic heart disease (CHD). CHD may manifest itself as myocardial infarction, angina pectoris, cardiac dysarrhythmias, congestive heart failure, and sudden death. CHD is frequently (erroneously) used synonymously with ischemic heart disease (IHD).

Coronary heart disease affects approximately 7 million Americans and is responsible for approximately 600,000 deaths in the United States annually (National Heart, Lung and Blood Institute, 1990). Almost half of these deaths occur suddenly, presumably without warning.

Until recently it was believed that CHD was uncommon among Blacks. Health care providers were of the opinion that somehow Blacks were immune to CHD; when chest pain occurred, it was commonly misdiagnosed as indigestion or hypertension. In a detailed review of the literature, it was pointed out (Gillum & Grant, 1982) that CHD is the major cause of death in Blacks and the death rates are higher in Black women than White women.

The National Center for Health Statistics data in 1984 indicate that CHD mortality rates are similar among Black and White men but that rates in women are greater among Blacks (Report of the Secretary's Task Force, 1986). However, other studies (e.g., Weisse, Abiuso & Thind, 1977; Keil, Loadholt, Weinrich, Sandifer & Boyle, 1984; Langford, Oberman, Borhani, Entwisle & Tung, 1984;

McDonough, Hames & Stulb, 1965) suggest that prevalence of CHD is higher for White than Black men and that prevalence of CHD in women of both races is about equal.

Acute myocardial infarction (MI) generally becomes manifest as severe chest pain and commonly results in hospital admission. As a result, surveillance of hospital admissions for this diagnosis provides useful information about prevalence and incidence of coronary artery disease.

Data from the National Hospital Discharge Surveys (NHDS) in 1973, 1975, 1978, and 1981 reveal that men and women over 45 years old maintained nearly constant rates of discharge from the hospital for acute myocardial infarction. During 1981, hospital discharge rates for Black men were about 45 percent of total rates for White men, whereas rates for Black women were approximately 70 percent of rates for White women. The Health Insurance Plan study also indicated that the annual age-adjusted incidence of first myocardial infarction in non-White men is half the rate of White men. The case-fatality rate was higher in non-Whites (i.e., 47.5% in non-Whites versus 35.5% in Whites). A higher incidence of acute myocardial infarction in Whites compared with Black men was also reported from Evans County (McDonough, Hames & Stulb, 1965; Sempos, Cooper, Kovar & McMillen, 1988), the Nashville study (Hagstrom, Federspiel & Ho, 1971), the Charleston Heart Study (Keil et al., 1984), and the Columbia University Study (Weisse et al., 1977). The incidence of acute myocardial infarction in women of both races was similar in these studies.

These reduced rates of hospital discharge for Blacks can be explained to a large extent by the fact that out-of-hospital deaths from CHD are more common in Blacks than among Whites. For example, in the Baltimore Study (Kuller, Cooper, Perper & Fisher, 1973), sudden death rates out of the hospital were somewhat higher for Black men than for White men.

RISK FACTORS

Numerous studies (Gillum & Grant, 1982; Kannel, 1987) from around the world have repeatedly shown that specific individual traits or "risk factors" are reliable predictors of future CHD. The major risk factors are cigarette smoking, abnormal blood lipids, and hypertension.

Cigarette Smoking

The National Health Interview Surveys (NHIS) of 1965 and 1976 indicate that increasing numbers of Black females began to smoke cigarettes between 1965 and 1976 (Kleinman, Feldman & Monk, 1979). The data indicate that the prevalence of moderate cigarette smoking in 1976 was higher among Black males than White males, whereas more White males were heavy smokers (greater than 25 per day). Both Black females and White females had similar prevalence rates, but more White females were heavy smokers. Table 2.1 shows the prevalence

Table 2.1
Cigarette Smoking, Ages 25 to 74 Years, 1976–1980

	No. of current smokers	No. of participants smoking 25 or more/day
White males	39.3	16.9
White females	33.1	7.3
Black males	50.4	8.5
Black females	31.1	3.8

Source: National Center for Health Statistics, 1991b (NHANES II).

of cigarette smoking in the National Health and Nutrition Examination Survey (NHANES) (Rowland & Roberts, 1982) to be similar to that in the National Health Interview Survey.

Serum Lipids

Many studies (e.g., Tyroler, Hames, Krishan, Heyden, Cooper & Cassel, 1975; Srinivasan, Frerichs, Webber & Berensen, 1976; Heyden, Heiss, Hames & Bartel, 1980; Tyroler, Glueck, Christensen & Kwiterovich, 1980; Morrison, Khoury, Mellies, Kelly, Howitz & Glueck, 1981) indicate that Blacks have higher levels of high-density lipoprotein (HDL) cholesterol and lower levels of low-density and very low-density lipoproteins (LDL) than Whites, an asset that may protect Blacks from CHD (Gordon, Castelli, Hjortland, Kannel & Dawber, 1977). However, in a random sample of 100 Black males and females in Framingham, Massachusetts, the results were different. Black males had a mean plasma total cholesterol level of 184, HDL cholesterol of 37.2, and triglycerides of 78 mg/dl. The corresponding levels for the 55 Black females in the study were a mean plasma total cholesterol of 192, HDL cholesterol of 50.4, and triglycerides of 49 mg/dl. These values for HDL cholesterol were significantly lower than the levels for a comparable sample of Framingham White males and females (Wilson, Savage, Castelli, Garrison, Donahue & Feinleib, 1983). The possibility that environmental factors may be having a negative impact on HDL cholesterol levels in these subjects needs to be investigated. Table 2.2 shows the mean serum cholesterol levels of White males and females compared with Black males and females (ages 25 to 74 years) in 1971–1975 and 1976–1980.

Table 2.2
Mean Serum Cholesterol Levels, Ages 25 to 74 Years

	1971–1975	1976–1980
White males	217.5	216.7
White females	221.4	219.9
Black males	225.7	214.9
Black females	221.2	219.0

Source: National Center for Health Statistics, 1991a (NHANES I), 1991b (NHANES II).

Hypertension

Hypertension is a well-recognized risk factor for CHD. Yet, many populations of Blacks with high prevalence rates of hypertension have surprisingly low prevalence rates of CHD. Examples of Black populations with high prevalence rates of hypertension and low prevalence rates of CHD include Blacks in Africa, the Caribbean, and, until recently, the United States. Japan is another country with high rates of hypertension and low rates of CHD (McDonough et al., 1965; Shaper, Hutt & Fejfar, 1974; Oalmann, Malcolm, Toca, Guzman & Strong, 1981; Miall, Kass, Ling & Stuart, 1962; Akinkugbe, 1976). Table 2.3 shows hypertension data from the NHANES II (1976–1980), in which 23.1 percent of Black males and 24.4 percent of Black females were hypertensive in 1976–1980. Prevalence rates of the magnitude shown in Table 2.3 would lead one to expect an enormous incidence of CHD, but this expectation has only recently been recognized. Either hypertension alone is not a significant risk factor in Blacks or some unknown factor partially ameliorates its impact. Epidemiologic studies have implicated high levels of HDL cholesterol as the ''protective factor.''

Diabetes Mellitus as a Risk Factor

It is well recognized that diabetes is associated with an increased risk of CHD. Females with diabetes experience CHD at a higher rate than nondiabetic females. Males with diabetes experience CHD at twice the rate of nondiabetic males (Stearns, Schlesinger & Rudy, 1947).

Data from the Evans County study suggest that the prevalence of diabetes among Black males is about equal to that among White males, but Black females have a higher prevalence rate than White females (Deubner, Wilkinson, Helms,

Table 2.3
Age-adjusted Rate (ages 25 to 74 years) for Elevated Blood Pressure (per 100)

	1971–1975	1976–1980
White males	18.0	16.0
White females	14.2	11.0
Black males	35.7	23.1
Black females	30.6	24.4

Source: National Center for Health Statistics, 1991a (NHANES I), 1991b (NHANES II).

Tyroler & Hames, 1980). A prospective cohort study of the risk of CHD associated with diabetes in Blacks is needed in order to quantify the risk and to better understand the relationships between the two processes.

In a retrospective study of risk factors in Blacks with M.I. admitted to Howard University Hospital in 1980–1981, a striking 50.9 percent of females were seen to be diabetic. The corresponding prevalence of diabetes for Black males admitted with M.I. was 25.3 percent. The literature indicates an average prevalence rate for diabetes among White women with CHD of approximately 21 percent, compared to a range of 10 percent to 20 percent for White males with CHD.

Significance of Risk Factor Data in Blacks

Gillum and Grant (Gillum & Grant, 1982) have pointed out that the dearth of prospective studies in the Black population raises uncertainty about the significance of various CHD risk factors in Blacks. According to NHANES, 7 of 10 Black males and 6 of 10 Black females had one or more of the three major risk factors in the late 1970s. This burden, together with the unmeasured risk of socioeconomic and psychosocial factors, places the Black American in a precarious situation with regard to CHD risk.

CLINICAL MANIFESTATIONS

The clinical manifestations of CHD apparently do not differ significantly from those seen in other ethnic groups. Clearly, individuals of lower educational attainment and/or various regional and cultural dialects may choose different words to express themselves when requested to describe a given complaint. Less well understood is the meaning and significance of a given symptom in the Black individual. One study (Langford et al., 1984) compared indexes of CHD and myocardial infarction for both races in the stepped-care cohort of the Hypertension Detection and Follow-up Program. A standardized Rose Questionnaire was used to elicit symptoms of angina pectoris and myocardial infarction and to inquire about the clinical diagnosis of myocardial infarction. It was found that angina pectoris was more prevalent in Blacks. In men of either race and White women, baseline prevalence of angina was associated with an approximate doubling of 5-year mortality. Curiously, a positive Rose Questionnaire outcome for angina pectoris was not predictive of subsequent mortality in Black women. Similar findings were reported in the Coronary Artery Surgery Study.

MEDICAL CARE OF BLACKS WITH CORONARY HEART DISEASE

One of the objectives of the U.S. Department of Health and Human Services, listed in *Healthy People 2000* (1990), is to reduce CHD deaths to no more than 100 per 100,000 people from the present age-adjusted baseline (1987) of 135 per 100,000. The baseline for Blacks is 163 deaths per 100,000 and the target for the year 2000 is 115 deaths per 100,000.

Efforts at prevention must begin with the control of known risk factors. Data derived from several studies confirm the clinical impression that extensive changes in the lifestyle of Blacks can be accomplished and that there is no reason to vary treatment of CHD from conventional approaches (Connett & Stamler, 1984). Reported poor medical prognosis and disappointing surgical results from several centers are probably related to factors such as inadequate sample size, duration and severity of illness, co-morbidity, and other factors associated with socioeconomic disadvantages.

Data from a study in Massachusetts (Wenneker & Epstein, 1989) indicate that Whites underwent one-third more coronary angiographies and more than twice as many coronary artery bypass graft procedures as Blacks, which suggests that sociocultural factors may adversely affect the quality of care of Black patients and that medical decisions are based on race. Whether socioeconomic status and lack of medical insurance influences the performance of angiograms and coronary artery bypass graft revascularizations in Blacks requires further investigation. More studies that contribute to an understanding of the pathogenesis of CHD and its control among Blacks should be initiated. The study of CHD control in Blacks must also be broadened to include cost of drug therapy for prevention, that is, antihypertensive and lipid-lowering medications and drugs for protection after myocardial infarction.

SUMMARY

Coronary artery disease is the leading cause of death for Blacks. This population appears to experience more than its share of deaths from this preventable disease. However, as economic, social, racial, and cultural barriers to medical care disappear in this country, it is reasonable to expect a dramatic and immediate decline in morbidity and mortality rates associated with CHD in Blacks.

REFERENCES

Akinkugbe, O. O. (1976). The epidemiology of hypertension in Africa. In Akinkugbe, O. O., editor, *Cardiovascular Disease in Africa,* p. 91. Geneva: Ciba-Geigy, Ltd.

Connett, J. E., & Stamler, J. (1984). Responses of black and white males to the special intervention program of the multiple risk factor intervention trial. *American Heart Journal, 108,* 839–848.

Deubner, D. C., Wilkinson, W. E., Helms, M. J., Tyroler, H. A., & Hames, C. G. (1980). Logistic model estimation of death attributable to risk factors for cardiovascular disease in Evans County, Georgia. *American Journal of Epidemiology, 112,* 135.

Frerichs, R. R., Srinivasan, S. R., Webber, L. S., Rieth, M. C., & Berenson, G. S. (1978). Serum lipids and lipoproteins at birth in a biracial population: The Bogalusa Heart Study. *Pediatric Research, 12,* 858.

Gillum, R. F., & Grant, C. T. (1982). Coronary heart disease in black populations. II. Risk factors. *American Heart Journal, 104,* 852.

Glueck, C. J., Heiss, G., Tyroler, H. A., Christensen, B., Kwiterovich, P. O., deGrott, I., Chase, G., Mowery, R., & Tamir, I. (1978). Black-white plasma lipoprotein differences in children. *Circulation, 58* (Supp. 2), 31.

Gordon, T., Castelli, W. P., Hjortland, M. C., Kannel, W. B., & Dawber, T. R. (1977). High-density lipoprotein as a protective factor against coronary heart disease: The Framingham Study. *American Journal of Medicine, 62,* 707.

Hagstrom, R. M., Federspiel, C. F., & Ho, Y. C. (1971). Incidence of myocardial infarction and sudden death from coronary heart disease in Nashville, Tennessee. *Circulation, 44,* 884–890.

Healthy People 2000. (1990) National health promotion and disease prevention objectives. DHHS Publication No. (PHS) 91-50213. Washington, DC: Government Printing Office. Conference edition.

Heyden, S., Heiss, G., Hames, C. G., & Bartel, A. G. (1980). Fasting triglycerides as predictors of total and CHD mortality in Evans County, Georgia. *Journal of Chronic Diseases, 33,* 275–282.

Kannel, W. B. (1987). Metabolic risk factors for coronary heart disease in women: Perspective from the Framingham Study. *American Heart Journal, 114,* 413–419.

Keil, J. E., Loadholt, C. B., Weinrich, M. C., Sandifer, S. H., & Boyle, E., Jr. (1984). Incidence of coronary heart disease in blacks in Charleston, South Carolina. *American Heart Journal, 108,* 779–786.

Kleinman, J. C., Feldman, J. J., & Monk, M. A. (1979). The effects of changes in smoking habits on coronary heart disease mortality. *American Journal of Public Health, 69,* 745.

Kuller, L. H., Cooper, M., Perper, J., & Fisher, R. (1973). Myocardial infarction and sudden death in an urban community. *Bulletin of New York Academy of Medicine, 49,* 532–543.

Langford, H. G., Oberman, A., Borhani, N. O., Entwisle, G., & Tung, B. (1984). Black-white comparison of indices of coronary heart disease and myocardial infarction in the stepped-care cohort of the Hypertension Detection and Follow-up Program. *American Heart Journal, 108,* 797–801.

McDonough, J. R., Hames, C. G., & Stulb, S. C. (1965). Coronary heart disease among Negroes and whites in Evans County, Georgia. *Journal of Chronic Diseases, 18,* 443–468.

Miall, W. E., Kass, E. H., Ling, J., & Stuart, K. L. (1962). Factors influencing arterial pressure in the general population in Jamaica. *British Medical Journal, 2,* 497.

Morrison, J. A., Khoury, P., Mellies, M., Kelly, K., Howitz, R., & Glueck, C. (1981). Lipid and lipoprotein distributions in black adults: The Cincinnati Lipid Research Clinic's Princeton School Study. *Journal of the American Medical Association, 245,* 939.

National Center for Health Statistics. (1991a). Biochemistry, serology, hematology peripheral blood slide in urinary findings ages 1–74 years. Public Use Tape Documentation (#4800), National Health and Nutrition Examination Survey I, 1971–1975 (machine readable data file and documentation). Reprinted October, 1991. Hyattsville, MD.

National Center for Health Statistics. (1991b). Hematology and biochemistry ages 6 months–74 years, version 2. Public Use Tape Documentation (#5411), National Health and Nutrition Examination Survey II, 1976–1980 (machine readable data file and documentation). Reprinted August, 1991. Hyattsville, MD.

National Heart, Lung and Blood Institute. (1990). Morbidity and Mortality Chartbook on Cardiovascular, Lung and Blood Disease. Washington, DC: U.S. Department of Health and Human Services, 1990.

Oalmann, M. C., Malcolm, G. T., Toca, V. T., Guzman, M. A., & Strong, J. P. (1981). Community pathology of atherosclerosis and coronary heart disease: Postmortem serum cholesterol and extent of coronary atherosclerosis. *American Journal of Epidemiology, 113,* 396.

Report of the Secretary's Task Force on Black and Minority Health. (1986). Executive Summary. U.S. Department of Health and Human Services, Publication No. 186-620–638:40716. Washington, DC: Government Printing Office.

Rowland, M., & Roberts, J. (1982). Blood pressure levels and hypertension in persons ages 6–74 years: United States, 1976–80. National Center for Health Statistics Advance Data, No. 84.

Sempos, C., Cooper, R., Kovar, M. G., & McMillen, M. (1988). Divergence of the recent trends in coronary mortality for the four major race-sex groups in the United States. *American Journal of Public Health, 78,* 1422–1427.

Shaper, A. G., Hutt, M. S. R., & Fejfar, Z. (1974). Cardiovascular disease in the tropics. *London British Medical Association,* p. 171.

Srinivasan, S. R., Frerichs, R. R., Webber, L. S., & Berensen, G. S. (1976). Serum lipoprotein profile in children from a biracial community: The Bogalusa Heart Study. *Circulation, 54,* 309.

Stearns, S., Schlesinger, M. J., & Rudy, A. (1947). Incidence and clinical significance of coronary artery disease in diabetes mellitus. *Archives of Internal Medicine, 80,* 463.

Tyroler, H. A., Hames, C. G., Krishan, I., Heyden, S., Cooper, G., & Cassel, J. C. (1975). Black-white differences in serum lipids and lipoprotein in Evans County. *Preventive Medicine, 4,* 541.

Tyroler, H. A., Glueck, C. J., Christensen, B., & Kwiterovich, P. O., (1980). Plasma high-density lipoprotein cholesterol comparisons in black and white populations. *Circulation, 62* (Supp. IV), 99.

Weisse, A. B., Abiuso, P. D., & Thind, I. S. (1977). Acute myocardial infarction in Newark, NJ: A study of racial incidence. *Archives of Internal Medicine, 137,* 1402–1405.

Wenneker, M. B., & Epstein, A. M. (1989). Racial inequalities in the use of procedures for patients with ischemic heart disease in Massachusetts. *Journal of the American Medical Association, 261,* 253–257.

Wilson, P. W. F., Savage, D. D., Castelli, W. P., Garrison, R. J., Donahue, R. P., & Feinleib, F. (1983). HDL-cholesterol in a sample of black adults: The Framingham Minority Study. *Metabolism, 274,* 161.

3

Cerebrovascular Disease in Blacks

Gary H. Friday

Cerebrovascular disease (stroke) rates are higher in Blacks than in Whites in the United States. This includes rates for both morbidity and mortality. This fact has been shown consistently over time and by different studies. Differences have been noted not only in rates of stroke but also in the location and type of stroke. This chapter discusses the epidemiology of the problem, current treatments for stroke and how they relate to stroke in Blacks, and current studies and future research needed to address the problem.

EPIDEMIOLOGY

Mortality Rates

Stroke is the third leading cause of death in the United States in both Blacks and Whites (Cooper, 1987). The stroke mortality rate measures the number of deaths caused by stroke, usually reported as deaths per 100,000 population per year. Stroke mortality rates in Blacks in the United States are approximately twice as high as those in Whites, as shown in Figure 3.1, and are among the highest in the world (Report of the Secretary's Task Force on Black and Minority Health, 1986b). In the younger age groups (25–64), the rate in Blacks is about three to five times as high as that in Whites (see Table 3.1).

Overall, Blacks die at a higher rate than Whites in the United States. Stroke is the single disease entity that accounts for most of the excess mortality rates for Blacks as compared with those for Whites (Otten, Teutsch, Williamson & Marks, 1990), with 28 percent of the mortality excess being due to stroke. Death secondary to hypertension and heart disease combined to account for another 29 percent of the mortality excesses.

Figure 3.1
**Death Rates (per 100,000) for Cerebrovascular Diseases According to Race and
Sex (all ages, age adjusted): United States, 1989**

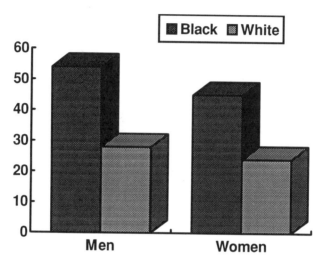

Source: Health, United States, 1991 (pp. 165–166). Department of Health and Human Services.
1992. DHHS Pub. No. (PHS) 92-1232, Hyattsville, MD: U.S. Government Printing Office.

The stroke mortality rate has been decreasing in the United States. However
the imbalance between Black and White Americans still remains (see Table 3.2).
The decline in the stroke mortality rate appears to be leveling off since 1985 in
Whites based on the Minnesota Heart Survey (McGovern, Burke, Sprafka, Xue,
Folsom & Blackburn, 1992). It is not known if mortality rates are also leveling
off for Blacks for that time period.

Incidence Rates

Higher incidence rates have been noted in Blacks as compared with Whites
in the United States (Gillum, 1988). Incidence rates in 1981 from the National
Hospital Discharge Survey were 652 per 100,000 for Blacks and 483 per 100,000
for Whites 35 to 74 years of age. The discharge diagnosis was not validated in
this study. However, a study in which diagnosis was validated, comparing the
incidence of hospitalized stroke over a four-year period (1984 to 1988), between
Blacks and Whites in the Lehigh Valley in Pennsylvania, showed that Blacks
had approximately twice the rate of Whites overall and 3 to 4 times the rate in
the younger age groups (Friday, Lai, Alter, Sobel, LaRue, Gil-Peralta, McCoy,
Levitt & Isack, 1989) (see Table 3.3). In a study of a New York City community
from 1983 to 1986, it was found that the annual stroke rate was approximately
twice as high in Blacks compared to Whites (Sacco, Hauser & Mohr, 1991). It

Table 3.1
Ratio of Stroke Mortality by Age and Race, 1989

	Black Men/ White Men	Black Women/ White Women
25–34	2.8	3.8
35–44	5.0	3.9
45–54	4.5	3.3
55–64	2.9	2.8
65–74	2.0	2.1
75–84	1.3	1.5
85+	0.9	0.8

Source: Health, United States, 1991 (pp. 165–166). Department of Health and Human Services. 1992. DHHS Pub. No. (PHS) 92-1232, Hyattsville, MD: U.S. Government Printing Office.

Table 3.2
Changes in Cerebrovascular Disease Death Rates, per 100,000, by Sex and Race (all ages, age adjusted), 1980 and 1989

	1980	1989	Change
U.S. Black (men)	78	54	24
U.S. White (men)	42	28	14
U.S. Black (women)	62	45	17
U.S. White (women)	35	24	9

Source: Health, United States, 1991 (pp. 165–166). Department of Health and Human Services. 1992. DHHS Pub. No. (PHS) 92-1232, Hyattsville, MD: U.S. Government Printing Office.

was reported that the annual age-adjusted stroke incidence per 100,000 for men 40 years of age or older to be 567 for Blacks and 326 for Whites and for women 40 years of age or older to be 716 for Blacks and 326 for Whites (see Figure 3.2). The results of these studies mirror the increased rates of mortality for

Table 3.3
Black Age-specific Observed and Expected (based on the White population)
Stroke Frequency in the Lehigh Valley

Age	Population	Strokes	Expected
<45	6,347	5	0.88
45-64	1,078	21	4.90
65-74	269	16	5.48
>75	142	3	7.28
Total	7,836	45	18.54

Source: Friday et al. (1989). Stroke in the Lehigh Valley: Racial/ethnic differences. *Neurology 39,* 1167. Copyright 1989 by Advanstar Communications, Inc. Adapted by permission.

Figure 3.2
Stroke Incidence (per 100,000) Comparing Race and Gender (age > or = 40)

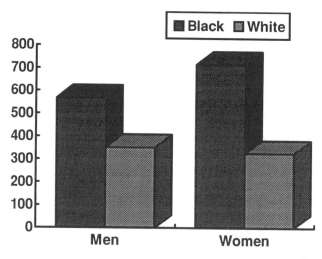

Source: "Hospitalized Stroke in Blacks and Hispanics in Northern Manhattan," R. L. Sacco, W. A. Hauser, and J. P. Mohr, 1991, *Stroke, 22,* p. 1493. Copyright 1991 by Stroke. Adapted by permission.

Blacks, suggesting that the higher stroke mortality rates are mostly due to higher incidence rates.

Prevalence Rates

The overall prevalence of stroke was found to be higher in Blacks than in Whites in the United States. The Evans County, Georgia, study (Heyman, Karp & Hayden, 1971) found the prevalence to be 41 per 1,000 versus 45 per 1,000 for White and Black men respectively, and 13 per 1,000 and 33 per 1,000 for White and Black women, respectively. Also, a study in Copiah County, Mississippi (Schoenberg, Anderson & Haerer, 1986), found a higher prevalence rate of stroke in Blacks as compared with Whites. These differences were not as great as seen in the incidence studies noted earlier, but this discrepancy could be secondary to a lower survival rate for Blacks with stroke, since prevalence studies would count only survivors of stroke.

Stroke Type

Different types of stroke have different outcomes. There are two main types of stroke: hemorrhagic (bleeding within or around the brain) and ischemic (lack of blood flow to the brain secondary usually to blockage of arteries). The hemorrhagic type of stroke has a worse outcome, with 40 percent to 50 percent early mortality rates (Broderick, Brott, Tomsick, Huster & Miller, 1992) versus approximately 17 percent for all types of stroke (Broderick, Phillips, Whisnant, O'Fallon & Bergstralh, 1989).

Subarachnoid hemorrhage (bleeding from a ruptured blood vessel on the surface of the brain) was recently noted to be 2.1 times more common in Blacks than Whites. This study was carried out in the Cincinnati metropolitan area (Broderick et al., 1992). They also found that intracerebral hemorrhage was 1.4 times more common in Blacks than in Whites. In addition, another study (Gross, Kase, Mohr, Cunningham & Baker, 1984), from southern Alabama, found that Blacks had a higher incidence of intracerebral hemorrhage. The study by Sacco et al. (1991), from New York City, also found a higher incidence of intracerebral and subarachnoid hemorrhage in Blacks.

In the Lehigh Valley study (Friday et al., 1989), it was also found that the types of ischemic stroke were different, with Blacks having a higher rate of lacunar stroke (deep strokes secondary to blockage of small arteries within the brain) and Whites having a higher rate of embolic stroke (stroke secondary to heart disease or disease of the large arteries in the neck). Also in the Lehigh Valley study, it was found that Blacks had fewer transient ischemic attacks (TIAs), which are very mild strokes in which the symptoms clear in less than 24 hours, than did Whites. These TIAs are the only clear warning signs of an impending stroke. The majority of TIAs are felt to be secondary to disease of the extracranial blood vessels in the neck. Case series in the United States have demonstrated that Whites have more disease of the extracranial blood vessels than do Blacks (Caplan, Gorelick & Hier, 1986; Gil-Peralta, Alter, Lai, Friday, Otero, Katz & Comerota, 1990). This may explain the lower rate of TIAs in Blacks compared to Whites.

Risk Factors for Stroke

There is no single clear cause for stroke, but a number of factors (other diseases and/or life-styles) have been identified that increase the risk of having a stroke. Some of these risk factors are present to a greater extent in Blacks than Whites in the United States.

The most widely studied and possibly the most important risk factor is hypertension. It has been shown that hypertension can increase risk of stroke (Kuller & Anderson, 1978) and that treatment of hypertension can reduce the occurrence of stroke (Veterans Administration Cooperative Study Group on Antihypertensive Agents, 1967, 1970). Blacks have a higher prevalence of hypertension (Kumanyika & Savage, 1986). In the Lehigh Valley study (Friday et al., 1989), a history of hypertension was found in 67 percent of Black and 56 percent of White stroke patients. Hypertension also develops earlier in Blacks (Kumanyika & Savage, 1986). This increased rate of hypertension helps explain some of the increased rate of stroke seen in Blacks as compared with Whites.

Diabetes mellitus has also been shown to increase the risk of stroke. In the Lehigh Valley study (Friday et al., 1989), diabetes mellitus was seen more often in Black (33%) than in White (26%) stroke patients. Prevalence of diabetes mellitus in the First National Health and Nutrition Examination Survey (NHANES I) was higher in Black men and women (6.7% and 8.8%, respectively), than in White men and women (5.5% and 5.0%, respectively) Kittner, White, Losonczy, Wolf & Hebel, 1990).

Smoking has been shown to be a risk factor for stroke in the Framingham Study, which looked at stroke incidence over a 26-year period in a small, predominantly White community (Wolf, D'Agostino, Kannel, Bonita & Belanger, 1988). The few data available for Blacks from the Multiple Risk Factor Intervention Trial (MRFIT) do not show a clear relationship between smoking and stroke (Neaton, Kuller, Wentworth & Borhani, 1984).

Heart disease is a risk factor for stroke, especially the presence of the cardiac arrhythmia, atrial fibrillation (Stroke Prevention in Atrial Fibrillation Investigators, 1992). In the Lehigh Valley study (Friday et al., 1989) Black patients with stroke had higher rates than Whites of a history of a prior myocardial infarction, 20 percent versus 16 percent, and other heart disease, 53 percent versus 48 percent, respectively.

Lower socioeconomic status is associated with a higher stroke mortality rate. In a study in Baltimore, Kuller and Seltser (1967) reported that both White and non-White men and women had higher stroke mortality rates in the lower half of the socioeconomic group. Further analysis by others has shown that social disorganization as evidenced by factors such as family instability, unemployment, lower percentage of home ownership, higher crime rates, and lower per-capita income were more strongly associated with a higher stroke mortality rate than was a lower socioeconomic status alone (Nesser, Tyroler & Cassel, 1971; James & Kleinbaum, 1976). Also, the rate of stroke among other ethnic groups with socioeconomic status similar to or even lower than Blacks, for example Hispanics in the Lehigh Valley and in New York City (Friday et al., 1989; Sacco et al., 1991), is closer to that of Whites than to Blacks.

Sickle cell anemia is an inherited anemia seen more commonly in Blacks than in Whites. Stroke occurs in approximately 10 percent of those with sickle cell anemia (Mandelbaum & Chutorian, 1984). However, because of the low incidence of sickle cell anemia, the overall contribution to the total number of strokes in Blacks is small. There is no evidence that sickle cell trait, which is more common than sickle cell anemia but rarely causes stroke (Reyes, 1989), substantially increases risk of stroke.

After taking into account increased rates of known risk factors for stroke in Blacks in the United States, the increased rate of stroke is not fully accounted for and other, yet-unidentified factors may be present (Kittner, White, Losonczy, Wolf & Habel, 1990; Otten et al., 1990). Several potential risk factors for stroke are under investigation. These include certain lipid factors and coagulation factors. These risk factors have not yet been studied to any great degree in Black Americans.

ETIOLOGY

There are theories that Blacks in the United States are genetically susceptible to developing hypertension and, as a result, also stroke. However, when atherosclerotic disease of the cerebral blood vessels (the underlying cause of the majority of strokes) has been evaluated comparing Whites and Blacks in the United States and West Africans (Resch, Williams, Lemercier & Loewenson, 1970), it was found that Blacks in the United States had disease of the cerebral blood vessels (atherosclerosis) that was closer to that seen in Whites than in West Africans. This finding suggests common environmental factors that both Blacks and Whites in the United States are exposed to, rather than any genetic factor relating to the etiology of stroke. Also, to date, no clear genetic cause has been found for the vast majority of strokes. Even though a family history of stroke has been suggested as a possible risk factor, no clear pattern is evident such as a recessive or dominant inheritance pattern. It is possible that since families can be subjected to the same environmental factors (e.g., socioeconomic status and/or diet), these common environmental factors rather than genetics could explain any increased risk within families.

It has also been suggested that the ancestors of Blacks in the United States who survived the passage from Africa to America were selected because of their better salt retention ability and, therefore, were less susceptible to death from dehydration (Grim, 1988). This ability to retain salt could also lead to an increased risk of hypertension. However, in Africa there is evidence that risk of hypertension seems to be related to environmental factors. For example when ethnic groups in Africa that normally would reside in rural areas where hypertension is rare move into more urban areas, high rates of hypertension are then seen, with a resultant increase in the stroke rate (Report of the Secretary's Task Force on Black and Minority Health, 1986a). Therefore, the question of genetic versus environmental causes for increased stroke rates in Blacks in the United States is not fully answered; however, the evidence seems to be in favor of environmental causes.

TREATMENT

The best treatment for stroke is to prevent its occurrence (primary prevention). Efforts to do this have been aimed largely at treatment of hypertension and heart disease. Also, TIAs are a warning for a major stroke, and their treatment can prevent the later occurrence of a major stroke. The mortality from stroke has been declining, and the latest decline has been attributed to treatment of hypertension. As mentioned earlier, the mortality has declined for both Blacks and Whites, at a slightly faster rate for Blacks, but the gap still remains. Mortality rates at present, however, seem to be leveling off.

Blacks have stroke at younger ages. This may be secondary to the occurrence of hypertension at younger ages. There is evidence that younger age may be associated with poorer compliance with hypertensive therapy (Caldwell, Cobb, Dowling & Dejongh, 1970). This poorer compliance in the young would, therefore, have a more negative impact on Blacks than Whites in regards to stroke prevention. Also young people, especially men, may have less access to medical care and, therefore, diagnosis and treatment of hypertension could be delayed.

Atrial fibrillation (a heart arrhythmia) has been shown to increase the risk of stroke (especially in those with hypertension and other heart disease). Preventive treatment is usually with the blood thinner sodium warfarin, which requires close medical monitoring of its effect. The use of warfarin has been studied in atrial fibrillation, but little is known about its side effects in Blacks with atrial fibrillation, who are more likely to be hypertensive and therefore possibly at greater risk for complications (such as brain hemorrhage). Also, because of the need for close medical monitoring, those patients who are poor or who are without health insurance may be unable to receive this medication.

TIAs, which are warning signs of more severe strokes, are generally treated with aspirin. In the Lehigh Valley Study (Friday et al., 1989), approximately 10 percent of strokes in Whites were preceded by TIAs; however, in Blacks only 2 percent of strokes were preceded by TIAs. Therefore, Blacks are less likely to be identified as at risk for stroke and therefore could not benefit from this treatment.

At the present time, there is no acute treatment for stroke (with the exception of subarachnoid hemorrhage) other than supportive therapy and therapy to prevent additional strokes. However, clinical trials are being conducted for potential acute therapies. Involvement of Blacks in these trials has not been well documented. In a recent trial of ganglioside treatment for acute stroke involving almost 300 patients, only 18 percent were Black (Alter, personal communication, 1992). The effect of therapy on this group could not be evaluated separately, because of the small numbers. The only acute treatment for stroke that is approved in the United States is nimodipine for subarachnoid hemorrhage (SAH). Blacks in the United States appear to have a different distribution of risk factors for SAH and therefore may respond differently to treatment (Dennis, 1989). A study is presently under way (Dennis, personal communication, 1991) to look at outcome of Blacks with SAH who were treated with nimodipine. Trials with nimodipine and other similar drugs have not shown clear effectiveness in treating the other types of stroke, which constitute more than 90 percent of the total number of strokes. But even in the preliminary published studies Blacks are usually not mentioned, and if they are mentioned, the numbers are usually too small for Blacks to be analyzed separately.

Another important treatment for stroke is rehabilitation after stroke (e.g., training people to walk again or to be able to dress themselves). In case studies reported from Duke University Medical Center in Durham, N.C. (Horner, Matchar, Divine & Feussner, 1991), Blacks suffered more initial functional impairment according to the Barthel Index, which measures daily activities such as walking, eating, and bathing. Their initial scores were only one-half those of White patients. There was also slower improvement for Black patients. The investigators felt that delayed health care and a "worse-risk profile" may have been reasons for the greater initial impairment in Blacks. They also felt that a "poorer social network" and a higher number of widowed patients among Black patients may have led to the slowed improvement. However, one wonders about differences in the availability and quality of rehabilitation services for Black as compared with White patients as also a possible contributing factor. There is little information on the availability of rehabilitation services for Black stroke patients as compared with White patients.

FUTURE DIRECTIONS

Studies in Progress

Currently, there are ongoing studies to look at the epidemiology of stroke in Blacks in the United States. A number of issues that were not addressed in earlier studies. In many studies, computed tomography scans were not normally done (especially before 1980), so diagnosis of stroke type and location were not as accurate as is possible today. Also, even when computed tomography scans were done, type of stroke was not always analyzed. Therefore, outcome based on type of stroke often was not evaluated. The contribution of different risk factors, combinations of risk factors in the same patient, and their relative weight for predicting increased risk of stroke, especially for black patients, require more extensive and controlled study.

At the present time, a case-control study of stroke and known and suspected risk factors for stroke is being carried out in Blacks in the southern United States (Gaines, personal communication, 1991). This study will examine racial differences in the frequency of particular stroke types and the effect of stroke risk factors. Knowing which types of stroke are more likely to occur and which risk factors are the most important would allow for more specific and appropriate allocation of public health care resources to address the problem of excessive numbers of stroke in Blacks.

A study is also presently underway in Blacks to evaluate SAH, one of the least common types of stroke, but one of the more deadly with a 30-50 percent mortality rate. As mentioned previously, this type of stroke occurs more frequently in Black than in White patients and appears to have a different risk factor profile and different outcome in Black patients. These differences, which were noted at Howard University Hospital (Dennis, 1989), are being examined in a broader study including other health centers around the United States.

A number of clinical trials for the acute treatment of stroke are underway but no clear plan for analysis of racial differences in outcome has been outlined. The guidelines of the Food and Drug Administration for clinical trials give general recommendations for diversity of the populations studied in drug treatment trials. However, these guidelines are not always followed, and there have been efforts to have clinical trials include more elderly and women (Gurwitz, Col & Avorn, 1992). Similar attention to adequate representation of Black patients in clinical trials of new drug therapies for stroke should be given.

Recommendations

Longitudinal studies similar to those conducted in Framingham, Massachussetts, and in Rochester, Minnesota, looking at risk factors for stroke in Black populations need to be conducted. This type of study could be used to identify additional risk factors and to confirm risk factors already identified for White patients that are not clear risk factors in Black patients. Longitudinal studies looking at control of risk factors and their effect on reducing stroke rates also need to be evaluated. Case control studies on less common types of stroke, such as SAH in which a longitudinal study may be impractical because of the large number of subjects required, are needed to try to identify possible preventive measures.

Studies of the effect of rehabilitation treatment and availability of such treatment to Black stroke patients need to be performed.

Risk factors for recurrent stroke have not been evaluated in Black patients. Even in White patients, there are few data, but it appears that control of known risk factors for initial stroke may not lead to prevention of recurrent strokes.

SUMMARY

It is clear that Blacks in the United States have a higher rate of stroke than do Whites, with a resultant excess of stroke mortality. At the present time, treatment of hypertension is the best means of preventing stroke and has led to a decrease of stroke mortality in both Blacks and Whites. However, stroke still remains the third leading cause of death in both Blacks and Whites and is the single most important disease that accounts for the excess mortality seen in Blacks as compared with Whites. Therefore, much work still needs to be done. In addition to improved treatment and prevention of hypertension, more work needs to be done to determine other methods of reducing the stroke rate, possibly by identifying other treatable risk factors for stroke. Also, more work needs to be done to ensure that acute treatments for stroke, both rehabilitation and drugs, include Blacks as well as Whites. As newer treatments arrive, improved availability and utilization of health care by Black patients become that much more important.

REFERENCES

Alter, Milton (personal communication, March 15, 1992).

Broderick, J. P., Brott, T., Tomsick, T., Huster, G., & Miller, R. (1992). The risk of subarachnoid and intracerebral hemorrhages in blacks as compared to whites. *New England Journal of Medicine, 326*, 733–736.

Broderick, J. P., Phillips, J. S., Whisnant, J. P., O'Fallon, W. M., & Bergstralh, E. J. (1989). Incidence rates of stroke in the eighties: The end of the decline in stroke? *Stroke, 20*, 577–582.

Caldwell, J. R., Cobb, S., Dowling, M., & Dejongh, D. (1970). The drop-out problem in antihypertensive treatment: A pilot study of social and emotional factors influencing a patient's ability to follow antihypertensive treatment. *Journal of Chronic Disease, 22*, 579–592.

Caplan, L. R., Gorelick, P. B., & Hier, D. B. (1986). Race, sex and occlusive cerebrovascular disease: A review. *Stroke, 17*, 648–655.

Cooper, E. S. (1987). Clinical cerebrovascular disease in hypertensive blacks. *Journal of Clinical Hypertension, 3*, 79S–84S.

Dennis, G. (1989). *Aneurysms in Afro-Americans.* Paper presented at the meeting of the Neurology/Neurosurgery Section of the National Medical Association, Orlando, FL.

Dennis, Gary (Personal communication, August 15, 1987).

Friday, G., Lai, S. M., Alter, M., Sobel, E., LaRue, L., Gil-Peralta, A., McCoy, R. L., Levitt, L. P., & Isack, T. (1989). Stroke in the Lehigh Valley: Racial/ethnic differences. *Neurology, 39*, 1165–1168.

Gaines, Kenneth (Personal communication, January 15, 1991).

Gil-Peralta, A., Alter, M., Lai, S. M., Friday, G., Otero, A., Katz, M., & Comerota, A. J. (1990). Duplex doppler and spectral flow analysis of racial differences in cerebrovascular atherosclerosis. *Stroke, 21*, 740–744.

Gillum, R. F. (1988). Stroke in blacks. *Stroke, 19*, 1–8.

Grim, C. E. (1988). On slavery, salt and high blood pressure in black Americans. *Clinical Research, 36,* 426A.

Gross, C. R., Kase, C. S., Mohr, J. P., Cunningham, S. C., & Baker, W. E. (1982). Stroke in South Alabama: Incidence and diagnostic features—a population-based study. *Stroke, 15,* 249–254.

Gurwitz, J. H., Col, N. F., & Avorn, J. (1992). The exclusion of the elderly and women from clinical trials in acute myocardial infarction. *Journal of the American Medical Association, 268,* 1417–1422.

Heyman, A., Karp, H. R., & Hayden, S. (1971). Cerebrovascular disease in the bi-racial population of Evans County, Georgia. *Stroke, 2,* 509–518.

Horner, R. D., Matchar, D. B., Divine, G. W., & Feussner, J. R. (1991). Racial variations in ischemic stroke-related physical and functional impairments. *Stroke, 22,* 1497–1501.

James, S. A., & Kleinbaum, D. G. (1976). Sociological stress and hypertension related mortality rates in North Carolina. *American Journal of Public Health, 66,* 354–358.

Kittner, S. J., White, L. R., Losonczy, K. G., Wolf, P. A., & Hebel, J. R. (1990). Black-white differences in stroke incidence in a national sample. *Journal of the American Medical Association, 264,* 1267–1270.

Kuller, L. H. (1986). Stroke report. In *Report of the Secretary's Task Force on Black and Minority Health, Cardiovascular and Cerebrovascular Disease.* (p. 478). Washington, DC: Department of Health and Human Services.

Kuller, L., & Anderson, H. (1978). Epidemiology of stroke. *Advances in Neurology, 19,* 282–311.

Kuller, L., & Seltser, R. (1967). Cerebrovascular disease mortality in Maryland. *American Journal of Epidemiology, 86,* 442–450.

Kumanyika, S. K., & Savage, D. D. (1986). Ischemic heart disease risk factors in black Americans. In *Report of the Secretary's Task Force on Black and Minority Health, Cardiovascular and Cerebrovascular Disease* (pp. 269–274). Washington, DC: Department of Health and Human Services.

Mandelbaum, D. E., & Chutorian, A. M. (1984). Neurological complications of the hemoglobinopathies. Part I. *Neurology and Neurosurgery, 23,* 3–7.

McGovern, P. G., Burke, G. L., Sprafka, J. M., Xue, S., Folsom, A. R., & Blackburn, H. (1992). Trends in mortality, morbidity, and risk factor levels for stroke from 1960 through 1990: The Minnesota Heart Survey. *Journal of the American Medical Association, 268,* 753–759.

Neaton, J. D., Kuller, L. H., Wentworth, D., & Borhani, N. O. (1984). Total and cardiovascular mortality in relation to cigarette smoking, serum cholesterol concentration, and diastolic blood pressure among black and white males followed up for five years. *American Heart Journal, 108,* 759–770.

Nesser, W. B., Tyroler, H. A., & Cassel, J. C. (1971). Social disorganization and stroke mortality in the black population of North Carolina. *American Journal of Epidemiology, 93,* 166–175.

Otten, M. W., Teutsch, S. M., Williamson, D. F., & Marks, J. S. (1990). The effect of known risk factors on the excess mortality of black adults in the United States. *Journal of the American Medical Association, 263,* 845–850.

Report of the Secretary's Task Force on Black and Minority Health, Cardiovascular and

Cerebrovascular Disease. (1986a). (pp. 27–28). Washington, DC: Department of Health and Human Services.

Report of the Secretary's Task Force on Black and Minority Health, Cardiovascular and Cerebrovascular Disease. (1986b). (p. 518). Washington, DC: Department of Health and Human Services.

Resch, J. A., Williams, A. O., Lemercier, G., & Loewenson, R. B. (1970). Comparative autopsy studies on cerebral atherosclerosis in Nigerian and Senegal Negroes, American Negroes and Caucasians. *Atherosclerosis, 12*, 401–407.

Reyes, M. G. (1989). Subcortical cerebral infarctions in sickle cell trait. *Journal of Neurology, Neurosurgery and Psychiatry, 52*, 516–518.

Sacco, R. L., Hauser, W. A., & Mohr, J. P. (1991). Hospitalized stroke in blacks and Hispanics in Northern Manhattan. *Stroke, 22*, 1491–1496.

Schoenberg, B. S., Anderson, D. W., & Haerer, A. F. (1986). Racial differences in the prevalence of stroke: Copiah County, Mississippi. *Archives of Neurology, 43*, 565–568.

Stroke Prevention in Atrial Fibrillation Investigators. (1992). Prediction of thromboembolism in atrial fibrillation: II. Echocardiographic features of patients at risk. *Annals of Internal Medicine, 116*, 6–12.

Veterans Administration Cooperative Study Group on Antihypertensive Agents. (1967). Effects of treatment on morbidity in hypertension: Results in patients with diastolic blood pressure averaging 115 through 129 mmHg. *Journal of the American Medical Association, 202*, 1028–1034.

Veterans Administration Cooperative Study Group on Antihypertensive Agents. (1970). Effects of treatment on morbidity in hypertension: Results in patients with diastolic blood pressure averaging 90 through 114 mmHg. *Journal of the American Medical Association, 213*, 1143–1152.

Wolf, P. A., D'Agostino, R. B., Kannel, W. B., Bonita, R., & Belanger, A. J. (1988). Cigarette smoking as a risk factor for stroke. *Journal of the American Medical Association, 259*, 1025–1029.

4

Hypertension: A Community Perspective

Lee R. Bone, Martha N. Hill, and David M. Levine

Hypertension is one of the most prevalent and best researched health conditions in Blacks. Despite dramatic improvements over the past three decades in the proportion of Blacks with diagnosed and controlled hypertension, undetected and/or uncontrolled hypertension remains one of the most important health challenges in the United States. The gap between the development of research findings and policy recommendations about the detection, evaluation, and treatment of hypertension and effective application of this information at the individual and community levels are the basis of the current hypertension control problem. To narrow this gap, efforts need to be focused not only at the individual and community levels but also at the interface between them. The solution to decreasing hypertension can be found in applying scientific knowledge about behavior, pathophysiology, and therapeutics to individuals and communities.

This chapter presents a discussion of the hypertension challenge primarily from the individual and community levels. The individual level includes persons and their interactions with family, friends, and health care providers. The community level includes geography, local institutions (i.e., churches, schools, and work sites), and the health care delivery system.

THE EPIDEMIOLOGY OF HYPERTENSION

Essential hypertension, also named primary hypertension and high blood pressure (HBP), is defined as sustained elevation of blood pressure (systolic ≥ 140 mmHg and/or diastolic ≥ 90 mmHg) or lower blood pressure and taking antihypertensive medication. Approximately 50 million Americans have hypertension, an estimated 10 million fewer than a decade ago (Joint National Committee, 1992). The prevalence of HBP is 30 percent higher in African Americans compared to Whites (38 percent vs 29 percent), and the rate increases with age in the United States (Report of the Secretary's Task Force on Black and Minority Health, 1986). In Blacks, HBP develops at an earlier age and is more severe than in Whites. Severely elevated levels (DBP $\geq$ 115 mmHg) of blood pressure (BP) are five times greater in Black males compared to White males and seven times more common in Black females than in their White counterparts (Subcommittee on Definition and Prevalence, 1985). The higher prevalence of HBP persists when controlled for age, adiposity, and socioeconomic status.

Cardiovascular diseases are the single largest contributing factor to the differential morbidity and mortality in Blacks. Mortality rates attributable to HBP increase with age and peak earlier in Blacks (Keil & Saunders, 1991). Nationally, heart disease and stroke are, respectively, the first and third leading causes of death for the total population, with Black males bearing the highest rates for all race/sex groups. The stroke mortality rate among Blacks is estimated to be 66 percent higher than among Whites (Hypertension Detection and Follow-Up Program Cooperative Research Group, 1982).

Complications of uncontrolled HBP, especially cerebral vascular accidents, left ventricular hypertrophy, congestive heart failure, acute myocardial infarction, and end-stage renal disease (ESRD), are more common in U.S. Blacks than in Whites. The economic costs of hypertension, its sequelae, and its treatment are high. Estimates of the cost of antihypertensive medication in 1989 were $2.9 billion. The costs of cerebrovascular disease, specifically rehabilitation and work years lost, were estimated in 1988 at $12.9 billion. Treatment for renal failure including dialysis and transportation cost Americans $2 billion in 1988. Dialysis treatment in 1989 cost $25,000 per year per patient (Shulman, 1991).

REVIEW OF CAUSATIVE AND TREATMENT FACTORS

Risk Factors: Individual Level

HBP is a multifactorial condition in which genetics, neural, humoral, vascular, cardiac, renal, nutritional, and psychosocial factors play interdependent roles. The familial aggregation of essential hypertension has been well documented in both Blacks and Whites; however, no studies to date have shown genetic differences between Blacks and Whites which explain the phenomenon (Gillum, 1979). Blacks, as compared to Whites, have greater sensitivity to sodium and experience lower plasma renin activity, suppression of the renin angiotensin system, and increased vascular reactivity to stress. Data from INTERSALT have not consistently shown a higher intake of sodium in Blacks compared to Whites; a lower intake of potassium in Blacks has been shown to result in a higher sodium-potassium ratio, which may explain the effect on blood pressure (Elliot, Dyer & Stamler, 1989).

Epidemiologic studies have identified life-style factors including obesity, amount and type of dietary fat intake, sodium and potassium intake, physical activity level, and use of alcohol as possible determinants of BP levels. Further, chronic psychological stress may also be important in the etiology of BP (Fredrikson & Mathews 1990). While it is acknowledged that genetic and biologic antecedents are necessary for the development of HBP, environmental, psychosocial, and behavioral factors are recognized as interacting with the former factors in the development of HBP.

Obesity is more prevalent in Blacks compared to Whites and correlates with increases in blood pressure especially with increasing age. In the population-based NHANES II (1987) the prevalence of obesity in Black females was 43.8 percent compared with 27.1 percent of total female population. Obesity may be explained by intake of secondary food items, i.e., snacking and finishing up after meals, and by lower levels of energy expenditure in Black females (Kumanyika, 1989). NHANES II data indicate higher levels of obesity in middle-aged (35–54 years) Black males compared to White males. Data from National Health Interview Survey (NHIS) (1985) indicates that the extent of physical activity in Black males is similar to that of White males. In considering obesity as a risk factor for HBP and cardiovascular disease it is important to distinguish between body fat and weight, which, although highly correlated, may represent differing metabolic processes and different cardiovascular disease risk mechanisms (Kumanyika, 1989).

The role of increasing levels of alcohol consumption and increasing levels of blood pressure has been demonstrated in cross-sectional and prospective studies (MacMahon, 1987). While agreement on the cardiac benefits of small amounts of alcohol has not been reached, there is no disputing the adverse effects of heavy alcohol consumption on blood pressure levels (Joint National Committee, 1988). Heavy alcohol consumption (more than 2 alcoholic beverages per day) has been associated with 5 percent of hypertension in individuals 18–49 years of age and 6 to 7 percent increase in individuals equal to or greater than 50 years of age (Moore, Levine, Southard, Entwistle & Shapiro, 1990).

The socioeconomic and political experience of Blacks directly influences the number and severity of psychosocial risk factors. Blacks' exposure to poverty is strongly related to economic insecurity, high unemployment, low occupational status, and low educational status. Low-income Blacks have reported more psychological distress than lower-income and high-income Whites and high-income Blacks, perhaps due to the combined burden of poverty and racism (Anderson, McNeilly & Myers, 1991). Additional psychosocial risk factors in Blacks are job-related stress, lack of social integration and social support, chronic anxiety, and exhaustion or fatigue. Coronary prone (Type A) behavioral risk factors characterized by competitiveness, impatience, excessive drive and hostility, as well as "John Henryism" (a behavior pattern of determination against overwhelming odds), have been found in Blacks (Livingston, Levine & Moore, 1991). The studies conducted to assess these factors and their association with cardiovascular risk and disease are difficult to interpret. There is a lack of knowledge about what these variables mean in terms of underlying biological processes and about ways in which individuals with different personalities, from different backgrounds and cultures, identify situations as stressful and handle stressful life events.

Health Care Utilization

Inadequate utilization of health care is a well-recognized problem that adversely affects BP control for Blacks and particularly for Black males. Access to health care is a particularly important problem for Blacks, where physical, logistical, structural, financial, and sociocultural factors all contribute to the problem. Barriers to care include failure to recognize culturally specific health care seeking patterns of Blacks, lack of continuity of providers, inadequate provider-patient communication, absence of and inconvenient transportation, long waiting times, inconvenient primary care locations and appointment times, absence of preappointment reminders, and insufficient follow-up efforts. In the Hypertension Detection and Follow-up Program (HDFP), patients were more likely to become inactive clinic attenders if they were young, Black, had a lower level of educational attainment, were unemployed, were cigarette smokers, and had lower baseline diastolic blood pressures (Smith, Curb, Hardy, Hawkins & Tyroler, 1982). Access to care is also influenced by financial barriers. Among the 35 million uninsured Americans, Blacks are approximately 1.5 times more likely than Whites to be uninsured (22 percent vs. 15 percent) (Long, 1987). Twenty percent of Blacks compared to 13 percent of Whites report no usual source of care (Amber & Dull, 1987). Furthermore, Blacks are more than twice as likely to receive care in hospital clinics or emergency rooms as compared to Whites (Collins, 1983). For these individuals, hypertension care and treatment are at best sporadic and, in urban areas, commonly provided as non-urgent care in emergency rooms.

Effective Interventions: Individual Level

Treatment for HBP is both nonpharmacologic (life-style modification) and pharmacologic. There is evidence indicating that at similar starting BP levels, Blacks, when provided equal access to therapy, will achieve similar declines in BP and lower incidence of cardiovascular disease than Whites (Ooi, Budner & Cohen, 1989). Clinical trials of drug treatment for diastolic hypertension have demonstrated the efficacy of drug treatment in preventing stroke, coronary heart disease, and all-cause mortality for Blacks as well as Whites. However, in major multicenter clinical trails, Blacks, particularly males, have benefitted less than Whites despite the trial-neutralizing issues of access, resources, and adherence enhancement (HDFP, 1982). The Systolic Hypertension in the Elderly Program (SHEP), which included Blacks, demonstrated the effectiveness of treating isolated systolic hypertension (systolic BP $\geq$ 160 mmHg) in persons 60+ years, with reductions in both cardiovascular and cerebrovascular morbidity in the treated group.

Nonpharmacologic treatment, or life-style modification, has an important role in the management of HBP and potentially in the primary prevention of HBP. Life-style modification recommendations include weight control, exercise, sodium reduction, increased potassium consumption, reduction of dietary saturated fat and cholesterol, and, if alcohol is consumed, intake of no more than one ounce of ethanol per day. Clinical trials, which included Blacks, have demonstrated positive and sustained effects of weight loss, exercise, sodium restriction, and dietary potassium supplementation on BP (TOHP, 1992). Life-style modifications are recommended for all stages of stepped care proposed by the 1992 Joint National Committee.

The advantages of nonpharmacologic approaches include reduced cost of medical treatment and minimal associated side-effects. However, these approaches may require referral for dietary counseling and do require additional provider time for assessment, explanation, education, support and reinforcement, particularly if the individual is attempting to make a change in a habitual behavior. Furthermore, for the patient, maintaining multiple behavior changes over time can be very difficult, especially if a supportive environment is absent.

The complications of HBP can be prevented, delayed, and/or minimized if BP control is maintained within normal limits. The most important factor related to inadequate BP control is poor adherence to recommended treatment and retention in care. The most extreme consequence of noncompliance includes death, which can be attributed, at least in part, to patient's failure to adhere to a medication regimen. Studies conducted in the 1980s indicated that compliance with antihypertensive medications ranged from a low of 39 percent to a high of 95 percent and varied by practice setting (Dunbar-Jacob, Dwyer & Dunning, 1991). Poor adherence, or noncompliance, remains a challenge because it is difficult to assess, is usually related to multiple factors, and changes over time. Patients may not comply due to misunderstanding of the illness condition and the importance of ongoing treatment, the asymptomatic nature of hypertension, and failure to remember to follow the treatment plan as prescribed. Another important reason for noncompliance may be the lack of continuous application of effective strategies to promote long-term patient adherence and behavior change. The quality of communication in the provider-patient relationship also has been shown to be very important in patient compliance with care and treatment (Roter, 1978).

The HDFP Program demonstrated that hypertension care and control is enhanced with extensive and continuous interventions to improve adherence that include responsive multidisciplinary provider teams that address patient concerns, extensive follow-up and supervision, and free medications, if needed. However, these and the aforementioned aspects of hypertension care have not been widely applied in practice settings where Blacks receive care. Furthermore, in some routine practice settings, where research findings have been integrated into practice, compliance rates have not improved. This may be because the applied strategies were too complex and not culturally relevant to Black patients.

Risk Factors: Community Level

Secondary prevention studies of HBP carried out at the community level, such as the population-based cardiovascular risk reduction studies of North Karelia, Stanford, Pawtucket and Minnesota, as well as the seven state coordination programs, have all demonstrated the feasibility and effectiveness of conducting broad-based comprehensive programs. These programs conducted educational-behavior change interventions based on multiple theoretical frameworks including social learning theory, diffusion theory, and community organization and action theories. Community-wide participation, skill building in problem solving and leadership, as well as ownership at all levels of planning and interventions, form the cornerstone of the conduct and sustainability of these programs. A recent review of community-based cardiovascular and cerebrovascular risk factor reduction programs noted that despite the health disparity between Blacks and Whites, few cardiovascular risk reduction programs directed to Blacks have been implemented and evaluated. Moreover, most programs directed toward Blacks have emphasized only one risk factor, and only a few have focused on multiple risk factors. They have been carried out in close collaboration with multiple health organizations and agencies, including members of the nonprofit sector, such as the American Heart Association. Strengths of these programs include their reliance on already existing infrastructures and the extensive involvement of volunteers and local community leaders in planning and implementing such programs. A particular strength is found in those programs carried out by the black churches. However, a major weakness in the descriptions of these programs is the absence of qualitative and quantitative evaluation components. Thus the ability to determine program effectiveness is limited.

Primary prevention of HBP at the community level is a global, long-range public health goal that offers the potential to interrupt and reduce the prevalence and costly management of hypertension and its complications. It can be accomplished by life-style modification, i.e. nonpharmacologic BP reduction interventions, directed toward the entire population to lower BP in those most likely to develop hypertension. The potential of this approach has been demonstrated in Trials of Hypertension Prevention Phase 1 (TOHP-1), which demonstrated significant reductions of BP with modest reductions in weight or in sodium intake over an 18-month follow-up period. In this and other studies, small changes in mean BP have translated into reduced incidence of hypertension. It has been estimated that the incidence of hypertension may be reduced by as much as 30–50 percent by these approaches (Stamler, 1991).

CASE STUDY: THE EAST BALTIMORE EXPERIENCE

The East Baltimore community was selected as the urban case study example for further discussion because of its long-term, multiphase HBP research and educational intervention programs. Its population has suffered from the highest rates of premature cardiovascular and cerebrovascular disease and death in the state of Maryland, primarily because of uncontrolled hypertension (Levine, Morisky & Bone, 1982). In East Baltimore, one-third of Black adults have HBP, yet less than half are on treatment and are achieving BP control (Southard, 1982). A 21-census tract area in East Baltimore, served by the Johns Hopkins Medical Institutions, was targeted for this program. Currently, the population is 88 percent Black with a median age of 25 years. Fifty-three percent of community residents are women. The average number of completed years of education is 10. Thirty-three percent of eligible adults are unemployed, and 50 percent have incomes below the poverty level.

In the first phase of the East Baltimore High Blood Pressure Control Program (1974–1979), a randomized intervention trial was conducted in a hospital-based outpatient clinic with a sample of 400 hypertensive patients from the East Baltimore community (Levine, Green & Deeds, 1979). This study was supported by the National Heart Lung and Blood Institute to determine the efficacy of behavioral-educational interventions to enhance hypertension care and control. The interventions, which were based upon the PRECEDE framework and provided state-of-the-art hypertension management to the intervention groups, utilized a factorial design to demonstrate the value of enhanced weight control, continuity of care, and adherence to treatment (Green, Levine, Wolle & Deeds, 1979).

The interventions included an exit interview at the end of the clinic visit to clarify the regimen and misperceptions about HBP; a family or peer support with the person to whom the patient turns for health advice, conducted during a home visit to enhance family support and reinforcement of patient adherence to dietary recommendations, medication taking and appointment keeping; and group sessions led by a trained health educator to enhance motivation and peer support. Those patients receiving all three interventions demonstrated the highest continuity of care, weight control, improvement in and adherence to medication taking, and BP control (79 percent in the treatment group vs. 38 percent in the control group). Moreover, these improvements were associated with a 36 percent decrease in hospitalization and a 65 percent decrease in five-year mortality rates from uncontrolled hypertension (Morisky et al., 1983).

In Phase II (1979–1982), the clinic and home-based clinical trial intervention strategies were disseminated throughout the East Baltimore community. This demonstration program, utilizing the PRECEDE framework (Green, Kreuter & Deeds, 1980) and testing coordination of existing provider and community resources, was part of a five-year National Heart, Lung and Blood Institute supported statewide HBP control program. Essential principles for community-based interventions applied in this program include (1) identification of subsets of the population with the greatest health needs, (2) development of coordinating structure made up of representatives from health care providers and community groups, (3) assessment of patterns and factors related to preventable and/or controllable morbidity and mortality, (4) selection of specific measurable health status goals and behavioral objectives, (5) design of multiple intervention strategies and evaluation methods, and (6) maximal community and provider participation and ownership to improve the sustainability of effective interventions (Levine, Becker & Bone, 1992).

An East Baltimore Community-Provider Task Force was formed to plan, implement, and evaluate the program. The Task Force was comprised of representatives from community agencies and organizations as well as representatives from the major providers of health care in the community, including the Johns Hopkins Medical Institutions. The chair of the Task Force, a community leader, was selected because of her extensive experience in the community and her commitment to improving health services in East Baltimore.

To improve the communities' access to HBP screening, monitoring, educational counseling, outreach, and follow-up, 27 community residents, selected by the Task Force, were trained and certified by the American Heart Association and Johns Hopkins as community health workers (CHWs). Their training included BP measurement, educational counseling in HBP and the other cardiovascular risk factors, and strategies for outreach and follow-up.

CHW services were provided from geographically dispersed community sites including two Mayor's Stations, a school, and two community multipurpose centers. Later in the program, they were selected from health care delivery sites and recreation centers. The introduction of CHWs was associated with enhanced continuity of care and adherence to treatment, with a 19 percent improvement in appointment keeping among patients receiving the CHW interventions (Bone, Levine & Parry, 1984), and improved BP control in males from 12 percent to 40 percent (Levine, Becker & Bone, 1992).

The third and ongoing phase of the program (1982–1995), supported by the Maryland Department of Health and Mental Hygiene and more recently by the Johns Hopkins Hospital, focuses on the high-risk Black male population. The primary target population are males 18–49 years old, who are least likely to be aware (59.4 percent), in care (39.6 percent) and achieving BP control (24.2 percent) (Bone, Levine, Parry, Morisky & Green, 1984).

Hospital emergency rooms are the primary site selected for interventions during this phase because 85 percent of the targeted Black male population have at least one visit to the emergency room per year. During this time salaried CHWs have been fully integrated into the Johns Hopkins Hospital Emergency Department to supplement and reinforce Emergency Room staff in HBP detection, referral, and follow up. The CHWs provide continuous reinforcement and facilitate continuity of care and adherence to treatment by tracking and providing outreach services to approximately 600 males over a 2-year time period. Significant positive effects of the CHW interventions include enhanced linkage with care, continuity of care, and BP control of 40 percent in men from the community (Levine & Bone, 1990).

Currently, a clinical trial, supported by the National Center for Nursing Research, is being conducted to systematically investigate whether educational-behavioral interventions, administered by a nurse-CHW team, can reduce uncontrolled HBP by increasing retention in care and adherence to therapy in East Baltimore Black males 18–49 years of age. Simultaneously, a larger community wide health promotion program is being implemented. This program is being carried out in an expanded geographical area of East Baltimore by the Johns Hopkins Center for Health Promotion in collaboration with Clergy United for Renewal of East Baltimore (CURE) (Levine, Becker & Bone, 1992). Additionally, the education of future practitioners of community public health is being expanded, as well as efforts to recruit and provide traineeships for Blacks. In the fall of 1992, the W. K. Kellogg Foundation funded a four-year program to improve the public health of the East Baltimore community by enhancing public health education, training and community-based practice. This partnership program includes CURE, the Baltimore City Health Department and school system, Health Care for the Homeless, and the Johns Hopkins University Schools of Public Health, Medicine and Nursing as well as the Johns Hopkins Health System.

RECOMMENDATIONS

Primary Prevention

Primary prevention efforts are needed if the incidence of hypertension in the United States population, particularly in Blacks, is to be reduced. Further investigation is critical if we are to learn the most effective and enduring methods to bring about behavior change to prevent HBP at the individual, provider, and community levels. Behavioral and educational interventions aimed at reducing salt intake and alcohol consumption, increasing physical activity, and reducing obesity, should be targeted toward children, adolescents, and young adults. The testing of family approaches to support and maintain life-style changes is needed.

Secondary Prevention

The social context within which Black patients live and receive health care needs to be better understood in order to have more effective BP control programs. Cultural relevance and sustainability of effective interventions are mandatory if interventions are to be effective over time. Care must be organized and delivered in all sites to include the following: working with the individual to understand and impact upon the barriers to care and treatment, enhancing provider responsiveness to patient concerns, reinforcement and support of the individual, and implementation of outreach and follow-up services.

Models for efficient and effective care of hypertension are based upon multidisciplinary approaches. Use of CHWs and nurse-run clinics are encouraged. Easily accessible illness prevention and health promotion centers located in high-risk communities also are encouraged. These centers, which can be staffed by a nurse and trained certified volunteer health workers from the community, can provide free services to supplement the provider system. These outreach services include screening, monitoring, educational counseling, referral, follow-up, and outreach.

Nonadherence to HBP treatment and continuing care are major barriers to the achievement of BP control, and they seriously compromise the efforts of community-wide programs. Continuing research on the application and sustainability of approaches that have been shown to be effective are needed. In addition, the reasons for noncompliant behavior, particularly for subsets of the population, such as Black males, are not fully understood. While studies have shown that multiple strategies are necessary, the best matching of patients with effective approaches and the best reinforcement strategy over a lifetime have not yet been studied, nor do we fully understand why individuals cycle in and out of adherent behavior. Furthermore, mechanisms for reimbursement for HBP monitoring and education outside of and within medical care need to be established.

Improving Detection

Early detection of HBP is feasible, especially if annual or biannual measurement of BP remains prevalent. However, providers must give attention to BP readings and make specific recommendations for primary as well as secondary prevention. Providers also must refer patients to follow-up educational counseling and treatment, if necessary, and monitor the benefits and risks to assure that the treatment is not worse than the disease.

Community Screening

Community-based screening for new-onset HBP in the general population is not needed. If held, community-based screening should be conducted in situations where high-risk populations can be reached, counseled, referred, and followed. It is important that all screenings are staffed, not only by individuals trained in accurate BP measurement but also by at least one health care professional experienced in assessment and counseling of individuals with HBP. This later recommendation is based upon the likelihood that previously diagnosed and treated individuals will be present at a screening for HBP monitoring and will need individualized educational counseling.

CONCLUSION

A comprehensive national strategy in research, education, and policy development has led to improvement in HBP control at the individual and community levels. The coordinated efforts of the National Heart Lung and Blood Institute, health professional organizations, the American Heart Association, the American Red Cross, the National Black Health Providers Task Force, and the Office of

Minority Health, as well as state and local health departments, have all contributed to the success of the National HBP Education Program.

Local and statewide initiatives have funded programs specifically to improve hypertension control and to reduce the associated risk factors. In many states, governor-appointed commissions and targeted funding for innovative strategies have reached Black hypertensives through churches, recreation centers, and outreach programs from hospitals and ambulatory care settings. Trained community health workers have been vital to the success of these programs. The extent to which these programs are community-based and owned has been shown to be strongly associated with their sustainability.

The importance of continuing support for these programs, both from the public and private sectors cannot be underestimated, especially in times of scarce resources and competitive demands for health care resources, for example, from other epidemics such as AIDS and tuberculosis. Of particular concern are the underinsured and uninsured Black subgroups with HBP who will need proactive advocates with creative approaches at the individual and community levels to bring and maintain them in continuing care and treatment. While there have been some improvements in the health status of U.S. Blacks, major gaps still exist between the health status of Blacks and Whites. These gaps are primarily related to poverty in resources, as well as spirit. The challenge is to ensure that community-based approaches reach high-risk subgroups and that existing policies reflect this priority.

NOTE

I would like to acknowledge the following individuals: Mary Davis, M.S.P.H., a doctoral candidate in the Department of Health Policy and Management, who assisted with the editing. In addition, Beverly Siegel, my secretary, who patiently typed all drafts and the final copy of the chapter.

REFERENCES

Anderson, N. B., McNeilly, M., & Myers, H. (1991). Autonomic reactivity and hypertension in Blacks: A review and proposed model. *Ethnicity and Disease, 1*, 154–170.

Amber, R. W., & Dull, H. B. (1987). *Closing the Gap: the Burden of Non-necessary Illness*. New York: Oxford University Press.

Bone, L. R., Levine, D. M., Parry, R. E., Morisky, D. E., & Green, L. W. (1984). Update on the factors associated with high blood pressure compliance. *Maryland State Medical Journal, 33*, 201–204.

Bone, L. R., Mamon, J., & Levine, D. M. (1989). Emergency department detection and follow up of high blood pressure: Use and effectiveness of community health workers. *American Journal of Emergency Medicine, 7*, 16–20.

Collins, J. G. (1983). Physician visits, volume and interval since last visit (U.S. 1980. DHHS Publication No. (PHS) 83-1572). National Center for Health Statistics. Washington, DC: Government Printing Office.

Dunbar-Jacob, J., Dwyer, K., & Dunning, E. J. (1991). Compliance with antihypertensive regimen: A review of the research in the 1980s. *Annals of Behavioral Medicine, 13*, 31–39.

Elliot, P., Dyer, A., & Stamler, R. (1989). The INTERSALT study: Result for 24-hour sodium and potassium, by age and sex. *Journal of Human Hypertension, 3*, 323.

Fredrikson, M., & Mathews, K. A. (1990). Cardiovascular responses to behavioral stress and hypertension: A metaanalytic review. *Annals of Behavioral Medicine, 12*, 30–39.

Gillum, R. F. (1979). Pathophysiology of hypertension in blacks and whites: A review of the basis of racial blood pressure differences. *Hypertension, 1*, 468–475.

Green, L. W., Levine, D. M., Wolle, J., & Deeds, S. G. (1979). Development of randomized patient education experiments with urban poor hypertensives. *Patient Counseling and Health Education, 1*, 106–111.

Green, L. W., Kreuter, M. W., and Deeds, S. G. (1980). *Health education planning: A diagnostic approach.* Palo Alto, Calif.: Mayfield Publishing Co.

Hypertension Detection and Follow-Up Program Cooperative Group (HDFP). (1982). Five-year findings of the hypertension detection and follow-up program III: Reduction in stroke incidence among persons with high blood pressure. *Journal of the American Medical Association, 247*, 633–638.

Joint National Committee. (1988). The 1988 report of the Joint National Committee on Detection, Evaluation and Treatment of High Blood Pressure.

Joint National Committee. (1992). The 1992 report of the Joint National Committee on Detection, Evaluation and Treatment of High Blood Pressure. (Draft)

Keil, J. E., & Saunders, E. (1991). Urban and rural differences in cardiovascular disease in blacks. In E. Saunders (Ed.), *Cardiovascular Disease in Blacks.* Philadelphia: F. A. Davis Co.

Kumanyika, S. K. (1989). The association between obesity and hypertension in Blacks. *Clinical Cardiology 12* (Supp. 4), 72–77.

Levine, D. M., Becker, D. M., & Bone, L. R. (1992). Narrowing the gap in health status of minority populations—Description of a community-academic medical center partnership. *American Journal of Preventive Medicine, 8*, 319–323.

Levine, D. M., & Bone, L. R. (1990). The impact of a planned health education approach on the control of hypertension in a high risk population. *Journal of Human Hypertension, 4*, 317–321.

Levine, D. M., Morisky, D. E., & Bone, L. R. (1982). Data-based planning for educational interventions through hypertension control programs for urban and rural populations in Maryland. *Public Health Reports, 97*, 109–112.

Levine, D. M., Green, L. W., & Deeds, S. G. (1979). Health education for hypertensive patients. *Journal of the American Medical Association, 241*, 1700–1703.

Livingston, I. L., Levine, D. M., & Moore, R. D. (1991). Social integration and black intraracial variation in blood pressure. *Ethnicity & Disease, 1*, 135–149.

Long, S. H. (1987). Public versus employment-related health insurance: Experience and implications for Black and Nonblack Americans. *Millbank Quarterly, 65*, 200–210.

MacMahon, S. (1987). Alcohol consumption and hypertension. *Hypertension, 9*, 111–121.

Moore, R. D., Levine, D. M., Southard, J., Entwistle, G., & Shapiro, S. (1990). Alcohol consumption and blood pressure in the 1992 Maryland Hypertension Survey. *American Journal of Hypertension, 3,* 1–7.

Morisky, D. E., Levine, D. M., Green, L. W., Shapiro, S., Russell, P. R., & Smith, C. (1983). Five-year blood pressure control and mortality following health education for hypertensive patients. *American Journal of Public Health, 73,* 153–162.

Ooi, W. L., Budner, N. S., & Cohen, H. (1989). Impact of race on treatment response and cardiovascular disease among hypertensives. *Hypertension, 14,* 227–234.

Report of the Secretary's Task Force on black and minority health. (1986). Volume 4: Cardiovascular and Cerebrovascular Disease (Parts 1 and 2). USDHHS, Washington, DC: Government Printing Office.

Roter, D. (1978). Patient participation in the patient-provider interaction: The effect of patient question asking on the quality of interaction, satisfaction and compliance. *Health Education Monographs, 50,* 281–315.

Shulman, N. B. (1991). Economic Issues Relating to Access to Medications. In E. Saunders (Ed.), *Cardiovascular Disease in Blacks* (pp. 75–82), Philadelphia: F. A. Davis Co.

Smith, E. O., Curb, J. D., Hardy, R. J., Hawkins, C. M., & Tyroler, H. A. (1982). Clinic attendance in the Hypertension, Detection and Followup Program. *Hypertension, 4,* 710–715.

Southard, J. (1982). *Final Report: State of Maryland demonstration of statewide coordination for the control of high blood pressure.* Baltimore: Maryland State Department of Health and Mental Hygiene. Stamler, R. (1991). Implications of the INTERSALT study. *Hypertension, 17*(1), (Supp. 1), 1–20.

Stamler, R. (1991). Implications of the INTERSALT study. *Hypertension, 17* (1), (Supp. 1), 1–20.

Subcommittee on Definition and Prevalence of the 1984 Joint National Committee. (1985). Hypertension prevalence and the status of awareness, treatment and control in the United States. *Hypertension, 7,* 457–468.

Systolic Hypertension in the Elderly Program Cooperative Research Group (1991). Preventing stroke by antihypertensive drug treatment in older persons with isolated hypertension: Final results of the systolic hypertension in the elderly program (SHEP). *Journal of the American Medical Association, 265,* 3255–3264.

Trials of Hypertension Prevention Collaborative Research Group (TOHP). (1992). The effects of nonpharmacologic interventions on blood pressure of persons with high normal levels. *Journal of the American Medical Association, 267,* 1213–1220.

United States National Committee on Vital and Health Statistics (1981). *National health interview survey/report of the National Committee on Vital and Health Statistics.* U.S. Department of Health and Human Services, Public Health Service, PHS 81-1160, Office of Health Research, Statistics and Technology, National Center for Health Statistics.

5

End-Stage Renal Disease

Camille A. Jones and Lawrence Y. Agodoa

End-stage renal disease (ESRD) occurs when the kidneys can no longer function sufficiently well to sustain life. Death is no longer an inevitable consequence of ESRD; individuals who develop ESRD can prolong their lives through the use of renal replacement therapy, consisting of kidney dialysis or kidney transplantation. However, renal replacement therapy does not restore the ESRD patient to perfect health. Even with renal replacement therapy, ESRD patients have dramatically reduced lifetimes compared to persons of the same age without ESRD. Part of the decreased life expectancy may be due to the high prevalence of other serious conditions coexisting at onset of ESRD, such as coronary artery disease (41.1%), congestive heart failure (40.8%), neoplasms (9%), and undernutrition (13.6%) (USRDS, 1992). Other life-threatening complications that can develop in ESRD patients include loss of the access site for dialysis, graft rejection in patients who have kidney transplants, severe infections, and new or recurrent cardiovascular and peripheral vascular disease.

In 1989, the monetary cost of providing renal replacement therapy to one patient for one year averaged $37,800, not including costs due to required travel, most drugs, or loss in productivity. Most ESRD patients would be unable to afford therapy if subsidized treatment was not available. Since 1977, the United States Government has financed renal replacement therapy for ESRD patients, through the Medicare system (USRDS, 1991). Patients who have survived at least 90 days past the time of their first treatment for ESRD are eligible for Medicare, in addition to those who are already enrolled by reason of age or disability.

The National Institute of Diabetes and Digestive and Kidney Diseases (NIDDK) and the Health Care Financing Administration (HCFA) collaborated in 1987 to develop the United States Renal Data System (USRDS) database.

This database contains information on 95 percent of treated ESRD patients in the United States, based on data from HCFA, the Veterans Administration Hospital, and other sources. The Annual Data Report of the USRDS presents nationally representative information on incidence, prevalence, mortality and survival for various subgroups of treated ESRD patients. The data are categorized by age, race, gender, and cause of ESRD. Much of the data presented in this chapter are derived from the 1991 *USRDS Annual Data Report,* containing information on patients who developed ESRD up to December 31, 1989.

Prevalence and Incidence of ESRD in Adults

The total size of the ESRD population (incident and prevalent patients) has increased steadily since the middle to late 1970s. In 1978, there were 39,784 Medicare ESRD patients; in 1989, there were 150,880 patients in the Medicare System.

African Americans (subsequently referred to as Blacks) are disproportionately represented in both the total (prevalent) ESRD pool and in the number of new (incident) patients who develop ESRD each year. In 1989, 30 percent of the 150,880 prevalent ESRD patients were Black. The 1989 unadjusted ESRD prevalence rates were 472 per million for Whites and 1,451 per million for Blacks. After adjusting for age and gender, the rates were 440 per million and 1,731 per million for Whites and Blacks, respectively.

During 1989, 41,317 new (incident) patients were treated for ESRD; of these, 11,566 (28%) were Black and 27,851 (67%) were White (USRDS 1991). The incidence rate for ESRD in the Black population is currently 3–4 times higher than that seen in the White population. Blacks have higher incidence rates of ESRD for three of the four major causes reported by the U.S. Renal Data System (Figure 5.1).

MAIN CAUSES OF ESRD IN ADULTS

End-stage renal disease can result from a number of disease conditions that directly and indirectly cause damage to the kidneys. The four diseases that are most commonly cited as the cause of ESRD in adults are diabetes mellitus, hypertension, glomerulonephritis, and cystic diseases of the kidney.

Diabetes Mellitus

Diabetes mellitus is a metabolic disorder characterized by impaired insulin secretion relative to physiologic requirements. Diabetes mellitus afflicts Blacks more frequently than Whites, with a prevalence rate of known diabetes of 32.3 per 1000 in Blacks compared to 23.8 per 1000 in Whites (Drury & Powell, 1987). The increased prevalence of diabetes in Blacks compared to Whites is consistent across age, gender, and income. Type II diabetes, or non-insulin-

Figure 5.1
ESRD Incidence Rate, 1987–89, by Diagnosis and Race, Adjusted for Age and Gender

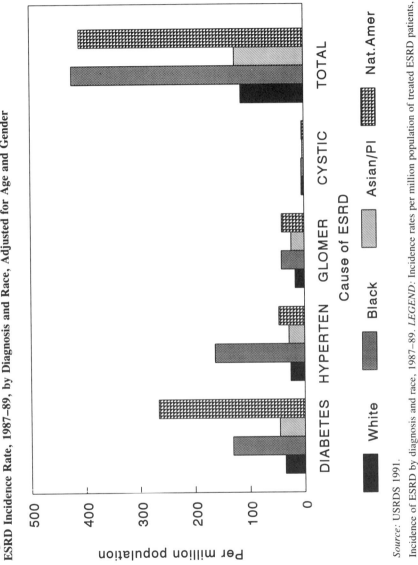

Source: USRDS 1991.

Incidence of ESRD by diagnosis and race, 1987–89. *LEGEND:* Incidence rates per million population of treated ESRD patients, by race, four major primary disease groups (diabetes, hypertension, glomerulonephritis, cystic kidney), and total, 1987–89. Adjusted for age and sex. Medicare patients only. Diabetes = diabetes mellitus, hyperten = hypertension, glomer = glomerulonephritis, cystic = cystic kidney diseases, Asian PI = Asian or Pacific Islander, Nat. Amer. = Native American.

dependent diabetes mellitus (NIDDM) is the predominant type of diabetes found in the black population.

Incidence of diabetic ESRD is higher in Blacks for all age groups (Figure 5.2). Black women have the highest rate of developing diabetic ESRD (143.2 per million population), compared to Black men, White men, and White women (115.6 per million, 39.3 per million, and 33.3 per million population respectively) (USRDS 1991). Between 1987 and 1989, the age- and gender-adjusted incidence rates of diabetic kidney failure were almost 4 times higher in Blacks than in Whites (Figure 5.1).

Several ecologic studies report that the higher prevalence of diabetes mellitus in Blacks does not completely explain the higher diabetic ESRD incidence rates in Blacks. When adjustment was made for the prevalence of diabetes in the Black population of southeastern Michigan (Cowie, 1989), the Black/White incidence ratio for diabetic ESRD remained high (rates of developing ESRD were 2.26 and 2.93 times higher for Black males and Black females compared to White males and White females respectively). A study from ESRD Network 9 (Kentucky and southwestern Ohio) showed that Blacks with NIDDM had increased risk of developing ESRD in Blacks compared to whites with NIDDM (RR = 4.9, 95% CI 3.6–6.5) (Stephens, Gillaspy, Clyne, Mejia & Pollak, 1990). A study from ESRD network 5 (Maryland) showed that adjusting for the higher prevalence of diabetes and hypertension in the Black community did not eliminate the increased risk of developing diabetic ESRD in Blacks (Brancati, Whittle, Whelton, Seidler & Klag, 1992).

Hypertension

Blacks tend to develop hypertension at younger ages than Whites and to have a higher prevalence of severe hypertension (Drizd, Dannenberg & Engel, 1986; Report of the Secretary's Task Force on Black and Minority Health, 1985). Blacks also tend to develop hypertensive kidney failure at a younger age than Whites (Figure 5.3). In 1988, the median age at onset of hypertensive ESRD was 59 years in Blacks, compared to 70 years in Whites (USRDS, 1992).

Several ecologic studies show that Blacks continue to have higher incidence rates of ESRD than Whites, even after adjusting for the higher prevalence of hypertension in the Black community (McClelland, Tuttle & Issa, 1988; Whittle, Whetton, Seidler & Klag, 1991). Among untreated hypertensive patients who enrolled in the Multiple Risk Factor Intervention Trial (MRFIT) Study and who achieved excellent control of diastolic blood pressure over the 6 years of follow-up, the Black patients showed progressive increases in mean serum creatinine over time, while the White patients did not (Walker et al., 1992). Systolic blood pressure was an important predictor of increasing creatinine in those patients in whom diastolic blood pressure was controlled. This study suggests that factors other than diastolic blood pressure level may affect the onset of kidney disease in Black hypertensive patients.

Figure 5.2
Diabetic ESRD Incidence Rate, 1986–89, by Age and Race, Adjusted for Gender

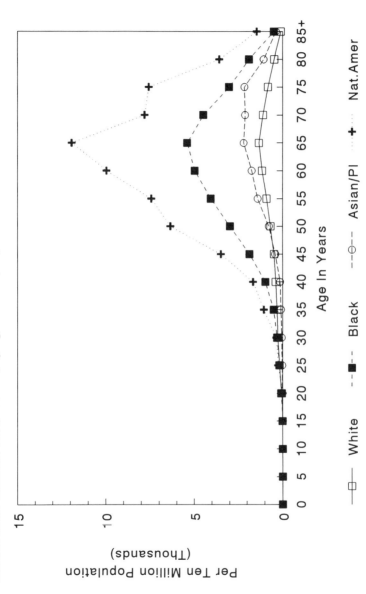

Source: USRDS 1991.

Diabetic ESRD incidence rates by age and race, 1986–1989. *LEGEND:* Average annual incidence rates per million population for patients with diabetes as cause of treated ESRD, by age and race, 1986–89. Adjusted for sex. Incidence rates are averaged for 1986 through 1989. Medicare patients only.

Figure 5.3
Hypertensive ESRD Incidence Rate, 1986–89, by Age and Race, Adjusted for Gender

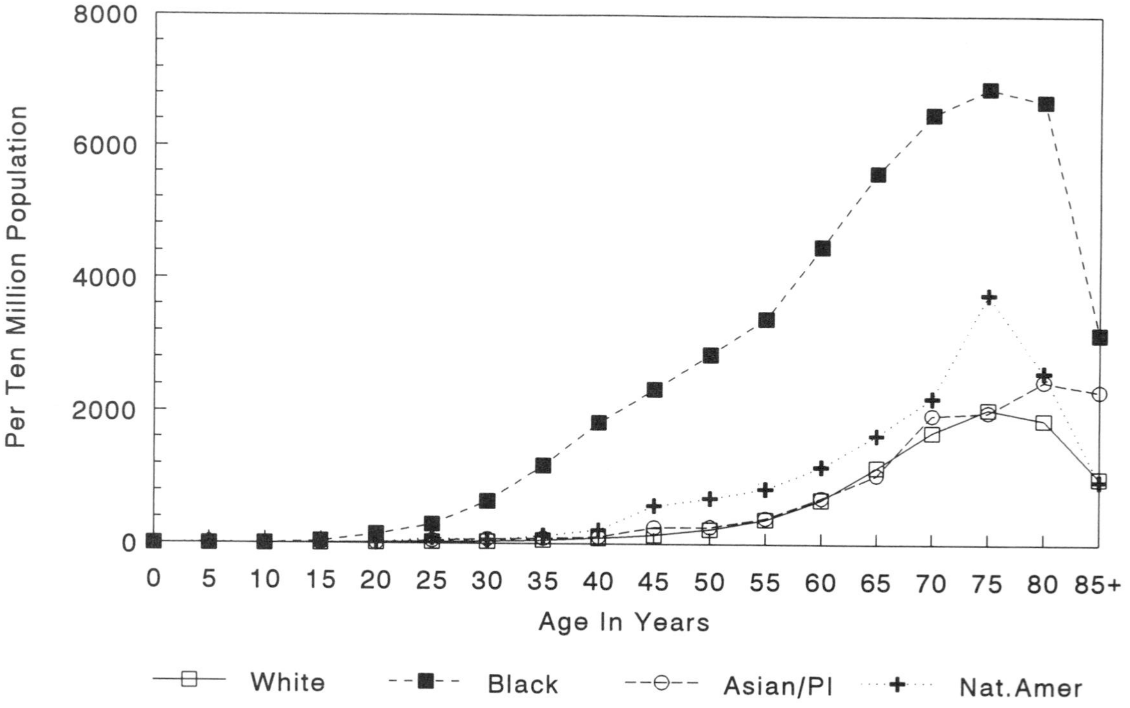

Source: USRDS 1991.

Hypertensive ESRD incidence rates by age and race, 1986–1989. *LEGEND:* Average annual incidence rates per million population for patients with hypertension as cause of treated ESRD, by age and race, 1986–89. Adjusted for sex. Incidence rates are averaged for 1986 through 1989. Medicare patients only.

Glomerulonephritis

Glomerulonephritis (GN) is an inflammatory condition of the kidney. It is usually associated with the deposition of antigen-antibody complexes in the kidney, in association with infection or autoimmune disease. Glomerulonephritis often causes excess protein loss in the urine, hypertension, and/or decline in kidney function.

From 1986 to 1989, 14.9 percent of the newly diagnosed ESRD patients had GN as the cause of their kidney failure. The incidence rate of ESRD due to GN has increased slowly; in 1989 the incidence rate was 22 per million (USRDS, 1991). Blacks have higher incidence rates of ESRD from GN than do Whites, beginning at age 10 and persisting for all ages thereafter (Figure 5.4).

Other Causes of ESRD

Cystic Kidney Diseases

These diseases, characterized by development of fluid-filled spaces (cysts) in the kidney, can occur from congenital, hereditary, or secondary causes. However, the most common cause of cystic kidney disease in adults is autosomal dominant polycystic kidney disease (ADPKD). ADPKD was the cause of ESRD for 3.6 percent of incident patients in 1989, with an annual ESRD incidence rate of 5 cases per million population. The age- and sex-adjusted incidence rates of ESRD due to cystic kidney diseases are equivalent in Blacks and Whites.

Obstructive Nephropathy

This occurs as a result of a blockage or constriction of the ureters or urethra, which in turn can cause increased pressure in the kidney and increased risk of infection and eventually can lead to kidney dysfunction. Obstructive uropathy and/or nephropathy is particularly a risk in infants and children who have congenital lesions, such as posterior urethral valves, and is also a risk in elderly men who may have enlargement of the prostate gland. Between 1986 and 1989, 2.5 percent of all new ESRD cases were ascribed to obstructive uropathy or nephropathy, with a median age at onset of 68 years; obstructive uropathy was the cause of ESRD in 1.3 percent of the Blacks and 3.5 percent of the Whites during this time (USRDS, 1991).

Interstitial Nephritis

This is a disease characterized by infiltration of the kidney by various types of white blood cells, leading eventually to permanent scarring and loss of kidney function. Interstitial nephritis has many causes, including drugs such as antibiotics, nonsteroidal anti-inflammatory drugs, and diuretics; infection; toxins; and collagen vascular diseases (Brenner & Rector, 1991). Between 1986 and 1989, interstitial nephritis was the cause of 3.7 percent of the new ESRD cases,

Figure 5.4
Glomerulonephritic ESRD Incidence Rate, 1986–89, by Age and Race, Adjusted for Gender

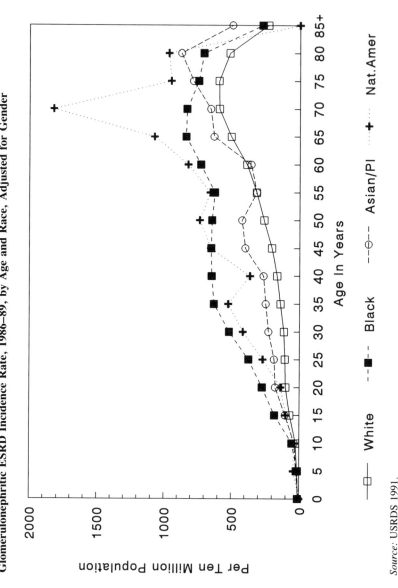

Source: USRDS 1991.

Glomerulonephritic ESRD incidence rates by age and race, 1986–89. *LEGEND:* Average annual incidence rates per million population for patients with glomerulonephritis as cause of treated ESRD, by age and race, 1986–89. Adjusted for sex. Incidence rates are averaged for 1986–89. Medicare patients only.

accounting for 2.1 percent of incident ESRD cases in Blacks and 4.5 percent in Whites.

Systemic Lupus Erythematosus (SLE)

This is an autoimmune disease in which 90 percent of patients are female. It is estimated that 35–90 percent of patients with SLE may eventually develop some type of clinical kidney disease, and a significant number of these patients eventually develop progressive disease leading to ESRD. SLE accounted for 2.2 percent of Black and 1.1 percent of White incident cases between 1986 and 1989 (USRDS, 1991). Early detection and aggressive treatment of lupus nephritis may slow or prevent the development of ESRD.

Sickle Cell Anemia

This is a disease caused by a type of blood hemoglobin that polymerizes inside the red blood cell, deforming the cell into a sickle shape, which leads to blockage of blood vessels due to the clumping of the sickled cells. Although nearly 7 percent of Blacks inherit the gene for sickle cell hemoglobin, and sickle cell disease is common in the Black population, ESRD due to sickle cell disease accounts for only 0.3 percent of the ESRD in Blacks.

HIV Infection

This disease is caused by infection with a retrovirus, which destroys CD4 + T-helper lymphocytes in the blood, causing impaired immunologic response to infectious agents. It is currently unknown how many of the HIV-infected persons with kidney involvement (proteinuria, nephrotic syndrome, and progressive kidney failure) will eventually progress to ESRD (Glassock, 1990). However, with the increasing duration of survival of AIDS patients this proportion will increase. Currently, HIV is the cause of ESRD in less than 0.1 percent of treated ESRD incident patients (USRDS, 1991).

PEDIATRIC ESRD

ESRD is much less common in children (ages 0–19 years) than in adults. The average yearly ESRD incidence rate between 1987 and 1989 was 15 per million in Black children, and 11 per million in White children; much of the difference is due to the two-fold higher incidence rate of ESRD in Black children aged 15–19 years old (Figure 5.5). In children, glomerulonephritis (38%), congenital/hereditary diseases (19%), collagen vascular diseases (10%), and urologic problems such as posterior urethral valves, which cause obstructive nephropathy (6%), are the major causes of ESRD. Black children have a higher percentage of ESRD due to lupus nephropathy, primary glomerulonephritis, hypertension, and sickle cell disease; White children have a higher percentage of ESRD due to cystic kidney disease and congenital/hereditary conditions (USRDS, 1991).

Pediatric patients are more likely to receive a transplant or to use continuous

Figure 5.5
Pediatric ESRD Incidence Rate, 1987–89, by Age and Race, Adjusted for Gender

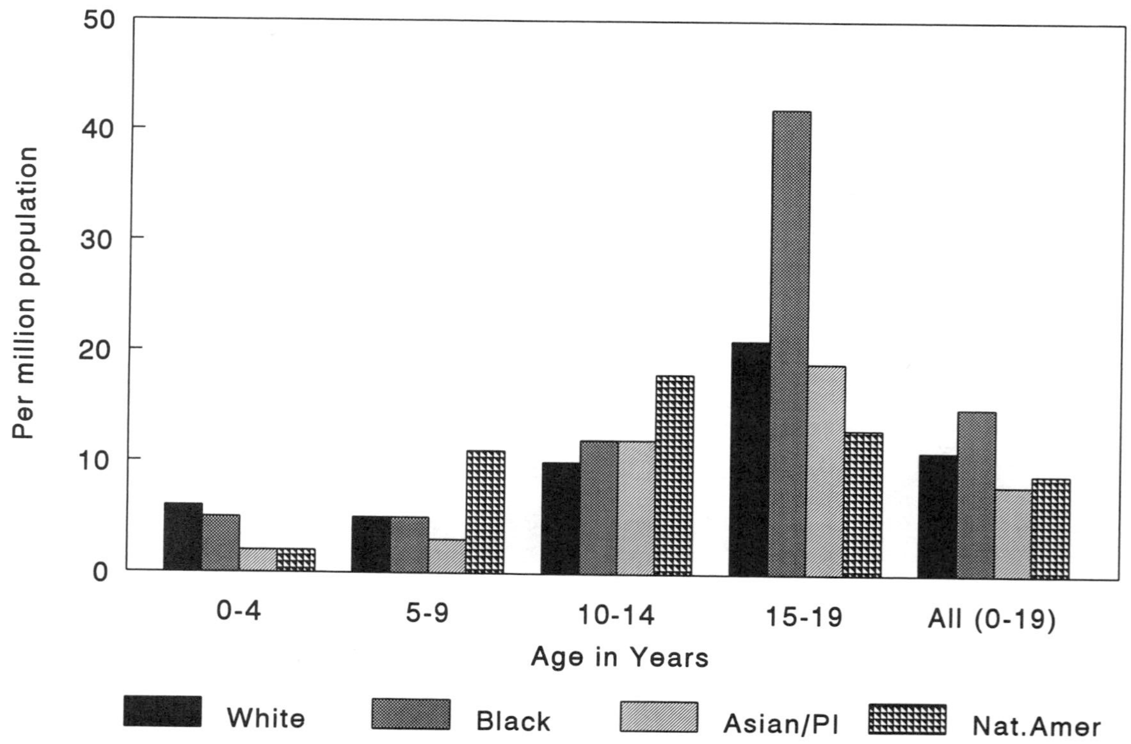

Source: USRDS 1991.

Pediatric ESRD incidence rate by age and race, 1987–89. *LEGEND:* Reported pediatric incidence per million population by age and race. Average rate per year, 1987–89, adjusted for sex. Total rates (0–19) adjusted for age and sex.

ambulatory peritoneal dialysis (CAPD) than are adult patients. During 1987–1989, 47 percent of pediatric patients received a transplant within one year of onset of ESRD. Both cadaveric kidney transplantation rates and living related kidney transplantation rates are higher for White children than for Black children. In addition, once transplanted, White children have 25–33 percent better survival of the kidney graft than do Black children.

MODALITIES OF THERAPY

Dialysis is a method of treatment whereby waste products are removed from the body by artificial means. Overall, 75 percent of ESRD patients are treated with dialysis of some type. Two forms of dialysis are widely used in this country, namely, hemodialysis and peritoneal dialysis. Hemodialysis is a treatment consisting of passing the patient's blood through tubes into an artificial kidney, which contains a semipermeable membrane allowing waste products and other toxic substances to diffuse from the blood into the dialysate fluid present on the other side of the membrane; the cleansed blood is then returned to the patient. A typical hemodialysis treatment lasts from 2.5 to 4 hours at a time and is performed 3 times a week.

Peritoneal dialysis consists of a slow lavage of the peritoneal cavity with dialysate fluid. Two major forms of peritoneal dialysis treatment are currently available. The majority of peritoneal dialysis patients use continuous ambulatory peritoneal dialysis (CAPD), whereby the dialysis fluid is infused from a bag, through permanent indwelling tubing, into the patient's peritoneal cavity. The fluid is allowed to stay in the peritoneal cavity for about 4 to 5 hours (dwell time), during which time waste products from the body diffuse into the fluid. At the end of the dwell time, the fluid containing the waste products is drained back into the empty bag, a fresh bag with clean dialysis fluid is attached to the tubing, and the cycle is repeated. Approximately 5 to 6 cycles are necessary each day. CAPD is usually performed by the patient or by a close relative. When patients are unable to perform CAPD, they can be hooked to a machine that pumps the fluid into the abdominal cavity, allows the fluid to dwell in the abdomen for a time, and then pumps the fluid out into a drain. Machine assisted peritoneal dialysis is usually performed for about 6 to 8 hours at a time and may be done 4 to 6 times a week.

Kidney Transplantation

Kidney transplantation consists of implantation of kidneys from living related donors or cadaveric donors. Cadaver kidneys are the most common source of kidneys for transplantation (78.7% of all kidney transplants).

A number of different factors, including age, race, and gender, affect access to kidney transplantation. Young ESRD patients receive kidney transplantation much more frequently than older patients, and males receive kidneys more frequently than females. Certain coexisting conditions at the time of diagnosis of ESRD, such as coronary artery disease, cardiac arrhythmias, congestive heart failure, and malnutrition, are associated with lower likelihood of receiving a kidney allograft. Other factors that influence access to transplantation include socioeconomic status, presence of antibodies to blood components, HLA status, blood type, and patient acceptance of transplantation (USRDS, 1991; Kasiske et al., 1991; Held, Pauly, Bovbjerg, Newmann & Salvatierra 1988; and Kjellstrand, 1988).

Overall, 25 percent of ESRD patients have currently functioning transplanted kidneys. Thirty percent of White ESRD patients have functioning kidney transplants, and 51 percent of Whites are being treated with in-center hemodialysis; in contrast, only 13 percent of Black ESRD patients have functioning kidney transplants, and 74 percent of Blacks are treated with in-center hemodialysis (USRDS, 1991).

SURVIVAL WITH ESRD

ESRD patients have a dramatically reduced life expectancy compared to persons of the same age without ESRD. At age 40 years, an ESRD patient has a life expectancy of 8.8 years compared to 37.4 years in the general population, and at age 59 the ESRD patient's life expectancy is 4.2 years compared to 20.4 years in the general population (USRDS, 1991). This decreased life expectancy is also seen in children. White children with ESRD aged 5–19 years old had a life expectancy of 12–20 years, compared to 15–17 years for Black children.

Given that the patient has survived at least 90 days since onset of ESRD, the overall probability of surviving one year was 79.1 percent in 1989, with better survival for Blacks (82.9%) than for Whites (77.1%) even after adjusting for differences in age, sex, and cause of ESRD. Mortality rates are significantly higher in Whites who develop diabetic or hypertensive ESRD at age 40 years or older (Table 5.1) compared to Blacks of similar age. The mortality rates for White patients with ESRD due to GN are higher than those for Black patients of similar age, for all ages below 60 years (Table 5.1). The reason for the survival differences between middle-aged and older Blacks and Whites is unclear.

SUMMARY AND DISCUSSION

End-stage kidney disease is an increasingly important health and economic problem in the United States. The escalating incidence rate of ESRD is seen in all racial groups. Blacks tend to develop ESRD at younger ages and to suffer a higher burden of ESRD than Whites. The higher ESRD incidence rates are not explained by the higher prevalence of diabetes and hypertension in the Black community.

Other factors that might affect the apparent pattern of incidence and survival in ESRD patients include (a) the effects of competitive mortality in middle-aged

Table 5.1
ESRD Patient Deaths per 1,000 Patient Years at Risk, by Age and Cause of ESRD

	Diabetes		Hypertension		Glomerulonephritis	
	Black	White	Black	White	Black	White
0-4	0.0	461.5	---	.	69.3	58.0
5-19	0.0	61.0	66.6	30.9	45.5	14.5
20-24	165.6	91.6	45.8	18.9	26.6	19.9
25-29	117.7	110.7	45.7	39.0	44.8	20.7
30-34	152.8	117.7	65.9	39.4	80.8	25.1
35-39	144.7	130.2	66.9	46.8	75.9	31.2
40-44	151.2	164.6	82.0	67.3	69.3	43.7
45-49	154.9	202.0	92.6	85.7	76.8	56.2
50-54	191.4	266.6	110.4	133.8	102.8	79.8
55-59	218.1	331.5	134.3	173.5	131.3	116.6
60-64	239.1	391.4	182.4	228.1	173.8	172.5
65-69	286.6	422.6	215.5	289.6	201.1	224.7
70-74	333.8	486.5	271.2	361.2	294.1	284.8
75-79	377.9	537.8	322.3	431.0	269.5	354.8
80-84	464.7	606.3	367.0	544.7	338.5	426.6
85+	481.9	690.6	446.8	625.9	551.3	581.0

Source: Adapted from USRDS 1991 Annual Data Report, Table D.14. Death rates are computed based on calendar year periods using the cohort of patients who are alive at the beginning of the year and whose first service date is before October of the previous year. The number of deaths and the number of years at risk are computed separately for each year, and then summed over the three years before the rates are computed. The rates are computed as the total number of deaths divided by the total number of person-years at risk. The rate is multiplied by 1,000 to give deaths per 1,000 patient years at risk. In computing death rates for dialysis patients, the period at risk is censored (truncated) at the date of transplant if the patient has had a transplant during the year.

and older patients, from the sequelae of hypertension and diabetes such as congestive heart failure, sudden death, stroke, and infection; (b) the undetected effects of socioeconomic status on incidence of and survival with ESRD; (c) the effect of changes in the age structure and disease characteristics of the U.S. population; and (d) the effect of increased numbers of dialysis and transplantation units on the apparent increased incidence of treated ESRD over time. The number of patients who develop ESRD but elect not to be treated is unknown.

Future research into the causes of excess ESRD in the Black population must take into account the current and past prevalence of hypertension and diabetes mellitus in the community, as well as investigating the possible effects of environmental, occupational, and genetic factors. Studies to evaluate kidney structure and function may be needed to rule out concurrent glomerulonephritis or other treatable kidney diseases in patients with a diagnosis of hypertensive or diabetic kidney disease. Longitudinal studies comparing incidence of kidney injury in Blacks and Whites, beginning at the time of diagnosis of hypertension or diabetes mellitus, are also needed.

It is important to develop new, more sensitive, inexpensive, and non-invasive tests to detect early kidney dysfunction. Measurement of early changes in kidney function should be performed in all epidemiologic trials involving drug therapy, the elderly, or patients with diabetes mellitus, hypertension, or cardiovascular disease.

Health education research is also needed, including developing new methods of teaching how to identify the risk factors for developing kidney disease, how to prevent it, and how to recognize it. These efforts should be targeted toward the populations that are at highest risk of developing ESRD.

Finally, while it is important to attempt to slow progression from kidney injury to end-stage kidney disease, a primary objective of research in patients with kidney disease should be to find ways to prevent onset of early kidney injury. From these research efforts, we may begin to stem the rising tide of kidney-related disease and death in this country.

NOTES

For comments, please contact: Camille Jones, M.D., M.P.H., Director, Epidemiology Program NIH / NIDDK / DKUHD, Room 3A-07B, 5333 Westbard Avenue, Bethesda, MD 20892. Phone (301)594-7586. Fax (301)594-7501.

The data reported here have been supplied by The United States Renal Data System (USRDS). The interpretation and reporting of these data are the responsibility of the author(s) and in no way should be seen as an official policy or interpretation of the United States government.

REFERENCES

Brancati, F. L., Whittle, J. C., Whelton, P. K., Seidler, A. J., and Klag, M. J. (1992).
    The excess incidence of diabetic end-stage renal disease among blacks: A pop-

ulation-based study of potential explanatory factors. *Journal of the American Medical Association, 268,* 3079–3084.

Brenner, B. M., and Rector, F. C. (1991). *The kidney* (4th Ed.). Philadelphia: W. B. Saunders Company.

Cowie, C. C., Port, F. K., Wolfe, R. A., Savage, P. J., Moll, P. P., and Hawthorne, V. M. (1989). Disparities in incidence of diabetic end-stage renal disease according to race and type of diabetes. *New England Journal of Medicine, 321,* 1074–1079.

Drizd, T., Dannenberg, A. L., and Engel, A. (1986). Blood pressure levels in persons 18–74 years of age in 1976–80, and trends in blood pressure from 1960–1980 in the United States. National Center for Health Statistics. *Vital and Health Statistics.* Series 11, No. 234. DHHS Pub. No. (PHS) 86–1684. Public Health Service, Washington, DC: Government Printing Office.

Drury, T. F., & Powell, A. L. (1987). Prevalence of known diabetes among black Americans. *Advance Data From Vital and Health Statistics.* No 130. DHHS Pub. No. (PHS) 87-1250. Hyattsville, MD: National Center for Health Statistics.

Glassock, R. J., moderator (1990). Human immunodeficiency virus (HIV) infection and the kidney. *Annals of Internal Medicine, 112,* 35–49.

Held, P. J., Pauly, M. V., Bovbjerg, J. D., Newmann, J., & Salvatierra, O. (1988). Access to kidney transplantation: Has the United States eliminated income and racial differences? *Archives of Internal Medicine, 148,* 2594–2600.

Kasiske, B. L., Neylan, J. F., Riggio, R. R., et al. (1991). The effect of race on access and outcome in transplantation. *New England Journal of Medicine, 324,* 302–307.

Kjellstrand, C. M. (1988). Age, sex, and race inequality in renal transplantation. *Archives of Internal Medicine, 148,* 1305–1309.

McClelland, W., Tuttle, E., & Issa, A. (1988). Racial differences in the incidence of hypertensive end-stage renal disease (ESRD) are not entirely explained by differences in the prevalence of hypertension. *American Journal of Kidney Disease, 12,* 285–290.

Report of the Secretary's Task Force on Black and Minority Health. (1985). Cardiovascular and Cerebrovascular Diseases, Volume IV. USDHHS, Washington, DC: Government Printing Office.

Stephens, G. W., Gillaspy, J. A., Clyne, D., Mejia, A., & Pollak, V. E. (1990). Racial differences in the incidence of end-stage renal disease in Types I and II diabetes mellitus. *American Journal of Kidney Disease, 15,* (June), 562–567.

U.S. Renal Data System (USRDS). (1991). *USRDS 1991 Annual Data Report,* National Institutes of Health, National Institute of Diabetes and Digestive and Kidney Diseases, Bethesda, MD.

U.S. Renal Data System (USRDS). (1992). *USRDS 1992 Annual Data Report,* National Institutes of Health, National Institute of Diabetes and Digestive and Kidney Diseases, Bethesda, MD.

Walker, W. G., Neaton, J. D., Cutler, J. A., Neuwirth, R., Cohen J. D., et al. (1992). Renal function change in hypertensive members of the Multiple Risk Factor Intervention Trial: Racial and treatment effects. *Journal of the American Medical Association, 268,* 3085–3091.

Whittle, J. C., Whelton, P. K., Seidler, A. J., & Klag, M. J. (1991). Does racial variation in risk factors explain black-white differences in the incidence of hypertensive end-stage renal disease? *Annuals of Internal Medicine, 151,* 1359–1364.

II

General Chronic Conditions

6

Cancer and Black Americans

Ki Moon Bang

Cancer accounts for one out of every five deaths in the United States. During the period 1979–1990, trends of cancer incidence and mortality rates have increased, with a more rapid increase for Blacks than Whites and a greater increase for men than women. In 1989, the age-adjusted cancer incidence rate was 401.2 per 100,000 for Blacks and 379.5 for Whites, approximately a 7 percent difference (NCI, 1992). In 1990, the mortality rate was 182 per 100,000 for Blacks compared with 131.5 for Whites (NCHS, 1993). The five-year survival rate for cancer in Blacks diagnosed from 1983 through 1988 was about 38.3 percent compared with 53.5 percent for Whites (NCI, 1992). A considerable part of this difference in survival can be attributed to late diagnoses.

Strategies for reducing cancer incidence and mortality in Blacks have been developed and intervention and prevention programs targeted for high-risk populations including Black Americans. The Department of Health and Human Services has established an objective of reducing cancer mortality to less than 130 deaths per 100,000 population by the year 2000 (*Healthy People 2000*, 1991). Achieving this goal depends on the development and implementation of cancer prevention and control strategies directed at specific populations.

Cancer rates where Blacks have significantly higher incidence and mortality rates include lung, esophagus, stomach, liver, prostate, larynx, cervix uteri, and multiple myeloma. The excessive incidence of these sites in Blacks might be explained by smoking, alcohol consumption, diet, socioeconomic status, and lack of medical care. These factors are associated with an increased risk of cancer, but the precise cause-effect relationship has not been well addressed. This paper reviews the epidemiology of cancer for Black Americans, i.e., current status and risk factors, and also proposes recommendations to reduce the incidence of cancer and related mortality rates.

DATA SOURCES

The data in this paper were derived from the latest available sources. Incidence and survival data were obtained from the Surveillance, Epidemiology and End Results (SEER) program of the National Cancer Institute (NCI, 1992). The National Cancer Institute collects data from nine population-based tumor registries on all newly diagnosed patients and follow-up information on persons previously diagnosed. The geographic areas that make up the SEER program's database represent approximately 9.6 percent of the U.S. population and cover approximately 8.3 percent of U.S. Blacks. The mortality data were obtained from the National Center for Health Statistics vital statistics system (NCHS, 1993). Information on each death occurring in the United States includes cause of death, age at death, gender, and geographic area of residence at time of death.

CANCER STATUS

Incidence

The American Cancer Society (or ACS) estimates that 1,130,000 Americans will be diagnosed with cancer in 1992. About 115,000 of these cases will be Black Americans (ACS, 1992). The age-adjusted incidence rate of cancer was 410.7 per 100,000 population for the period 1985–1989 based on the SEER program. The overall incidence in Blacks rose 17.4 percent, while for Whites it increased 17 percent during the period 1973–1989 (Table 6.1) (NCI, 1992). However, the magnitude of the overall cancer incidence rate among Blacks is about 6 percent higher than among Whites in 1989. During the period 1985–1989, the age-adjusted incidence rate for Black males was 535 per 100,000 population compared with 442.6 for White males. In the case of females, the rate for Black females was 327 per 100,000 population compared with 344.1 for White females (Figure 6.1).

The top five rank-ordered sites for cancer incidence include the lung, prostate, breast, colon, and pancreas. The overall age-adjusted incidence rate of lung cancer is 78.1 per 100,000 population during the period 1985–1989. The percent change of lung cancer incidence over this time interval is 31.4 percent, and the estimated annual percentage change is 2.3 percent. The percentage change over the time interval is 18.6 percent for males, compared with 108.8 percent for females. Black men have a lung cancer rate three times higher than that of women and almost two times higher that of White men (Table 6.2). Prostate cancer incidence is the second highest in Blacks. The incidence rate is 55.9 per 100,000 population and higher than in Whites. Black American men have a higher risk for developing prostate cancer than Whites.

In 1989, female breast cancer incidence rate in Blacks was 87.6 per 100,000 population compared with 108.2 in White females. Black women over 65 years have much higher incidence (342.1/100,000) of breast cancer than Black women

Table 6.1
Age-adjusted Cancer Incidence Rates by Race and Sex, 1979–1989

Year	Blacks			Whites		
	Both	Males	Females	Both	Males	Females
1979	374.2	482.8	298.0	341.3	400.7	307.8
1980	392.2	512.1	306.4	346.4	407.8	311.2
1981	395.7	530.1	300.2	352.6	412.1	319.0
1982	391.0	519.6	300.3	353.1	412.5	319.8
1983	409.0	539.1	319.2	359.4	420.9	324.0
1984	412.4	542.5	323.0	365.8	424.9	332.5
1985	410.2	535.2	325.1	374.1	430.2	342.5
1986	410.9	532.4	328.7	375.3	436.0	340.2
1987	416.1	546.7	328.3	388.8	453.9	350.9
1988	415.4	536.0	334.5	383.8	447.7	346.5
1989	401.2	524.4	319.3	379.5	444.4	340.2

Source: National Cancer Institute, 1992.

*Rates are per 100,000 population and are age-adjusted to the 1970 U.S. standard population.

less than 65 years (65.1/100,000). Colon cancer incidence rate in Blacks is 40.1 per 100,000 compared with 35.5 for Whites during the period 1985–1989. Black men experience higher incidence of colon cancer than that of Black women. The percentage change in colon cancer during the period 1973–89 is 31.3 percent increase; 39.4 percent for men and 26.3 percent for women. Pancreas cancer incidence is 14.3 per 100,000 population compared with 8.9 for Whites. The pancreas incidence rate is higher for men (16.3 per 100,000) than for women (12.9 per 100,000).

Mortality

The total number of cancer death was 57,077 in 1990 compared with 42,981 in 1979 (NCHS, 1993). The overall age-adjusted mortality rates increased 9.4 percent, from 166.4 per 100,000 population in 1979 to 182.0 in 1990 (Table 6.3) (NCHS, 1993). The increase is higher for males (11.9%) than for females

Figure 6.1
Cancer Incidence and Mortality (1985–1989) and Relative Survival Rates (1983–1988) by Race and Sex

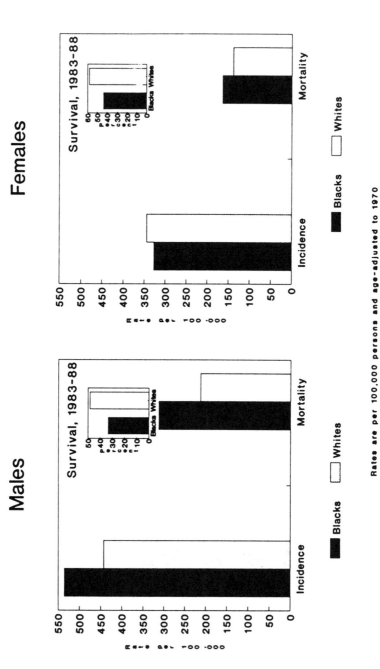

Source: National Cancer Institute, 1992.

Table 6.2
Age-adjusted Incidence Rate by Primary Cancer Site, 1985–1989

Site	Blacks			Whites		
	Both	Males	Females	Both	Males	Females
All sites	410.7	535.0	327.0	380.4	442.6	344.1
Lung	78.1	127.3	42.3	57.2	81.9	39.1
Prostate	55.9	139.7	–	40.3	98.8	–
Breast	52.9	1.4	92.5	60.7	0.8	110.8
Colon/ Rectum	52.2	60.5	46.4	50.0	61.0	42.1
Colon	40.1	45.9	36.1	35.5	41.8	31.1
Rectum	12.1	14.7	10.3	14.5	19.2	11.0
Pancreas	14.3	16.3	12.9	8.9	10.5	7.7
Corpus uteri	8.2	–	14.3	12.1	–	22.0

Source: National Cancer Institute, 1992.

*Incidence rates per 100,000 population are adjusted to the 1970 U.S. standard population.

(9.7%) during this period. The age-adjusted mortality rate for those aged 55 and over increased while it substantially decreased for those less than 55 years.

For major cancer sites, age-adjusted mortality rates per 100,000 population are 59.5 for lung cancer, 23.5 for colon and rectum, 17.5 for breast, 18.7 for prostate, and 11.9 for pancreas during the period 1973–1989 (NCI, 1992). Trends in cancer mortality rates during the period 1973–1989 are summarized in Figure 6.2. During this period, cancer sites where mortality rates increased more than 10 percent include the lung, prostate, breast, kidney, multiple myeloma, and larynx. The cancer sites with the decreased mortality rates were the stomach, cervix uteri, corpus and uterus, urinary bladder, and testis.

Differences between Blacks and Whites

The overall difference in cancer incidence and mortality between Blacks and Whites is summarized in Figure 6.3. For all sites combined, Blacks experience 10 percent higher cancer incidence and 30 percent higher mortality than Whites. Individual cancer sites for which there are particularly notable excesses in incidence and mortality in Blacks are esophagus, cervix uteri, larynx, prostate,

Table 6.3
Age-adjusted Cancer Mortality Rates by Race and Sex, 1979–1990

Year	Blacks			Whites		
	Both	Males	Females	Both	Males	Females
1979	166.4	221.8	125.1	127.8	158.7	105.7
1980	172.1	229.9	129.7	129.6	160.5	107.7
1981	171.2	231.4	127.3	128.6	158.5	107.4
1982	173.3	234.2	129.2	129.7	159.7	108.4
1983	175.2	236.9	130.9	129.8	159.7	108.7
1984	177.7	241.7	132.1	130.7	160.0	110.0
1985	176.6	239.9	131.8	131.2	160.4	110.5
1986	177.0	239.0	133.7	131.0	160.2	110.3
1987	177.2	240.0	133.9	130.8	160.1	110.0
1988	177.1	240.4	133.5	130.8	159.6	110.4
1989	179.4	246.2	133.5	131.2	159.4	111.1
1990	182.0	248.1	137.2	131.5	160.3	111.2

Source: National Center for Health Statistics, Vital Statistics System, 1993.

*Rates are per 100,000 population and are age-adjusted to the 1970 U.S. population.

stomach, lung (males), multiple myeloma, oral cavity, and liver. The cancer sites for which Blacks have less incidence and mortality than Whites are breast, leukemia, ovary, non-Hodgkin's, testis, brain and melanoma of skin.

Cancer survival rates are different between Blacks and Whites based on the data from SEER areas (Figure 6.1). The overall 5-year survival rates during the period 1983–1988 was 38.3 for Blacks compared with 53.5 for Whites. The survival rate for males was 33.4 compared with 43.6 for females (NCI, 1992). Blacks have more favorable survival than Whites for cancers of the brain and multiple myeloma. Cancer rates for which Whites have more than a 10 percent point in survival than Blacks are colon/rectum, oval cavity, larynx, melanoma, female breast, cervix uteri, corpus uteri, and prostate and urinary bladder.

In examining survival trends, it is desirable to observe changes in survival rates as related to the stage of disease at diagnosis. The stage can be classified as localized or regional cancer. Survival rate is much better in cases of localized

Figure 6.2
Trends in Cancer Mortality Rates in the United States by Race, 1973–1989

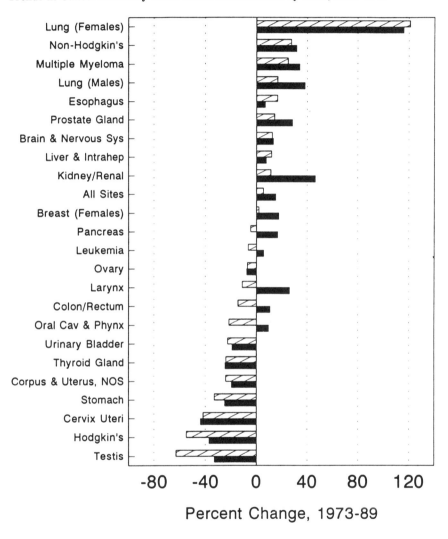

Source: National Cancer Institute, 1992.

Figure 6.3
SEER Cancer Incidence and Mortality Rates in the United States, 1985–1989:
Ratio of Black Rate to White Rate (All Ages)

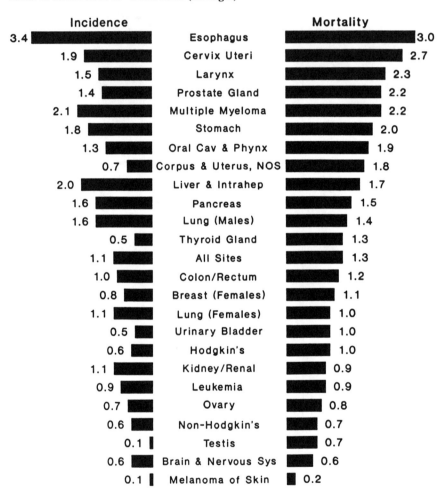

Ratio: (Black Rate)/(White Rate)
Rates Are Age-Adjusted to 1970 Standard

Source: National Cancer Institute, 1992.

cancer than regional cancer. For example, a vast difference is the 5-year survival rate of stomach cancer, which was observed according to stage, i.e., 87 percent for localized versus 12 percent for regional (Bang, White, Gause & Leffall, 1988). One of the reasons for poor survival in Blacks may be that the disease is diagnosed and treated at a late stage (White, Enterline, Alam & Moore, 1981). Low socioeconomic status can be a strong determinant of poor survival rates in Blacks (Bang, 1987). Also, the observed difference in survival rates between Blacks and Whites may be attributed to a number of factors including, but not limited to, less adequate medical care, cancer treatment, and cancer screening programs for Blacks than for Whites (Bang, White, Gause & Leffall, 1988).

RISK FACTORS

Multiple risk factors contribute to cancer in Blacks Americans. The major risk factors include: (1) life-style factors, (2) occupational/environmental exposure, (3) genetic predisposition, and (4) socioeconomic status. A discussion of these factors follows.

Life-style Factors

Life-style factors include cigarette smoking, alcohol consumption, and eating habits. The higher cancer incidence for Blacks might be the result of life-style (Baquet, Horm, Gibbs & Greenwald, 1991; McWhorter, Schatzkin, Horm & Brown, 1989; Hargreaves, Baquet & Gamshadzahi, 1989; Bang, White, Gause & Leffall, 1988; Gullatte, 1989). Higher cancer rates in the lung, head and neck, stomach, liver, and esophagus in Blacks can be attributed exclusively to smoking and drinking. Other risk factors include inadequate diet and obesity.

Smoking

Smoking accounts for 30 percent of all cancer deaths. Smoking is a risk factor for the lung, lip, tongue, mouth, larynx, esophagus, bladder, pancreas, and cervix uteri. Smoking is the most preventable cause of cancer death in our society. It is estimated that cigarette smoking is responsible for 87 percent of lung cancer: 90 percent for men and 79 percent for women (ACS, 1992). Currently, it is estimated that there are approximately 50 million smokers in the United States. From 1976 to 1987, males (20 years and older) who smoked dropped from 42 percent of the population to 32 percent, while smoking among women decreased from 32 percent to 27 percent.

Smoking prevalence is different between Blacks and Whites. In 1987, the Centers for Disease Control reported that 32.5 percent of Black males in the United States smoked compared with 29.3 percent of White males (CDC, 1987). For those between the ages of 25 and 34 years, 49.5 percent of Black men smoked compared with 32.4 percent of White men. When Black and White women were compared, 25.1 percent of Black women compared with 23.7

percent of White women smoked. At ages 25 to 34, however, the percentage of Black women who smoked was 30.9 percent compared with 29.1 percent for White women. For the ages 35 to 44 years the smoking prevalence was 36.4 percent for Black compared with 27.6 percent of White women. Smoking rates are higher among Black blue-collar workers and people with few years of education. The higher prevalence of smoking in Blacks is associated with an increased risk of lung cancer. A recent issue concerns the health effects of passive smoking. The U.S. Environmental Protection Agency report on the respiratory health effects of passive smoking indicates that secondhand smoke is responsible for approximately 3,000 lung cancer deaths per year in nonsmoking adults (EPA, 1992).

Drinking

Drinking has been reported to be associated with colon, breast, prostate, and esophageal cancers. The National Health and Nutrition Examination Survey (NHANES), conducted by the National Center for Health Statistics, showed that Black men report heavier drinking than do White men of comparable age (Mettlin, 1980). The incidence rate of esophageal cancer in Blacks is almost four times higher than in Whites. One of the reasons for this might be a higher alcohol consumption rate among Blacks than Whites. A recent case-control study by the National Cancer Institute showed that the major factors responsible for the excess of esophageal cancer in the District of Columbia was alcohol consumption, and the risk increased with the amount of ethanol consumed and was highest among drinkers of hard liquor (Potter, Morris & Blot, 1981). Besides esophageal cancer, alcohol consumption is associated with cancer of the larynx, stomach, colon/rectum, pancreas and breast.

Diet

The estimated proportion of cancer deaths attributed to diet is 35 percent overall, with a range of 10 to 70 percent depending on the type of cancer. (Surgeon General's Report on Nutrition and Health, 1988). Prior research has examined the role diet and nutrition may play in the development of cancer. Poor eating habits and the nutritional status of Black Americans are a national problem that could contribute to higher incidence and mortality rates from cancer. Blacks have different eating patterns than Whites. The NHANES data showed that Blacks consume higher levels of fats and fewer vegetables than Whites. Among men aged 18 to 44 years, 37 percent of Blacks report that they usually eat fruits and vegetables two or more times a day compared with 53 percent of Whites (Mettlin, 1980). Numerous studies have shown that daily consumption of vegetables and fruits is associated with a decreased risk of lung, prostate, bladder, esophagus, and stomach cancers.

Obesity

Dietary consumption is directly related to excessive body weight and cancer. Diets high in fat and low in fiber and obesity are associated with various cancers, particularly colon, breast, and prostate cancers. Recent survey data suggest that Blacks consume diets high in fat (Hargreaves, Baquet & Gamshadzahi, 1989). High-fiber diets may reduce risk of colon cancer. A diet high in fat may be a risk factor for colon, breast, and prostate cancers (ACS, 1992). Both obesity and the various nutritional deficiency states are potentially favorable for cancer growth. Obesity is associated with cancers of the endometrium, breast, colon, and ovary (Hargreaves et al., 1989). Cellular immune deficiency, a possible outcome of protein-calories malnutrition and zinc deficiency, may facilitate the development of head, neck, and gastric cancers (Hargreaves et al., 1989).

Occupational/Environmental Risk Factors

The contribution of occupational exposure to the cause of cancer in Blacks may be even greater than 4 percent of all cancer deaths that have been estimated (Doll & Peto, 1981; Report of the Secretary's Task Force, 1985). For many historical reasons, Blacks are believed to have higher occupational exposures compared with Whites because of placement in less skilled and more hazardous jobs. Various occupational hazards, especially ionizing radiation and chemicals like asbestos, benzene, chromium, lead, nickel, beta-naphthylamine, bischloromethyl ether, and vinyl chloride, are known to cause cancer (Frumkin & Levy, 1983).

Asbestos, another known carcinogen, is known to cause lung cancer. Previous epidemiologic studies have documented the carcinogenic effects of exposure to asbestos in the workplace. These data provide the basis for assessing the potential impact of general environmental asbestos exposures in the form of insulation for new buildings and asbestos-contained water (Decouflé, 1982). Ambient air pollution has been identified as carcinogenic for humans. Among the many organic particulates in polluted air, polycyclic aromatic hydrocarbons have been most intensively studied for potential carcinogenicity. Among carcinogenic polycyclic organic compounds identified in the air, benzo(a)pyrene is known to be the most potent carcinogen in humans. The sources of benzo(a)pyrene are inefficient, smoldering combustors of carbonaceous solid fuels, such as home boilers, coke ovens, and smoky coal refuse and forest fires (Shy & Struba, 1982).

Familial Predisposition and Genetic Factors

The aggregation of cancer in families is a long-observed and well-documented phenomenon, but it is still subject to debate. The large bowel is the site of more familial and heritable cancers than perhaps any other site. This is evidenced by occurrence of the disease in relatives of patients at rates three to four times greater than in some control groups. Specifically, what is seen are the numerous inherited polyposis syndromes that have long been associated with the familial occurrence of large-bowel cancer (Anderson, 1982). Other genetic evidence comes from the occurrence of gastric carcinoma as an associated neoplasm in several inherited disorders, including diffuse gastrointestinal polyposis, juvenile polyposis, hereditary adenocarcinomatosis, and Torre's syndrome (Anderson, 1978). This list also includes ataxia telangiectasis (Frais, 1979). Gastric cancer may also aggregate in families as the sole neoplasm. An example is Napoleon Bonaparte's family, in which his father, his sister, and he himself were documented as having stomach cancer, and his paternal grandfather was suspected of having the neoplasm as well (Sokoloff, 1938).

The role for genetic predisposition in cancer is most evident by familial transmission of retinoblastoma, dysplastic nervus syndrome, multiple endocrine neoplasia, and polyposis coli, where there is essentially a 100 percent chance of developing cancer in one's lifetime for persons who have inherited the trait (Shields, 1993). The Li-Fraumeni cancer family syndrome is among the most dramatic because family members are at risk for multiorgan cancers including breast, bone sarcomas, brain, leukemia, and adrenocortical neoplasm (Li, 1990; Garber et al., 1991), which suggests a germ-line mutation accounting for the multiorgan involvement. These inheritable syndromes involve genetic sequences for proto-oncogenics and tumor suppressor genes, metabolic capacity to activate or detoxify carcinogens, and the repair of DNA damage.

Socioeconomic Status

Socioeconomic status is an important factor in cancer incidence, survival, and mortality. The poor have less ability to practice good health habits and less access to good health care. Because of poor health habits, the incidence of cancer is high (Bang, White, Gause & Leffall, 1988). Low socioeconomic status correlates with poor survival rates from cancer (Smith, Shipley & Rose, 1990; Lipworth, Abelin & Connelly 1970). A study in the District of Columbia showed that cancer mortality in the southeastern area of the city was greater than in the northwestern area (White & Parker, 1981). People who live in the northwestern section have higher socioeconomic status than those in the southeastern section. Another epidemiologic study showed that the incidence of lung cancer was found in Blacks with lower income and less education (Devesa & Diamond, 1982).

It appears that Blacks tend to be less knowledgeable about cancer than Whites. In 1980, an American Cancer Society study of Black Americans' attitude toward cancer was conducted by EVAXX, Inc., a Black-owned evaluation organization (EVAXX, 1981). The study indicated that Blacks believe cancer is the main concern of Whites, while hypertension and sickle cell disease are the primary health concerns of Blacks. In particular, the study revealed that lower-income Blacks are less likely to have specific cancer tests and are less familiar with them. The study also showed that 69 percent of Blacks, as compared with 55 percent of Whites, think that they are not likely to get cancer, and that only 25 percent of Blacks, as compared with 54 percent of Whites, could name five to seven of cancer's seven warning signs.

RECOMMENDATIONS

Epidemiologic Studies

Numerous descriptive studies have adequately documented differences in incidence and mortality between Blacks and Whites. However, more comprehensive epidemiologic studies should be conducted to identify etiologic factors associated with higher rates of cancer of the prostate, esophagus, pancreas, multiple myeloma, and lung. A large population-based case-control study of pancreas, esophageal, prostate cancers, and multiple myeloma is in progress to evaluate the excess risk of these cancers among Blacks (Baquet & Gibbs, 1992). A comparison of Blacks and Whites should take into account socioeconomic or occupational difference. Additionally, biochemical and genetic epidemiologic studies should be conducted using case-control designs.

Basic Research and Clinical Trials

Basic laboratory research projects are needed to determine the risk factors of cancer sites that disproportionately affect Blacks. Cancer sites that should be examined for this research include the prostate and multiple myeloma. These sites have a high incidence of cancer for Blacks. A recent internal NCI breast cancer work group was formed to study breast cancer in Black women, and one of its objectives is to analyze potential molecular markers (Baquet & Gibbs, 1992).

More research on cellular oncogenes is needed. Oncogenes are genes that are specifically turned on for only a brief moment during the cell cycle, and they become altered by mutations. Also, oncogenes may operate continuously, thereby resulting in unregulated cell growth.

Life-Style Change and Risk Reduction

Life-style factors can increase an individual's risk of developing cancer. Therefore, life-style factors that are related to cancer incidence and mortality should be changed, and risk reduction activities should be performed. The Department of Health and Human Services established the year 2000 objectives for cancer reduction as follows: (1) reduce cigarette smoking to a prevalence of no more than 18 percent among Blacks aged 20 years and older, (2) reduce dietary fat intake to an average of 30 percent of calories or less and average saturated fat intake to less than 10 percent of calories among people aged 2 and older, and (3) increase complex carbohydrate and fiber-containing foods in the diets of adults to 5 or more daily servings for vegetables and fruits and to 6 or more daily servings for grain products (*Healthy People 2000*, 1991).

Socioeconomic status is related to cancer incidence and mortality. However, the exact interaction between socioeconomic status and cancer is not known.

Further research is required to specify and define the relationship of socioeconomic status to cancer incidence and survival. Since lower socioeconomic factors have been known to be associated with the risk of various cancers, cancer education is essential to reduce the risk of cancer in Blacks. NCI developed education materials and services for special populations as well as for the general population. The Cancer Prevention Awareness Program for Black Americans was developed to provide cancer information through the mass media and intermediary organizations. The Cancer Information Service is a nationwide program that offers current information about cancer prevention and treatment. By using the toll-free telephone number 1-800-4-CANCER, a variety of cancer information can be obtained (Baquet and Gibbs, 1992); it is to be hoped that it will be utilized.

Cancer prevention studies should be conducted to identify the factors related to reducing cancer incidence and mortality. One of the largest cancer prevention studies ever carried out in the United States is the American Cancer Society's Cancer Prevention Study II (ACS, 1992). This prospective study has been conducted since 1982 to examine the habits and exposures of more than one million Americans. The goal of this study is to identify those factors that affect a person's chance of developing cancer by comparing mortality rates in various exposed groups. Results from this study showed that exercise was associated with reduced cancer mortality; that among women, smokers die of lung cancer at a rate 12 times that of nonsmokers; and that men who smoke have an increased risk of myeloid leukemia (ACS, 1992).

Psychosocial and Behavioral Research

Research on behavioral modifications is having a significant impact on symptoms of cancer and its treatment. Research with humans on the role of stress has centered on either the ability of stress to cause cancer or the role of stress during the disease in encouraging a preexisting cancer to spread more rapidly. Although there are many studies about bereaved people who developed cancer following the deaths of their spouses, there is no scientific report to support this evidence. Experimental stress can alter immunity and cancer growth in animals, with stress generally favoring increased tumor growth in most experimental studies (Allen & Brickman, 1983). Whether or not these observed changes in laboratory measures of immunity have clinical relevance to resistance to human cancer growth remains to be proved. Stress is just beginning to be scientifically investigated for its potential association with cancer.

CONCLUSION

It is clear that the overall trend in cancer incidence and mortality among Blacks has been increasing for several decades. The overall cancer mortality for Blacks is approximately 30 percent higher than that for Whites. The reasons for these disparities are complex and involve issues related to differential exposures and risk factors. However, risk factors that may explain the large difference in cancer rates between Blacks and Whites include: (1) smoking habits, (2) alcohol consumption, (3) dietary habits, (4) exposure to occupational/environmental carcinogens, and (5) low socioeconomic status.

The burden of cancer is disproportionately distributed among Blacks compared with Whites in the United States. One of the major goals of the year 2000 objectives for the nation is to reduce health disparities among Americans. To reduce cancer incidence and mortality in Blacks, national cooperative efforts including research collaboration, intervention studies, epidemiologic and clinical trials, basic research, training, education, and information distribution must be continued. NCI should take a national leadership role to implement cancer prevention and control activities in the Black population. Furthermore, there should be cooperative agreements between various sectors, for example, the federal government, Black medical schools, professional organizations, and pharmaceutical companies regarding research and education. Also, culturally appropriate cancer control, prevention strategies and guidelines for the Black community should be developed. Medical and related personnel must, while emphasizing the importance of primary and secondary prevention, use innovative and effective approaches to focus their efforts toward educating the poor on the signs, symptoms, and dangers of cancer.

REFERENCES

Allen, W., & Brickman, M. (1983). Stress, personality, and cancer. In E. H. Rosenbaum (Ed.), *Can you prevent cancer?* (pp. 213–222). St. Louis: C. V. Mosby Company.

Anderson, D. E. (1978). Familial cancer and cancer families. *Seminars in Oncology, 5,* 11–16.

Anderson, D. E. (1982). Familial predisposition. In Schottenfeld, D., & Fraumeni, J., Jr. (Eds.), *Cancer Epidemiology and Prevention* (pp. 318–335). Philadelphia: W. B. Saunders Company.

American Cancer Society (ACS). (1992). *Cancer Facts and Figures 1992.* New York: American Cancer Society.

Bang, K. M., Perlin, E., & Sampson, C. C. (1987). Increased cancer risks in Blacks: A look at the factors. *Journal of National Medical Association, 79,* 383–388.

Bang, K. M., White, J. E., Gause, B. L., & Leffall, L. D., Jr. (1988). Evaluation of recent trends in cancer mortality and incidence among Blacks. *Cancer, 61,* 1255–1261.

Baquet, C. R., & Gibbs, T. (1992). Cancers and Black Americans. In R. L. Braithwaite and S. E. Taylor (Eds.), *Health Issues in the Black community,* San Francisco: Josey-Bass.

Baquet, C. R., Horm, J. W., Gibbs, T., & Greenwald, P. (1991). Socioeconomic factors and cancer incidence among Blacks and whites. *Journal of National Cancer Institute, 83,* 551–557.

Centers for Disease Control (CDC). (1987). Cigarette smoking in the United States. *Morbidity and Mortality Weekly Report, 36,* 581–585.

Decouflé, P. (1982). Occupation. In D. A. Schottenfeld & J. Fraumeni, Jr. (Eds.), *Cancer Epidemiology and Prevention* (pp. 318–335). Philadelphia: W. B. Saunders Company.

Devesa, S. S., & Diamond, F. L. (1982). Socioeconomic and racial difference in lung cancer incidence. *American Journal of Epidemiology, 118,* 818–831.

Doll, R., & Peto, R. (1981). The causes of cancer: Quantitative estimates of available risk of cancer in the United States today. *Journal of National Cancer Institute, 66,* 1192–1308.

Environmental Protection Agency (EPA). (1992). *Respiratory health effects of passive smoking: Lung cancer and other disorders.* Washington, DC: U.S. Environmental Protection Agency, Office of Health and Environmental Assessment, Office of Atmospheric and Indoor Air Programs, Publication No. EPA/600/8–90/006F.

EVAXX, Inc. (1981). Black Americans' attitudes toward cancer and cancer tests: Highlights of a study. *CA, 31*(4), 212–218.

Frais, M. A. (1979). Gastric adenocarcinoma due to ataxia-telangiectasis (Louis-Bar Syndrome). *Journal of Medical Genetics, 4,* 160–161.

Frumkin, H., & Levy, B. S. (1983). Carcinogens. In B. S. Levy and D. H. Wegman (Eds.), *Occupational Health* (pp. 145–175). Boston: Little Brown.

Garber, J. E., Goldstein, A. M., Kantor, A. F., Dreyfus, M. G., Fraumeni, J. F., Jr., & Li, F. P. (1991). Follow-up study of twenty-four families with Li-Fraumeni syndrome. *Cancer Research, 51,* 6094–6097.

Gullatte, M. M. (1989). Cancer prevention and early detection in Black Americans: Colon and rectum. *Journal of National Black Nurses Association, 3,* 49–56.

Hargreaves, M. K., Baquet, C., & Gamshadzahi, A. (1989). Diet, nutritional status, and cancer risk in American Blacks. *Nutrition and Cancer, 12,* 1–28.

Healthy People 2000. (1991). National health promotion and disease prevention objectives. DHHS Publication No. (PHS) 91-50212. Washington, DC: Government Printing Office.

Li, F. P. (1990). Familial cancer syndrome and clusters. *Current Problems in Cancer, 14,* 73–114.

Lipworth, L., Abelin, T., & Connelly, R. R. (1970). Socioeconomic factors in the prognosis of cancer patients. *Journal of Chronic Disease, 23,* 105–116.

McWhorter, W. P., Schatzkin, A. G., Horm, J. W., & Brown, C. C. (1989). Contribution of socioeconomic status to Black/white differences in cancer incidence. *Cancer, 63,* 982–987.

Mettlin, C. (1980). Nutritional habits of Blacks and Whites. *Preventive Medicine, 9,* 601–606.

National Cancer Institute (NCI). (1992). *Cancer statistics review 1973–1989.* NIH Publication Number 92-2789.

National Center for Health Statistics (NCHS). (1993). Vital Statistics of the United States 1990. U.S. Department of Health and Human Services (unpublished).

Potter, L. M., Morris, L. E., & Blot, W. J. (1981). Esophageal cancer among Black men in Washington, D.C: Alcohol, tobacco, and other risk factors. *Journal of National Cancer Institute, 67,* 777–783.

Report of the Secretary's Task Force on black and minority health. (1985). Volume 1: Executive summary. U. S. Department of Health and Human Services, Washington, DC: Government Printing Office.

Shields, P. G. (1993). Inherited factors and environmental exposures in cancer risk. *Journal of Occupational Medicine, 35,* 34–41.

Smith, C. D., Shipley, M. J., & Rose, G. (1990). Magnitude and causes of socioeconomic differentials in mortality: Future evidence from the Whitehall study. *Journal of Epidemiology and Community Health, 44,* 265–270.

Sokoloff, B. (1938). Predisposition to cancer in the Bonaparte family. *American Journal of Surgery, 11,* 673–678.

Shy, C. M., & Struba, R. J. (1982). Air and water pollution. In D. Schottenfeld and J. Fraumeni, Jr. (Eds.), *Cancer Epidemiology and Prevention* (pp. 336–363). Philadelphia: W. B. Saunders Company.

Surgeon General's report on nutrition and health. (1988). U.S. Department of Health and Human Services. Publication No. (PHS) 88-50210, Washington, DC: Government Printing Office.

White, J. E., & Parker, D. (1981). The distribution of cancer mortality in Washington, DC, 1971–76. Cancer Coordinating Council for Metropolitan Washington, Washington, D.C.

White, J. E., Enterline, J. P., Alam, Z., & Moore, F. M. (1981). Cancer among Blacks in the United States: Recognizing the problem. In A. I. Helleb (Ed.), *Cancer among Black Populations* (pp. 35–53). New York: Alan R. Liss.

7

Diabetes Mellitus in the African-American Population

Eugene S. Tull, Mohammed H. Makame, and
Jeffrey M. Roseman

INTRODUCTION

The 1986 report of the Secretary's Task Force on Black and Minority Health
called attention to the alarming excess morbidity and mortality from chronic
illnesses such as non-insulin-dependent diabetes mellitus (NIDDM), cancer, and
heart disease that exists in minorities in the United States. In addition to the
added disease burden, limited research in the area of minority health has exacerbated the problem in the African-American population by reducing the
knowledge necessary for understanding the causative factors and planning effective intervention strategies.

Diabetes mellitus, one of the diseases targeted for increased research focus
among minorities, continues to have devastating consequences on the African-
American population. It is estimated that approximately 1.8 million African
Americans are affected with the disease (Report of the Secretary's Task Force
on Black and Minority Health, 1985). Moreover, the prevalence and mortality
from diabetes are nearly twice as high among African Americans as in the U.S.
White population (CDC, 1990). Thus, there remains a critical need for research
designed to elucidate the factors contributing to the increased diabetes-related
morbidity and mortality in this ethnic group. In this chapter, we review the
limited data on the occurrence and impact of diabetes mellitus in the African-
American population and provide recommendations for future research and
control.

Classification and Diagnosis

Diabetes mellitus is a heterogenous group of disorders that are characterized
by an abnormal increase in the level of blood glucose. When studies are con-

ducted to assess the epidemiology and public health impact of diabetes mellitus on the African-American population, non-insulin-dependent diabetes mellitus (NIDDM) and insulin-dependent diabetes mellitus (IDDM) are most often considered. However, other forms of glucose intolerance have also been studied, including impaired glucose tolerance (IGT), gestational diabetes (GDM), and other atypical diabetes syndromes. Classification of these diabetes subtypes is generally based on criteria published by the National Diabetes Data Group (NDDG) (1979) and the World Health Organization (WHO) (1980). The diagnosis of diabetes is established by a finding of a fasting plasma glucose (FBS) value greater than 140 mg/dl or a value of 200 mg/dl two hours after a 75-gram glucose challenge on the oral glucose tolerance test (OGGT) (NDDG, 1979; WHO, 1980, 1985, p. 10–24). Characteristics and distinguishing features of the different diabetes subtypes appear in Table 7.1.

FACTORS INFLUENCING THE OCCURRENCE OF DIABETES

Important factors influencing the occurrence of diabetes mellitus in African Americans include personal characteristics such as genetics, age, sex, and history of glucose intolerance (IGT, GDM). Other life-style factors such as physical activity and obesity, which are associated with changing socioeconomic and cultural climates within countries, greatly affect the risk of developing the disease. Although the exact etiological interactions remain debatable, it is certain that a combination of most of these factors is responsible for precipitating the disease.

Genetics

An individual's risk of developing diabetes mellitus is to a great extent influenced by his/her genetic background. Individuals who are first-degree relatives of diabetes patients are at marked increased risk of developing the disease compared to unrelated individuals in the general population (Tuomilehto, Tuomilehto-Wolf, Zimmet, Alberti & Keen, 1992). First-degree relatives of NIDDM patients have a risk of about 5 to 10 percent of developing diabetes before age 65 (Tuomilehto et al., 1992). For IDDM, the risk to first-degree relatives has been estimated at around 3 to 10 percent by the age of 30 years (W.H.O. Multinational, 1991). Evidence from studies of identical twins indicate a concordance rate of about 90 percent for NIDDM and 50 percent for IDDM, indicating that the influence of genetics is greater in the former than in the latter (Barnett, Eff, Leslie & Pyke, 1981). The search for the genetic reasons that rates of diabetes vary in different ethnic groups has led to hypotheses that seek to account for the observed frequencies of NIDDM and IDDM in African Americans.

Table 7.1
Diabetes Subtypes Occurring in Black Populations, Plasma Glucose Values (WHO) for Diagnosis in Epidemiological Studies, and Description of Subtypes

TYPE	Clinical Diagnosis (WHO)	Description
[a]IDDM	FBS $\geq$ 140 mg/dl 2 hr OGTT $\geq$ 200 mg/dl	Also known as Type 1, commonly found in adolescence; characterized by abrupt onset of symptoms, insulinopenia, and ketosis; may have subclinical period lasting many years (Gorsuch et al., 1981); genes of HLA loci, autoimmunity, and viral infections may play role in etiology (Trucco & Dorman, 1987).
[b]NIDDM	FBS $\geq$ 140 mg/dl 2 hr OGTT $\geq$ 200 mg/dl	Also known as Type 2, comprises 90% of all diabetes cases; usually develops prior to age 40; patients are typically overweight, not prone to ketosis (NDDG, 1979); genetics and obesity are strongly associated with etiology (Permutt, 1990).
[c]IGT	FBS < 140 mg/dl 2 hr OGTT 141-199 mg/dl	Associated with an increased risk of developing overt diabetes; 2-3% of IGT patients will proceed to frank diabetes, almost always NIDDM (NDDG, 1979).
[d]GDM	FBS $\geq$ 140 mg/dl 2 hr OGTT $\geq$ 200 mg/dl	Occurrence of diabetes during pregnancy with return to normal tolerance after delivery; associated with increased risk of developing diabetes.
[e]PDPD	FBS $\geq$ 140 mg/dl 2 hr OGTT $\geq$ 200 mg/dl	Characteristic features include: BMI[f] < 19kg/M^2 body weight, insulin requirement > 1.5 Units/kg, no evidence of pancreatic calcification (WHO, 1985); ketosis resistant; its existence remains controversial.
[g]FCPD	FBS $\geq$ 140 mg/dl 2 hr OGGT $\geq$ 200 mg/dl	Characteristic features similar to PDPD with positive evidence of pancreatic calcification.
[h]ATYPICAL	FBS $\geq$ 140 mg/dl 2 hr OGGT $\geq$ 200 mg/dl	Diabetes syndromes characterized by periods of euglycemic remission; described by Winter et al. (1987) as atypical diabetes in young African Americans; by Morrison (1981) in Jamaica as phasic insulin dependence; also described among other black populations in U.S. (Banerji & Lebovitz, 1990) and Africa (Abu-Bakare, Taylor, Gill & Alberti, 1986).

[a] Insulin-Dependent Diabetes Mellitus; [b] Noninsulin-Dependent Diabetes Mellitus; [c] Impaired Glucose Tolerance; [d] Gestational Diabetes Mellitus; [e] Protein Deficient Pancreatic Diabetes; [f] Body Mass Index; [g] Fibrocalculus Pancreatic Diabetes; [h] Atypical Diabetes Subtypes.

Thrifty Gene Hypothesis

Neel (1962) suggested that populations exposed to periodic famines would through natural selection increase the frequency of genetic traits, "thrifty genes," that predispose to energy conservation. These genes would increase survival during times of famine by allowing for adept storage of fat in times of abundance. In the absence of feast and famine cycles, in times of continued abundance, these genes would become disadvantageous, predisposing to the development of obesity and an increased frequency of NIDDM. This hypothesis would be consistent with the observation of much higher rates of diabetes and obesity among African Americans and urban Africans compared to Black Africans residing in traditional environments.

Racial Admixture Hypothesis

MacDonald (1975) hypothesized that the frequency of IDDM might be higher in U.S. Black children compared to Black African children because IDDM susceptibility genes, more common in the U.S. White population, had become admixed into the Black population. In support of this hypothesis, using seven genetic markers, Reitnauer et al. (1982) demonstrated that African-American IDDM patients had more White admixture than nondiabetic African-American controls. Tull, Roseman, and Christian (1991), using grandparental race as a measure of admixture among African Americans in the U.S. Virgin Islands, also found that IDDM cases had more White ancestry than controls.

Genes of the HLA complex of Chromosome 6, involved in immunological rejection of foreign cells (Friedman & Failkow, 1982), are genetic factors that may be increased by admixture. African Americans with IDDM have been observed to have similar HLA allelic associations to those found in U.S. Whites, particularly for HLA-DR3 and DR4 (Reitnauer et al., 1981; Dunston, Henry, Christian, Ofuso & Callender, 1989). MacDonald et al. (1986), however, when studying Black IDDM patients in Nigeria (the ancestral home of many African Americans) found an association of HLA-DR3 but did not find the increased frequency of DR4 that is typically found in U.S. Black and White children. Assuming that the Nigerian patients had little or no White admixture, he suggested that the Caucasian-derived susceptibility determinant in the gene pool of African Americans is HLA-DR4 associated (MacDonald, 1988).

Epidemiologic Transition

In recent years, researchers have observed that the prevalence of NIDDM is increasing around the world (Alberti, 1986). This trend is consistent with the concept of the epidemiologic transition, whereby, as societies become more industrialized, infant mortality and death from infectious diseases decrease and life expectancy increases, along with a greater prevalence of and mortality from chronic diseases (Omran, 1983). The increasing rates of chronic diseases are usually preceded by dietary and other life-style changes that result from economic development. Often, non-insulin-dependent diabetes mellitus is the first chronic disease to increase in frequency with changes in life-style and industrialization.

From 1963 to 1985, the rates of known diabetes in the United States doubled for Whites, but tripled for African Americans (Drury & Powell, 1987). While the rate for Black females remained consistently higher than for the other three race-sex categories, a dramatic change occurred among African-American males. African-American males had a lower rate than White males from 1963 to 1973; but, after 1975, there was a crossover such that the rate for Black males became higher than the rate for White males. What were the factors responsible for these changes?

It is possible that the crossover among African-American males might reflect an increase in the proportion of diagnosed to undiagnosed cases or an increased survival of Black men. The overall changes observed during the 22-year period are likely the result of improving economic conditions and increased life expectancy, together with changes in diet, levels of physical activity, and patterns of obesity. Unlike island populations in the Pacific (Zimmet, Taylor & Whitehouse, 1982), the specific relationship between changes in the level of life-style risk factors and the development of NIDDM in African Americans remains obscure.

Age and Sex

In most populations the prevalence of diabetes varies with age and sex. For African Americans, the peak age range for diagnosis of IDDM is approximately 15–19 years of age (LaPorte et al., 1986; Wagenknecht, Roseman & Alexander, 1989), while NIDDM occurs more frequently after age 56, when it is three times more common than in the White population (Roseman, 1985). African-American females are more likely to develop IDDM compared to Black men (Wagenknecht et al., 1989) and are 1.2, 1.5, and 2.0 times more likely to develop NIDDM than Black men, White women, and White men, respectively (Harris, 1990). The sex differential for IDDM may be due to differences in susceptibility or exposure to etiologic agents (Dahlquist et al., 1985). Differences in NIDDM by gender may be due to differences in the levels of associated risk factors such as obesity and physical activity.

Socioeconomic Status (SES)

Racial differences in disease rates may reflect socioeconomic differences. In the United States socioeconomic status and the frequency of NIDDM have an inverse relationship (Drury & Powell, 1987). The impact of SES on NIDDM rates among African Americans may be especially strong, as 30.7 percent of African Americans live in poverty compared to 10 percent of White Americans (Johnson & Darley, 1992). Studies relating socioeconomic status to the development of IDDM have been inconsistent. Some studies found a positive association (Christau et al., 1977). Others have found a negative (Colle et al., 1984) or no association at all (Wagenknecht et al., 1989). It seems unlikely that socioeconomic status contributes significantly to racial differences in the frequency of IDDM in the United States.

Obesity

Obesity, generally measured as body-mass index (BMI) (weight in Kilograms/ height in meters^2), is a major risk factor for NIDDM (Broseay, 1988). Overweight is a serious problem for the African-American female, with the level of obesity (i.e., BMI > 27.3) being greater than 50 percent among women older than age 45 (Van Itallie, 1985). Compared to White women, African-American women are more obese at every decade from age 20 to 65. African-American men show a similar pattern of obesity (i.e., BMI > 27.8) with age when compared to White men, except for ages 35 to 55, when they are more obese (Van Italie, 1985).

The development of NIDDM is not only influenced by the presence of obesity but also by where the body fat is distributed. The risk of developing NIDDM is greater for individuals with central or android obesity (excess fat in the upper part of the body) (Hartz, Rupley, Kalkhoff & Rimm, 1983). African Americans have been reported to have a greater tendency to store more fat in the trunk than Whites, which could explain part of the excess prevalence of NIDDM in the Black population (Kumanyika, 1988).

Physical Activity

There is evidence that physical inactivity is an independent risk factor for developing NIDDM (Taylor et al., 1984). Conversely, exercise may be a strong protective factor against the development of the disease (Kriska et al., 1991; Helmrich, Ragland, Leung & Paffenbarger, 1991). In general there is an inverse relationship between levels of obesity and physical activity. Therefore, higher levels of obesity among U.S. Blacks compared to Whites suggest that decreased levels of physical activity among African Americans may contribute to their higher rate of diabetes.

Insulin Resistance

The risk of developing NIDDM is positively associated with fasting levels of circulating insulin (Sicree, Zimmet, King & Coventry, 1987). It has been shown that insulin resistance, characterized by hyperinsulinemia, can predate the development of NIDDM for years (Bogardus et al., 1987). In addition to diabetes, insulin resistance underlies a number of interrelated disorders including hypertension, body fat mass and distribution, and serum lipid abnormalities (Ferrannini, Haffner, Mitchell & Stern, 1991). This has prompted speculation (Zimmet,

1992) that hyperinsulinemia and/or insulin resistance may be the phenotypic expression of the "thrifty genotype" proposed by Neel (1962).

Impaired Glucose Tolerance (IGT) and Gestational Diabetes

Impaired glucose tolerance (IGT) and gestational diabetes mellitus (GDM) are two forms of glucose intolerance that are strong risk factors for developing NIDDM and IDDM. Gestational diabetes refers to the development of diabetes during pregnancy and a subsequent return to normal tolerance following parturition, while IGT is the category of glucose tolerance where fasting glucose values are between normal and diabetic. Approximately 50 percent of African-American women with glucose intolerance during pregnancy might be expected to develop diabetes over a 20-year period compared to about 10 percent of women who have normal tolerance during pregnancy (O'Sullivan & Mahan, 1968). The risk of developing overt diabetes among individuals with IGT is related to the severity of impaired tolerance and presence of other risk factors, including a positive family history of diabetes and obesity (Harris, 1989). A number of risk factors for GDM have been identified among African-American women, including age, gravidity, hypertension, obesity, and family history of diabetes (Roseman et al., 1991).

INCIDENCE AND PREVALENCE OF DIABETES MELLITUS

Non-Insulin-Dependent Diabetes Mellitus

The earliest estimates, based on national samples, of the occurrence of diabetes in African Americans came from data collected on male World War II registrants age 18–45, which suggested that the prevalence of diabetes was greater in White (3.0%) than Black males (1.4%) (Marble, 1949). Because these data were collected over age ranges with a preponderance of distribution toward younger age, where diabetes rates may primarily reflect insulin-dependent diabetes mellitus, they may not present a true picture of the prevalence of NIDDM in the races at that time. More recent and reliable data from the National Center for Health Statistics indicate that, in the United States, the prevalence of known diabetes is higher among African Americans than White Americans (5.3% vs 3.1%), particularly among individuals age 45–64, when the rate for Blacks is 50.6 percent higher (Harris, 1990). The prevalence of diabetes increases with age for U.S. Black adults and is approximately 1.2 times higher for females (Harris, 1990). Among African Americans, the prevalence of diabetes is inversely related to educational attainment and is highest among individuals in the lowest income group (Drury & Powell, 1987).

Insulin-Dependent Diabetes Mellitus

The prevalence of insulin-dependent diabetes mellitus follows a different racial pattern from that of NIDDM: White children have about twice the rate of Black children. Estimates of the prevalence of IDDM in African-American children have usually been less than 0.15 percent (Rosenbaum, 1967; National Center for Health Statistics, 1977). Recent data from population-based registries indicate that the incidence of IDDM among African-American children younger than 15 varies dramatically, with a range of 3.3 to 11.8 per 100,000 (see Figure 7.0). Corresponding rates for White children are nearly twice as high, ranging from 12.3 to 16.9 per 100,000 (LaPorte et al., 1986; Wagenknecht et al., 1989; Lipman, 1991).

These data indicate that, across the United States, there is much greater variability in the incidence of IDDM for African-American children than White children. It is possible the variability in IDDM incidence among African-American children might result from variations in degree of White admixture in the various registry locations. There is evidence that White admixture varies by geographic region in the United States with greater admixture in northern areas than in the south (Reed, 1969). This is consistent with the trend for more European-American genetic admixture (21.2%) in Allegheny County, Pennsylvania (Chakraborty, Mohammed, Nwankwo & Ferrel, 1992), where the incidence of IDDM in African Americans is higher (11.8/100,000), than in Jefferson County, Alabama, where genetic admixture is 17.9 percent (Reitnauer et al., 1982) and the incidence of IDDM is lower (4.4/100,000) (see Figure 7.1).

Atypical Diabetes

Atypical diabetic syndromes, characterized by normoglycemic remission with subsequent periods of hyperglycemic relapse, usually requiring insulin for glycemic control, have been described in African-American and other Black populations. Winter et al. (1987), reported an atypical diabetes in young African Americans that presents with features typical of IDDM but lacks the HLA associations characteristic of the disease. The insulin dependence in this syndrome was intermittent or gradually declined throughout the course of the illness. Diabetic syndromes presenting in adulthood with similar phasic insulin dependence have also been reported (Morrison, 1981; Banerji & Lebovitz, 1990). While other forms of diabetes including protein deficient pancreatic diabetes and fibrocalculus pancreatic diabetes occur in some Black African populations (Abu-Bakare, Taylor, Gill & Alberti, 1986), to date they have not been shown to be significant for African Americans.

DIABETES MORTALITY

Today, diabetes mellitus is the third most frequent cause of death from disease among African Americans. When compared to their White counterparts, the

Figure 7.1
Age-adjusted (0–14) Incidence of Insulin-Dependent Diabetes

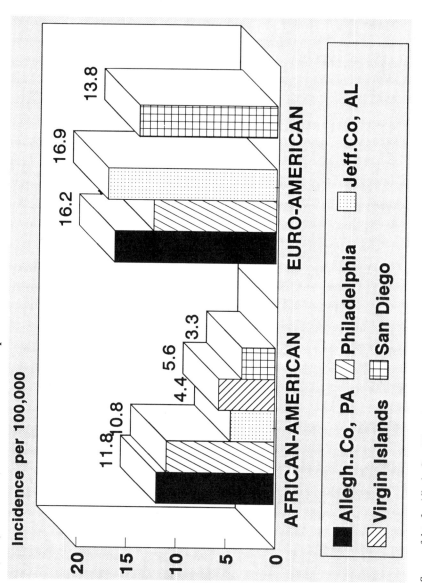

Source of data for Allegh. Co., PA = (LaPorte et al., 1986); Philadelphia, PA = (Lipman, 1991); US Virgin Islands = (Tull et al., 1991); San Diego, CA = (Lorenzi et al., 1985); Jeff. Co., AL = (Wagenknecht et al., 1989).

relative risk of death from diabetes is 1.9 for U.S. Black males and 2.5 for Black females (Report of the Secretary's Task Force on Black and Minority Health, 1985). Data on mortality specific to IDDM indicate that compared to Whites with the disease, African Americans have a death rate 2.0 to 2.5 times greater (Tull, LaPorte, Vergona, Gower & Makame, 1992).

Higher rates of diabetes mortality in African Americans compared to the White population may in part be due to their higher prevalence of diabetes. When mortality among individuals who have developed diabetes is considered, however, it appears that African Americans have a lower mortality rate than Whites with the disease (Harris, 1990). In recent years, there has been a leveling off in the rate of mortality from diabetes for both races (NCHS 1988; Harris, 1990).

DIABETIC COMPLICATIONS

Chronic diabetes mellitus is associated with a number of devastating complications that diminish the quality of life and lead to premature mortality. These include hypertension, diabetic retinopathy, neuropathy, nephropathy, and macrovascular complications.

In the United States, African Americans with diabetes have higher rates of hypertension than Whites (NCHS, 1982). The consistency of high rates of hypertension among African Americans and Afro-Caribbean populations (Grell, 1983) has led to the hypothesis that Western Hemisphere Blacks are descendants of a highly selected group of Africans who were efficient at retaining salt, which allowed them to maintain sodium homeostasis and survive the long sea voyages from Africa (Grim, 1988). Recent evidence suggests that high rates of hypertension among African Americans might be related to hyperinsulinemia and abnormal renal Na^+ transport (Douglas, 1990).

Data on the frequency and impact of other diabetes-associated complications are limited. However, retinopathy, neuropathy, and stroke appear to be more frequent in African Americans than Whites with diabetes (Roseman, 1985). The rate of lower extremity amputations (generally due to gangrene and ulceration) resulting from diabetes has been reported to be significantly greater (2.3 times) among U.S. Blacks than Whites (Most & Sinnock, 1983). Incidence rates of diabetic end-stage renal disease (ESRD) have been shown to be 2.9 to 5.6 times greater for African Americans than for Whites (Smith, Svetkey & Dennis, 1991). After developing ESRD however, U.S. Blacks appear to survive longer than Whites (Cowie et al., 1992). There is also some suggestion that certain cardiovascular complications including angina and heart attack may occur less frequently among African Americans than among Whites with diabetes (Harris, 1990).

It has been suggested that the overall higher rates of diabetes complications among African Americans might be related to poorer metabolic control (Delmater, Albrecht, Postellon & Gutai, 1991). In addition, the high rate of hypertension among African Americans with diabetes may exacerbate or hasten the onset of other complications such as retinopathy and nephropathy (i.e. gradual degeneration of the kidney's vital blood-cleaning system). Other important risk factors for diabetes complications include age of onset, education, cigarette smoking, socioeconomic status, and access to medical care (Roseman, 1985).

ADDRESSING THE PROBLEM

Today, diabetes mellitus remains a serious problem confronting the African-American population. High diabetes mortality rates reflect only part of the problem. The prospect of increasing diabetes prevalence rates casts an ominous shadow over the future for the African-American community. The morbidity associated with diabetic complications places a tremendous financial burden on individuals and communities least able to bear the cost of such an illness. Clearly, the challenge of addressing the problem of diabetes mellitus in the African-American population is great and will require a multidisciplinary approach involving government, researchers, educators, and members of the African-American community.

Health Promotion

Of primary importance is the need for dissemination of information about diabetes and its consequences into the African-American community. An uninformed African-American community may tend to underestimate the diabetes problem or to pay less attention to the signs and symptoms of its onset. This may result in delayed diagnosis or care, thereby increasing the likelihood of rapid onset of complications. Thus, culturally sensitive strategies designed to intervene and educate African Americans about the behavioral and environmental risk factors for diabetes and its complications are essential. Clearly, in order for African Americans to take steps to reduce the diabetes-associated morbidity and mortality in their communities they must have the ability to make informed decisions about the disease.

Cooperative Efforts for Provision of Health Services

Rates of diabetes mortality and complications may depend on the availability and continuity of care. There is some indication that African Americans with diabetes may be underserved with respect to medical care (Harris, 1990). Careful study of this problem is required, and innovative solutions must be developed. The African-American community must also become empowered to expect and demand the necessary care they deserve. To affect such change, community-based institutions, such as the church, can develop programs for using the health professionals within their congregations to provide care or counseling to diabetics and their families. Organizations concerned with minorities, such as the Urban

League, can include diabetes and other health problems in their national agendas to generate concern and action at the community and national levels.

Governmental agencies and institutions engaged in training health professionals, such as medical schools and schools of public health, should institute action to increase the pool of African Americans in the professions concerned with the care of individuals with diabetes. Federal agencies, such as the National Institutes of Health, may also provide special grant programs to encourage submission of research grants to study diabetes in African Americans and to enhance the development of minority researchers in the area.

Research

The limited data currently available on diabetes among African Americans raise many questions but deliver few answers about the etiology and natural history of diabetes and its complications in this ethnic group. To date, few studies of diabetes in the United States have incorporated representative samples of African Americans. This shortcoming must be addressed if future studies are to yield valid conclusions about the factors responsible for the occurrence of the disease in the African-American population. In the Report of the Secretary's Task Force on Black and Minority Health (1985), a number of research priority areas for addressing the health disparity between Black and White Americans were identified. These areas are particularly relevant to diabetes mellitus and include the following: (1) research into risk-factor identification, (2) research into risk-factor prevalence, (3) research into health education interventions, (4) research into prevention services interventions, (5) research into treatment services, and (6) research into sociocultural factors and health outcomes. The identification of these target areas for research and other recent efforts by the Department of Health and Human Services to promote the study of diabetes in the African-American population (Sullivan, 1990) are important steps toward addressing the gap in our knowledge of how diabetes affects African Americans. In the future we must translate the knowledge gained from new and ongoing studies into effective preventive action.

NOTE

Please address all correspondence to: Dr. Eugene S. Tull, Rangos Research Center, Fifth Floor, 3460 5th Avenue, Pittsburgh, PA 15213.

REFERENCES

Alberti, K.G.G.M. (1986). World aspects of diabetes. *Diabetic Medicine, 3,* 103–105.
Abu-Bakare, A., Taylor, R., Gill, G. V. and Alberti, K.G.G.M. (1986). Tropical or malnutrition-related diabetes: A real syndrome? *Lancet, 1,* 1135–1138.
Banerji, M. A., & Lebovitz, H. E. (1990). Remission in non-insulin-dependent diabetes

mellitus: Clinical characteristics of remission and relapse in black patients. *Medicine, 69,* 176–185.

Barnett, A. H., Eff, C., Leslie, R. D. G., & Pyke, D. A. (1981). Diabetes in identical twins, a study of 200 pairs. *Diabetologia, 20,* 87–93.

Bogardus, C., Lillioja, S., Foley, J., Christin, L., Freymond, D., Nyomba, B., Bennett, P. H., Reaven, G., & Salans, L. (1987). Insulin resistance predicts the development of non-insulin dependent diabetes mellitus in Pima Indians. *Diabetes, 36* (Supp.1), 47A.

Broseay, J. D. (1988). Native Americans. *Diabetes Forecast, 4,* 42–48.

Centers for Disease Control (CDC). (1990). Diabetes surveillance: Annual 1990 report. U.S. Department of Health and Human Services, Centers for Disease Control, Division of Diabetes Translation, Atlanta GA.

Chakraborty, R., Mohammed, K. I., Nwankwo, M., & Ferrel, R. E. (1992). Caucasian genes in African-Americans. *American Journal of Human Genetics, 50,* 145–155.

Christau, B., Kroman, H., Anderson, O., Christy, M., Buxchard, K., Arnung, K., Kristensen, I., Petersen, J., Steinrud, J., & Nerup, J. (1977). Incidence, seasonal, and geographic patterns of juvenile onset insulin-dependent diabetes mellitus in Denmark. *Diabetologia, 13,* 281–284.

Colle, E., Siemiatycki, J., West, R., Belmonte, M. M., Crepeau, M. P., Poirier, R., & Wilkins, J. (1984). Incidence of juvenile onset diabetes in Montreal—demonstration of ethnic differences and socioeconomic class differences. *Journal of Chronic Disease, 34,* 611–616.

Cowie, C. C., Port, F. K., & Rust, K. F. (1992). Survival differences between black and white diabetic subjects with end-stage renal disease. *Diabetes, 41* (Supp. 1), 7A.

Dahlquist, G., Blom, L., Holgren, G., Hogglof, B., Larsson, Y., Sterky, G., & Wall, S. (1985). The epidemiology of diabetes in Swedish children 0–14 years: A six year prospective study. *Diabetologia, 28,* 802–808.

Delmater, A. M., Albrecht, D. R., Postellon, D. C., & Gutai, J. P. (1991). Racial differences in metabolic control of children and adolescents with type 1 diabetes mellitus. *Diabetes Care, 14,* 20–25.

Douglas, J. G. (1990). Hypertension and diabetes in blacks. *Diabetes Care, 13* (Supp. 4), 1191–1195.

Drury, T. F., & Powell, A. L. (1987). Prevalence of known diabetes among black Americans. (U.S. Department of Health and Human Services publication No. (PHS) 87-1250. Government Printing Office.

Dunston, G. M., Henry, L. W., Christian, J., Ofosu, M. D., & Callender, C. O. (1989). HLA-DR3, DQ heterogeneity in American blacks is associated with susceptibility and resistance to insulin-dependent diabetes mellitus. *Transplantation Proceedings, 21,* 653–655.

Ferrannini, E., Haffner, S. M., Mitchell, B. D., & Stern, M. P. (1991). Hyperinsulinemia: The key feature of a cardiovascular and metabolic syndrome. *Diabetologia, 34,* 416–422.

Friedman, J. M., & Failkow, J. (1982). Genetics. In B. N. Broduff & S. J. Bleicher (Eds.), *Diabetes Mellitus and Obesity* (pp. 364–373). Baltimore, MD: Williams/Wilkins.

Grell, G. A. C. (1983). Hypertension in the West Indies. *Postgraduate Medical Journal, 59,* 616–621.

Grim, C. E. (1988). On slavery, salt and the greater prevalence of hypertension in black Americans. *Clinical Research, 36,* 426A.

Harris, M. I. (1989). Impaired glucose tolerance in the U.S. population. *Diabetes Care, 12,* 464–474.

Harris, M. I. (1990). Noninsulin-dependent diabetes mellitus in black and white Americans. *Diabetes Metabolism Review, 6,* 71–90.

Hartz, A. J., Rupley, D. C., Jr., Kalkhoff, R., & Rimm, A. A. (1983). Relationship of obesity to diabetes: Influence of obesity and body fat distribution. *Preventive Medicine, 12,* 351–357.

Helmrich, S. P., Ragland, D. R., Leung, R. W., & Paffenbarger, R. S. (1991). Physical activity and reduced occurrence of non-insulin-dependent diabetes mellitus. *New England Journal of Medicine, 325,* 147–152.

Johnson, O., & Darley, V. (1992). *Information Please Almanac* (IPA) (p. 805). Boston: Houghton Mifflin Company.

Kriska, A. M., Knowler, W. C., LaPorte, R. E., Pettitt, D. J., Saad, M. F., Nelson, R. G., & Bennett, P. H. (1991). Association between physical activity, plasma glucose concentrations, and body mass index, in the Pima Indians. *Diabetes, 40* (Supp. 1), 1211A.

Kumanyika, S. (1988). Obesity in black women. *Epidemiology Review, 9,* 31–50.

Laporte, R. E., Tajima, N., Dorman, J. S., Cruickshanks, K. J., Eberhardt, M. S., Rabin, B. S., Atchinson, R. W., Wagner, D. K., Becker, D. J., Orchard, T. J., Selemenda, C. W., Kuller, L. A., & Drash, A. L. (1986). Differences between blacks and whites in the epidemiology of insulin-dependent diabetes mellitus in Allegheny County, Pennsylvania. *American Journal of Epidemiology, 123,* 592–603.

Lipman, T. H. (1991). The epidemiology of Type 1 diabetes in children 0–14 years of age in Philadelphia. Doctoral dissertation, University of Pennsylvania, Pennsylvania.

Lorenzi, M., Cogliero, E., & Schmidt, N. J. (1985). Racial differences in incidence of juvenile-onset type 1 diabetes: Epidemiologic studies in southern California. *Diabetologia, 28,* 734–738.

MacDonald, M. J. (1975). Lower frequency of diabetes among hospitalized Negro than white children. Theoretical implications. *Acta Genet Med Gamelol, 24,* 119–126.

MacDonald, M. J. (1988). Speculation on the evolution of insulin-dependent diabetes genes. *Metabolism, 37,* 1182–1184.

MacDonald, M. J., Famuyiwa, O. O., Nwabuelo, I. A., Bella, A. F., Junaid, T. A., Marrari, M., & Duquesnoy, R. J. (1986). HLA-DR associations in black type 1 diabetics in Nigeria: Further support for models of inheritance. *Diabetes, 35,* 583–589.

Marble, A. (1949). Diabetes mellitus in the U.S. Army in World War II. *The Military Surgeon, 105,* 357–363.

Morrison, E. Y. (1981). Diabetes mellitus—a third syndrome (Phasic Insulin Dependence). *International Diabetes Federation Bulletin, 26,* 6.

Most, R. S., & Sinnock, P. (1983). The epidemiology of lower extremity amputations in diabetic individuals. *Diabetes Care, 6,* 87–91.

National Center for Health Statistics (NCHS). (1988). Advance report of final mortality statistics, 1986, Monthly Vital Statistics Report No. 6. U.S. Department of Health and Human Services publication No. (PHS) 88-1120. Washington, DC: Government Printing Office.

National Center for Health Statistics (NCHS). (1977). Prevalence of chronic conditions of the genitourinary, nervous, endocrine, metabolic, blood and blood forming systems and of other selected chronic conditions. Vital and Health Statistics No. 109. Washington, DC: Government Printing Office.

National Center for Health Statistics (NCHS). (1982). Blood pressure levels and hypertension in persons ages 6–74: United States 1976–1980. U.S. Department of Health and Human Services publication No. (PHS) 82-1250. Washington, DC: Government Printing Office.

National Diabetes Data Group (NDDG). (1979). Classification and diagnosis of diabetes mellitus and other categories of glucose intolerance. *Diabetes, 26*, 1039–1057.

Neel, J. V. (1962). Diabetes mellitus—A ''thrifty genotype'' rendered detrimental by ''progress''? *American Journal of Human Genetics, 14*, 353–362.

Omran, A. R. (1983). The epidemiologic transition theory: A preliminary update. *Journal of Tropical Pediatrics, 29*, 305–316.

O'Sullivan, J. B., & Mahan, C. M. (1968). Prospective study of 352 young patients with chemical diabetes. *New England Journal of Medicine, 278*, 1038–1041.

Reed, E. T. (1969). Caucasian genes in American Negroes. *Science, 165*, 762–768.

Reitnauer, P. J., Go, R. C. P., Acton, R. T., Murphy, C. C., Budowle, B., Barger, B. O., & Roseman, J. M. (1982). Evidence of genetic admixture as a determinant in the occurrence of insulin-dependent diabetes mellitus. *Diabetes, 31*, 532–537.

Reitnauer, P. J., Roseman, J. M., Barger, B. D., Murphy, C. C., Kirk, K. A., & Acton, R. F. (1981). HLA associations with insulin-dependent diabetes mellitus in a sample of the American Black population. *Tissue Antigens, 17*, 286–293.

Report of the Secretary's Task Force on Black and Minority Health. (1985). Volume 1: Executive Summary. DHHS Publication No. 017-090-00078. Washington, DC: Government Printing Office.

Roseman, J. M. (1985). Diabetes in black Americans. In M. I. Harris (Ed.). *Diabetes in America* (pp. 1–24). U.S. Department of Health and Human Services publication No. NIH 85-1468. Washington, DC: Government Printing Office.

Roseman, J. M., Go, R. C. P., Perkins, L. L., Barger, B. D., Beel, D. A., Goldenberg, R. L., DuBard, M. B., Huddlestone, J. F., Sedacek, C. M., & Acton, R. T. (1991). Gestational diabetes among African American women. *Diabetes and Metabolism Review, 7*, 93–104.

Rosenbaum, P. (1967). Juvenile diabetes at Charity Hospital. *Journal of Louisiana State Medical Society, 199*, 389.

Sicree, R. A., Zimmet, Z., King, O. M., & Coventry, J. S. (1987). Plasma insulin response among Nauruans: Prediction of deterioration in glucose tolerance over 6 years. *Diabetes, 36*, 179–186.

Smith, S. R., Svetkey, L. P., & Dennis, V. W. (1991). Racial differences in the incidence and progression of renal diseases. *Kidney International, 40*, 815–822.

Sullivan, L. (1990). Opening remarks. *Diabetes Care, 13* (Supp. 4), 1143.

Taylor, R., Ram, P., Zimmet, P., Raper, R., & Ringrose, H. (1984). Physical activity and the prevalence of diabetes in Melanesian and Indian men in Fiji. *Diabetologia, 27*, 578–582.

Tull, E. S., LaPorte, R. E., Vergona, R. E., Gower, I., & Makame, M. H. (1992). A two-fold excess mortality among African American IDDM cases compared with

Whites: The Diabetes Epidemiology Research International experience. *Diabetes, 41* (Supp. 1), 35A.

Tull, E. S., Roseman, J. M., & Christian, C. L. E. (1991). Epidemiology of childhood IDDM in the U.S. Virgin Islands from 1979–1988: Evidence for an epidemic in the early 1980s and variation by degree of racial admixture. *Diabetes Care, 14,* 558–564.

Tuomilehto, J., Tuomilehto-Wolf, E., Zimmet, P., Alberti, K. G. G. M., & Keen, H. (1992). Primary prevention of Diabetes mellitus. In K. G. G. M. Alberti, R. A. Defionzo, H. Keen, & P. Zimmet (Eds.), *International textbook of diabetes mellitus* (pp. 1656–1673). Chichester: John Wiley & Sons.

Van Itallie, T. B. (1985). Health implications of overweight and obesity in the United States. *Annals of Internal Medicine, 103,* 983–988.

Wagenknecht, L. E., Roseman, J. M., & Alexander, W. J. (1989). Epidemiology of IDDM in black and white children in Jefferson County, Alabama, 1979–1985. *Diabetes, 38,* 629–633.

Winter, W. E., Maclaren, N. K., Riley, W. J., Clarke, D. W., Kappy, S., & Spillar, R. P. (1987). Maturity-onset diabetes of youth in black Americans. *New England Journal of Medicine, 316,* 285–291.

World Health Organization. (1985). Diabetes mellitus: Report of a W.H.O. study group. Technical Report, Series no. 727, pp. 10–24. Geneva: World Health Organization.

World Health Organization. (1980). Report of expert committee on diabetes mellitus. Technical Report, Series no. 646. Geneva: World Health Organization.

WHO Multinational Project for Childhood Diabetes. (1991). Familial insulin-dependent diabetes mellitus (IDDM) epidemiology: Standardization of data for the DIA-MOND Project. *World Health Organization Bulletin OMS, 69,* 767–777.

Zimmet, P., Taylor, R., & Whitehouse, S. (1982). Prevalence of impaired glucose tolerance, and diabetes mellitus in various Pacific populations, according to new criteria. *Bulletin of the World Health Organization, 60,* 279–282.

Zimmet, P. (1992). Kelly West Lecture 1991: Challenges in diabetes epidemiology— From west to the rest. *Diabetes Care, 15,* 232–251.

8

Chronic Obstructive Pulmonary Disease in Blacks

Ki Moon Bang

INTRODUCTION

Chronic obstructive pulmonary disease (COPD) is the fifth leading cause of death and a major cause of chronic morbidity and disability in the United States (DHHS, 1991; Feinleib, Rosenberg, Collins, Delozier, Pokras & Chevarley, 1989). It is a significant cause of morbidity and mortality in Blacks (Mays, 1975; *Healthy People 2000*, 1991). Nearly 80,000 people die each year because of this condition, and cigarette smoking accounts for 82 percent of these deaths (Office on Smoking, 1989). Mortality rates from COPD have paralleled those for lung cancer and have increased progressively over the last 25 years. If the 1978–87 trend (18.7 per 100,000 population) continues, the mortality rate for COPD will reach 26 to 28 deaths per 100,000 population in the year 2000.

The Department of Health and Human Services has established an objective of reducing COPD deaths to less than 25 per 100,000 population by the year 2000 (*Healthy People 2000*, 1991). In 1990, the COPD death rate per 100,000 population in Blacks was 26.5 for males and 10.7 for females (NCHS, 1993). Although published studies indicate racial differences in COPD, there remains a need for more research in this area. This paper reviews the epidemiology of COPD in Black Americans and examines the risk factors for COPD in Blacks that may explain racial differences in COPD.

EPIDEMIOLOGY OF COPD

Definition

In this paper, the term COPD includes rubrics 490 to 496 of the ninth revision of the International Classification of Diseases (ICD-9). COPD consists of bronchitis (ICD-9 490–491), emphysema (ICD-9 492), asthma (ICD-9 493), and other conditions (ICD-9 494–496). COPD is clinically defined as obstructive airways disease manifested by a forced expiratory volume in one second (FEV_1) that is less than 65 percent of the predicted value (Higgins, Keller, Landis, Beaty, Burrows, Demets et al., 1984).

Mortality

In 1990, there were nearly 87,000 deaths from COPD in the United States (NCHS, 1993). Of the total deaths, 3,600 were attributed to bronchitis, 15,700 to emphysema, 4,800 to asthma, and 62,600 to other COPD and allied conditions. The age-adjusted COPD mortality rate was 19.7 per 100,000 population, and the rate for males was 27.2 compared with 14.7 for females. COPD mortality is disproportionately distributed at older ages. Approximately 96 percent of the deaths from COPD in 1990 occurred in people over the age of 55. Although men and women have similar rates of COPD prior to 55 years of age, men have higher rates than women after age 55.

Table 8.1 shows deaths and age-adjusted mortality rates of COPD in 1990. The age-adjusted mortality rate for Blacks was 16.9 compared with 20.1 for Whites. Mortality rates for asthma in Blacks was 3.4 per 100,000 population compared with 1.2 in Whites, and there were no sex differences in either race. Mortality rates for bronchitis and emphysema in Whites were higher than in Blacks.

Different mortality trends for COPD existed between Blacks and Whites during the period 1979–1990, as shown in Table 8.2. The age-adjusted mortality rate in Blacks rose 52.3 percent compared with 34.9 percent in Whites during this period. The increase for COPD death rates was 94.5 percent for Black females and 42.5 percent for Black males.

When all races are looked at by age group during the period 1979–1990, the mortality rate increased by 21.6 percent for those 55 to 64 years of age, by 30.3 percent for those 65 to 74 years of age, by 60 percent for those 75 to 84 years of age, and by 88.2 percent for those more than 85 years of age. (These data for the population as a whole are not reported in Table 8.3.) As seen in Table 8.3, which reports age-specific rates by race, rates for those 35 years and older were higher in Blacks than in Whites. The percentage change of the age-specific rates during this period was greater for Blacks than for Whites. In particular, the percentage changes for persons aged 85 years and over in Blacks was a 127 percent increase compared with an 88 percent increase in Whites.

Table 8.4 shows the age-adjusted mortality rate for bronchitis, emphysema, and asthma in Blacks. The mortality for bronchitis and emphysema in Blacks was stable during the period 1979–1990, but the mortality for asthma increased by 78.9 percent during this period.

Table 8.1
Deaths and Age-adjusted Mortality Rates* of Chronic Obstructive Pulmonary Disease in 1990

	Deaths			Rates per 100,000		
Category	Total	Male	Female	Total	Male	Female
			Blacks:			
Total	5,655	3,628	2,027	16.9	26.5	10.7
Bronchitis	190	125	65	0.5	0.9	0.3
Emphysema	763	552	211	2.3	4.1	1.1
Asthma	986	460	526	3.4	3.5	3.3
Other**	3,716	2,491	1,225	10.7	17.9	6.0
			Whites:			
Total	80,179	45,234	34,945	20.1	27.4	15.2
Bronchitis	3,365	1,726	1,639	0.8	1.0	0.6
Emphysema	14,828	8,769	6,059	3.9	5.5	2.8
Asthma	3,696	1,358	2,338	1.2	1.0	1.3
Other**	8,290	33,381	24,909	14.2	19.9	10.4

Source: NCHS, Vital Statistics System, 1993.

*Rates are per 100,000 population and are adjusted to the United States population as enumerated in 1940.

**Other COPD.

Prevalence

Prevalence estimates of COPD are available from the data obtained through national surveys of the National Center for Health Statistics (NCHS). These surveys include the annual National Health Interview Survey (NHIS) and the periodic National Health and Nutrition Examination Survey (NHANES). NHIS presents 1-year-period prevalence, which is equivalent to point prevalence for

Table 8.2

Age-adjusted Mortality Rates of Chronic Obstructive Pulmonary Disease by Race and Sex, 1979–1990*

Year	Black			White		
	Total	Male	Female	Total	Male	Female
1979	11.1	18.6	5.5	14.9	25.0	8.0
1980	12.5	20.9	6.3	16.3	26.7	9.2
1981	12.6	21.4	6.4	16.8	26.9	9.9
1982	12.8	20.6	7.4	16.6	26.3	10.1
1983	13.9	22.7	7.7	17.9	27.8	11.3
1984	14.4	23.4	8.1	18.2	27.7	11.8
1985	15.3	24.6	8.8	19.2	28.7	12.9
1986	15.7	25.6	9.0	19.3	28.3	13.3
1987	15.9	25.2	9.6	19.3	27.7	13.7
1988	17.1	27.4	10.2	20.0	28.2	14.5
1989	17.2	26.5	11.1	19.9	27.2	15.2
1990	16.9	26.5	10.7	20.1	27.4	15.2

Source: National Center for Health Statistics, Vital Statistics System, 1993.

*Rates are per 100,000 population and are adjusted to the U.S. population as enumerated in 1940.

chronic diseases (NCHS, 1986). NHANES may provide cumulative or lifetime prevalence because of several years' survey period (NCHS, 1981).

In the 1970 NHIS, asthma rates per 1,000 were 36.4 for Blacks compared with 27.9 for Whites among persons less than 6 years old. For ages 6 to 16 years, the rates were 25.2 for Blacks compared with 26.3 for Whites; and for ages 4 to 64 years, the rates were 44.5 for Blacks compared with 31.9 for Whites. Between 1979 and 1981, asthma ranked fourth among Blacks and eighth among Whites in prevalence of 19 conditions on the NHIS checklist (NCHS, 1986). Asthma prevalence rates per 1,000 were 31 for Whites and 32 for nonwhites. In the case of chronic bronchitis and emphysema, the prevalence rates for Blacks and Whites were similar. During the period 1982–85, the average annual prevalence rates were higher in Whites than in Blacks, except for asthma (Gillum, 1990). Large racial differences occurred only for chronic bronchitis and emphysema. Table 8.5 shows the prevalence rates per 1,000 persons of reported

Table 8.3
**Age-specific Death Rate per 100,000 Population of Chronic Obstructive
Pulmonary Disease, 1979 and 1990, by Race**

Age group	Black			White		
(Years)	1979	1990	% Change	1979	1990	% Change
35-44	4.3	4.5	+4.7%	1.4	1.3	-7.1%
45-54	13.4	16.2	+20.9%	9.0	8.5	-5.6%
55-64	35.4	48.2	+36.2%	41.1	49.9	+21.4%
65-74	70.8	113.8	+60.7%	122.3	158.1	+29.3%
75-84	101.7	201.9	+98.5%	210.0	333.7	+58.9%
85 +	106.4	241.7	+127.2%	239.0	449.4	+88.0%

Source: National Center for Health Statistics, Vital Statistics System, 1993.

chronic respiratory conditions in Blacks and Whites. These reports were based on the 1975–87 NHIS (NCHS, 1990). The prevalence rate was higher for Blacks than for Whites only for asthma. For chronic bronchitis and hay fever or allergic rhinitis without asthma, the prevalence rates were higher for Whites than for Blacks.

A recent study on the spirometry data obtained from NHANES I reported that prevalence of COPD in Blacks was 5.4 percent—3.7 percent for males and 6.7 percent for females. The prevalence was significantly higher with age for both males and females (Bang, 1993). NHANES I spirometry was performed using an electronic spirometer on all examinees aged 25 to 74 years in the detailed sample (NCHS, 1978). In NHANES I, sex ratios (male/female) for history of chronic bronchitis or emphysema were 0.5 for Blacks and 0.9 for Whites, ages 35 to 74. For asthma, the ratio was 0.6 for Blacks and 1.0 for Whites (Gillum, 1990). The reason for the higher ratio in Blacks may be related to Black women's immune defenses and familial or genetic factors or other related risk factors.

RISK FACTORS

Age and Sex

COPD mortality rate increases with age. In 1990, COPD mortality rate for ages 75 to 84 years was 321.1 per 100,000 population compared with 152.5 for

Table 8.4
Age-adjusted Mortality Rates* of Chronic Obstructive Pulmonary Disease for Blacks, 1979–1990

	COPD Category		
Year	Bronchitis	Emphysema	Asthma
1979	0.6	2.4	1.9
1980	0.7	2.3	2.2
1981	0.6	2.3	2.3
1982	0.6	2.0	2.5
1983	0.6	2.1	2.8
1984	0.5	2.1	2.6
1985	0.5	2.3	2.9
1986	0.5	2.3	3.0
1987	0.5	2.3	3.3
1988	0.6	2.5	3.6
1989	0.6	2.3	3.3
1990	0.5	2.3	3.4

Source: National Center for Health Statistics, Vital Statistics System, 1993.

*Rates are per 100,000 population and are adjusted to the U.S. population as enumerated in 1940.

ages 65 to 74, 48.9 for ages 55 to 64, 9.1 for ages 45 to 54, and 1.6 for ages 35 to 44. Many studies have shown that ventilatory lung function increases with age to about ages 25 to 30 years and then declines progressively. The decline is usually considered to be linear, though some studies have suggested that there may be interactions with age and height (Higgins, 1980).

In 1990, sex ratios (male/female) of age-adjusted mortality rates for COPD were 2.5 in Blacks and 1.8 in Whites. For asthma, the ratios were 1.1 in Blacks and 1.2 in Whites (NCHS, 1993).

Cigarette Smoking

Cigarette smoking is a major risk factor for COPD. Numerous papers show that cigarette smokers have higher death rates from chronic bronchitis, emphy-

Table 8.5
Average Number of the Prevalent Reported Chronic Respiratory Conditions per 1,000 Persons by Race, 1985–1987

	Black	White
Asthma	42.2	39.6
Chronic bronchitis	35.3	53.5
Hay fever or allergic rhinitis without asthma	59.8	95.4

Source: National Center for Health Statistics, "Health of Black and White Americans," 1990.

sema, and asthma than nonsmokers. Differences between cigarette smokers and nonsmokers increase as cigarette consumption increases. Pipe and cigar smokers have higher morbidity and mortality rates for COPD than nonsmokers (Higgins, 1984). There is a significant relationship between the number of cigarettes smoked per day and decrement of pulmonary function (Benowitz, Hall & Herning, 1983).

Trends in cigarette-smoking prevalence have been published for Blacks and Whites (CDC, 1987; NCHS, 1989; Fiore, Novotny, Pierce, Hatziandreu, Patal & Davis, 1989; Novotny, Warner, Kendrick & Remington, 1988). In 1987, 43 percent of Black men aged 45 and older smoked cigarettes compared with 30 percent of White men (NCHS, 1989). Black women aged 20 to 24 smoked more than Black men the same age (Fiore et al., 1989).

Although the importance of cigarette smoking as a cause of COPD is clearly known, some facets of the health effects are not fully understood. The health effects of cigarette smoking are not of equal frequency and severity in all smokers. The cigarette smoke-COPD relationship may be influenced by personal factors as well as by other environmental hazards.

The effect of involuntary exposure to cigarette smoke also has attracted recent attention. Passive smoking was reported to be significantly related to lower FEV_1 and forced vital capacity (FVC) values among French women (Kauffmann, Dockery, Speizer & Ferris, 1989). Mean levels of ventilatory lung function were significantly lower and prevalence rates of respiratory symptoms and disease higher in nonsmoking wives of smoking husbands, and in nonsmoking children of smoking parents than in nonsmoking households (USDHEW, 1979; Lefioe, Ashley, Pederson & Keays, 1984). Although the effect of passive smoking appears to be small, it is important to investigate the effect of involuntary exposure of smoking in relation to COPD.

Although smoking prevalence is higher in Blacks than in Whites, lower COPD mortality and morbidity are reported in Blacks compared with Whites. These differences in race-related prevalence and health outcomes may enhance understanding of the pathophysiology and etiology of COPD and the effects of smoking (see Gillum, 1990; Novotny et al., 1988).

Environmental/Occupational Exposures

Many studies have shown the adverse effects of pollution on the respiratory tract. Temporal and spatial variations in mortality, morbidity, the prevalence of respiratory symptoms, lung functions values, and sickness absence from work have been shown to correlate with various indices of pollution in different populations. Past studies have examined the acute effects of daily air pollution concentrations on daily morbidity and mortality. Some of the earlier studies were initiated in London in 1958. In these studies moderately high correlations (r = 0.6) were seen between daily concentrations of smoke and sulfur dioxide and daily morbidity and mortality (Higgins, 1980). Presently, Blacks have more exposure experience to air pollution than Whites. In 1980, Blacks (59.7%) were more likely than Whites (27%) to live in central cities, where air pollution exposure is usually greater than in rural areas. Relatedly, indoor air pollution and passive smoking effects may be associated with the increased risk of COPD, especially asthma, in Blacks.

Death rates for chronic respiratory diseases are higher than expected among men in certain occupations and industries. Epidemiologic surveys have shown that exposures at work to cotton, hemp, or grain dust; fire fighting and work involving exposure to asbestos are associated with respiratory symptoms and reduced lung function. Comparison of prevalence rates of respiratory symptoms and mean levels of FEV_1 in miners and nonminers in West Virginia showed that respiratory function was poorest in miners who smoked and best in nonsmoking nonminers (Higgins, 1970). Interaction between certain occupational hazards and cigarette smoking results in increased rates of COPD. Blacks may have been employed more frequently than Whites in occupations with the above-mentioned and other health hazards. In 1984, 9.6 percent of all employed persons were Black. Of these employed persons, 14.3 percent were operators and laborers, 5.7 percent managers and professionals, and 8 percent technical workers, sales, and administrative support personnel (U.S. Bureau of the Census, 1985).

Genetic Factors

Several reports show the familial occurrence of COPD (Higgins & Keller, 1975; Hubert, Fabsitz & Feinleib, 1982; Cohen, Ball, Bias, Brashears, Chase, Diamond et al., 1975). It has been reported that COPD patients have a higher frequency of Pi variant phenotypes than those without lung disease (Cohen et al., 1975). Also, alphal-antitrypsin deficiency (PiZ homozygote) was reported to be less frequent in Blacks than Whites (Lieberman, Gaidulis & Roberts, 1976;

Young, Headings, Henderson, Bose & Hackney, 1978). No study has reported on familial aggregation of COPD or pulmonary function in Blacks, although familial aggregation was reported on for Whites (Redline, Tishler, Lewitter, Tager, Munoz & Speizer, 1987). Bronchial asthma probably results from the interaction of multiple gene loci with one or more factors in the environment (NIH, 1981).

Ventilatory capacity and bronchial reactivity show some degree of familial similarity in Whites (NIH, 1981). Bronchial reactivity shows patterns consistent with genetic effects in twin and sibling studies (NIH, 1981). However, no studies are found of racial difference in mucociliary flow and other host factors. However, greater reactivity might be expected in Blacks given their higher rates of asthma.

Infection

Patients with COPD are more susceptible to respiratory infections. For example, persons with chronic bronchitis usually have a history of frequent attacks of pneumonia and pleurisy. However, the role of infectious agents in recurrent exacerbations of chronic bronchitis is uncertain. There is a significant increase in bacterial, viral, and mycoplasmal pathogens during exacerbations. The extent to which respiratory infections contribute to the initiation of COPD is less certain (Speizer & Tager, 1979), but several studies report that childhood respiratory illness may be associated with reduced lung function at older ages (USDHEW, 1979). Incidence rates of obstructive airways disease and chronic bronchitis were higher in those with a history of respiratory tract infections in Tecumseh (Higgins, 1984).

Influenza and pneumonia mortality rates are reported to be higher in Blacks than in Whites (Gillum & Liu, 1984). NHANES I showed that Black children aged 1 to 5 years had more episodes of pneumonia than white children. At ages 6 to 11, 12.9 percent of Black girls compared with 9.5 percent of White girls had a history of treatment for pneumonia (Gillum, 1991).

Allergies

A recent study based on the data from NHANES III-Phase I survey, 1988–1991 reported that Blacks have higher allergen reactivity than Whites and Mexican Americans (Bang, Gergen & Turkeltaub, 1993). The prevalence of asthma in children and young adults was higher in Blacks than in Whites. In NHANES I, a history of treatment for allergens other than asthma was more prevalent in White children ages 1 to 11 than in Black children of similar ages. These findings may be explained by a different presentation of atopy in Blacks compared to Whites or differential access to medical care resulting in diagnosis of more severe forms of atopy in Blacks compared to Whites (Witting, McLaughlen, Leifer & Belloit, 1978).

The relationship between allergies and COPD has not been clearly determined. There are a number of questions to be resolved. For example, is the reported association between higher blood eosinophil count and both lower level and faster decline of pulmonary function among nonsmokers a reflection of an adverse effect of environmental antigens on allergies? Do allergies have a significant impact on lung growth and development during childhood? If so, does this influence the risk of COPD in later life? Research in these areas will hopefully provide important insights into the pathogenesis of COPD.

Other Risk Factors

Other potential risk factors include socioeconomic status, nutrition, alcohol consumption, and climate. However, these factors are less important than the risk factors discussed before.

Chronic bronchitis, emphysema, and asthma were reported to be more frequent in persons with low socioeconomic status. Low socioeconomic status may be important in explaining the higher asthma mortality in Blacks (Evans, Mullally, Wilson, Gergen, Rosenberg, Grauman et al., 1987). Several surveys have noted a higher prevalence of respiratory symptoms, chronic bronchitis, and lower ventilatory lung function in less-educated persons (Higgins, 1980).

Periodontal disease has been shown to be inversely related to FEV in men and women. Upper abdominal surgery, especially when performed in an emergency, is also associated with an increased risk of chronic respiratory disease (Higgins, 1980).

CONCLUSION

The apparent continuing rise in COPD mortality among Blacks requires more attention and further investigation to determine to what extent the rise is real and to what extent it is an artifact of changing fashion and practices in diagnosis and exposures to environmental/occupational risk factors. Population-based studies have shown that age and cigarette smoking are risk factors for COPD in Blacks. Other potential risk factors for COPD, previously discussed, should be investigated using comprehensive epidemiologic approaches. Since NHANES I was a cross-sectional study, longitudinal studies of changes in lung function and the development of respiratory symptoms with increasing age in Black smokers and nonsmokers are needed. These studies must utilize state-of-the-art statistical, epidemiological, and other methodologies. Repeated measurements of the prevalence of COPD are required in order to monitor secular changes on morbidity. The data from NHANES III, which have been collected since 1988, will be an important source of this information for COPD studies in the future.

Prevention and treatment of COPD in Blacks are important areas of scientific pursuit. The higher prevalence of cigarette smoking in Blacks (versus Whites) is associated with a higher prevalence of and mortality from asthma. Therefore, smoking prevention and cessation programs for Blacks should be expanded at the national, state, and local levels. With cessation of smoking, the rate of pulmonary functional loss declines, but lost function cannot be regained. However, timely smoking cessation (e.g., through effective health promotion/education campaigns, especially in the black community) can prevent the development of symptomatic disease (*Healthy People 2000*, 1991).

Reduction of air pollution is clearly desirable. Strict enforcement of the National Ambient Air Quality standards in the United States should contribute to the elimination of general air pollution as a factor in the development and progression of respiratory disease.

Greater regulatory and enforcement policies are needed for federal, state and local governments. For example, more stringent control of occupational exposures should be mandated by the Occupational Safety and Health and Mining Safety and Health Acts. Also, legislative requirements to restrict the use of potentially hazardous materials used in occupations should help to ultimately eliminate occupational irritants as risk factors in COPD.

Lastly, prompt and adequate treatment of acute respiratory infection and of exacerbations of chronic bronchitis and asthma will reduce COPD mortality and also reduce the economic costs associated with loss from work. If these and other related issues are addressed, the COPD-related morbidity and mortality associated with the population in general and the Black population in particular (especially for asthma-related health outcomes) will be significantly controlled.

REFERENCES

Bang, K. M. (1993). Prevalence of chronic obstructive pulmonary disease in blacks. *Journal of the National Medical Association, 85,* 51–55.

Bang, K. M., Gergen, P., & Turkeltaub, P. (1993). Allergen skin-test reactivity in a United States national sample: Results from phase 1 of the third National Health and Nutrition Examination Survey (NHANES III), 1988–1991. Proceedings of the 1993 annual meeting of American Academy of Allergy & Immunology, Chicago, Illinois.

Benowitz, N. K., Hall, S. M., & Herning, R. I. (1983). Smokers of low-yield cigarettes do not consume less nicotine. *New England Journal of Medicine, 309,* 139–142.

Centers for Disease Control (CDC). (1987). Cigarette smoking among blacks and other minority population. *Mortality & Morbidity Weekly Report, 36,* 404–407.

Cohen, B. H., Ball, W. C., Bias, W. B., Brashears, S., Chase, G. A., Diamond, E. L., Hsu, S. H., Kreiss, P., Levy, D. A., Menkes, H. A., Permutt, S., & Tockman, M. S. (1975). Genetic-epidemiologic study of chronic obstructive pulmonary disease. *Johns Hopkins Medical Journal, 137,* 95–104.

Evans, R., III, Mullally, P. I., Wilson, R. W., Gergen, P. J., Rosenberg, H. M., Grauman, J. S., Chevarley, F. M., & Feinleib, M. (1987). National trends in mortality and morbidity of asthma in the USA: Prevalence, hospitalization, and death from asthma over two decades, 1965–1984. *Chest, 91* (supp.), 65s–74s.

Feinleib, M., Rosenberg, H., Collins, J. G., Delozier, J. E., Pokras, R., & Chevarley,

F. M. (1989). Trends in COPD morbidity and mortality in the United States. *American Review of Respiratory Disease, 140*, s9–s18.

Fiore, M. C., Novotny, T. E., Pierce, J. P., Hatziandreu, E. J., Patal, K. M., & Davis, R. M. (1989). Trends in cigarette smoking in the United States: The changing influence of gender and race. *Journal of the American Medical Association, 261*, 49–55.

Gillum, G. F., & Liu, K. C. (1984). Coronary heart disease mortality in United States blacks, 1940–1978: Trends and unanswered questions. *American Heart Journal, 108*, 728–732.

Gillum, G. F. (1990). Chronic obstructive pulmonary disease in blacks and whites: Mortality and morbidity. *Journal of the National Medical Association, 82*, 417–428.

Gillum, G. F. (1991). Chronic obstructive pulmonary disease in blacks and whites: Pulmonary function norms and risk factors. *Journal of the National Medical Association, 83*, 393–401.

Healthy People 2000. (1991). National health promotion and disease prevention objectives. DHHS Publication No. (PHS) 91-50213. Washington, DC: Government Printing Office.

Higgins, I. (1970). Occupational factor in chronic bronchitis and emphysema. In N. G. M. Orie & R. Van Der Lende (Eds.), Bronchitis III: *Proceedings of the third international symposium on bronchitis*. Springfield, IL.: Charles C. Thomas.

Higgins, I. (1980). Respiratory disease. In J. M. Last (Ed.), *Public health and preventive medicine* (11th ed.). New York: Appleton-Century-Crofts.

Higgins, M. (1984). Epidemiology of COPD: State of the art. *Chest, 85*, 35–85.

Higgins, M. W., & Keller, J. B. (1975). Familial occurrence of chronic respiratory disease and familial resemblance in ventilatory capacity. *Journal of Chronic Disease, 28*, 239–251.

Higgins, M. W., Keller, J. B., Landis, J. R., Beaty, T. H., Burrows, B., Demets, D., Diem, J. E., Higgins, I. T. T., Lakatos, E., Lebowitz, M. D., Menkes, H., Speizer, F. E., Tager, I. B., & Weill, H. (1984). Risk of chronic obstructive pulmonary disease. *American Review of Respiratory Disease, 130*, 380–385.

Hubert, H. B., Fabsitz, R. R., & Feinleib, M. (1982). Genetic and environmental influences on pulmonary function in adult twins. *American Review of Respiratory Disease, 125*, 409–415.

Kauffmann, F., Dockery, D. W., Speizer, F. E., & Ferris, B. G. (1989). Respiratory symptoms and lung function in relation to passive smoking: A comparative study of American and French women. *International Journal of Epidemiology, 18*, 334–344.

Lefioe, N. M., Ashley, M. J., Pederson, L. I., & Keays, J. J. (1984). The health risks of passive smoking. *Chest, 1*, 90–95.

Lieberman, J., Gaidulis, L., & Roberts, L. (1976). Racial distribution of alpha1-antitrypsin variants among junior high school students. *American Review of Respiratory Disease, 114*, 1194–1198.

Mays, E. E. Pulmonary diseases. (1975). In R. A. William (Ed.), *Textbook of black-related diseases* (pp. 429–436). New York: McGraw-Hill Book Company.

National Center for Health Statistics (NCHS). (1978). Plan and operation of the NHANES I. Augmentation survey of adults 25–74 years, United States, 1974–75. *Vital and*

Health Statistics, USDHHS, DHEW Publication No. (PHS) 78-1314; Series 1, No. 14. Washington, DC: Government Printing Office.

National Center for Health Statistics. (1981). Plan and operation of the second National Health and Nutrition Examination Survey, 1976–80. *Vital and Health Statistics,* DHHS Publication No. (PHS) 81-1317, Series 1, No. 15. Washington, DC: Government Printing Office.

National Center for Health Statistics. (1986). Prevalence of selected chronic conditions, United States, 1979–81. *Vital and Health Statistics,* DHHS Publication No. (PHS) 86-1583, Series 10, No. 155. Washington, DC: Government Printing Office.

National Center for Health Statistics. (1989). *Health United States 1988.* DHHS Publication No. (PHS) 89-1232. Washington, DC: Government Printing Office.

National Center for Health Statistics. (1990). Health of black and white Americans, 1985–87. *Vital Health Statistics,* DHHS Publication No. (PHS) 90-1599. Washington, DC: Government Printing Office.

National Center for Health Statistics. (1993). Vital Statistics of the United States 1990. USDHHS (unpublished).

National Institutes of Health (NIH). (1981). *Epidemiology of Respiratory Disease Task Force Report.* NIH Publication 82-2019. Bethesda, MD: Government Printing Office.

Novotny, T. E., Warner, K. E., Kendrick, J. S., & Remington, P. L. (1988). Smoking by blacks and whites: Socioeconomic and demographic differences. *American Journal of Public Health, 78,* 1187–1189.

Office on Smoking and Health. (1989). *Reducing the health consequences of smoking: 25 years of progress. A report of the Surgeon General.* DHHS Publication No. (CDC) 89-8411. Washington, DC: Government Printing Office.

Redline, S., Tishler, P. V., Lewitter, F. I., Tager, I. B., Munoz, A., & Speizer, F. E. (1987). Assessment of genetic and nongenetic influences on pulmonary function: A twin study. *American Review of Respiratory Disease, 135,* 217–222.

Speizer, F. E., & Tager, I. B. (1979). Epidemiology of chronic mucus hypersecretion and obstructive airways disease. *Epidemiologic Review, 1,* 124–142.

U.S. Bureau of the Census. (1985). *Statistical abstract of the United States,* 106th Edition. Washington, DC: Government Printing Office, 19, 402–403.

U.S. DHHS. (1979). *Smoking and Health. A report of the Surgeon General.* DHHS Publication No. (PHS) 79-50066. Washington, DC: Government Printing Office.

Witting, H. J., McLaughlen, E. T., Leifer, K. L., & Belloit, J. D. (1978). Risk factors for the development of allergic disease: Analysis of 2190 patient records. *Annals of Allergy, 41,* 84–88.

Young, R. C., Headings, V. E., Henderson, A. L., Bose, S., & Hackney, R. L., Jr. (1978). Protease inhibitor profile of black Americans with and without chronic cardiopulmonary disease. *Journal of National Medical Association, 70,* 849–856.

9

Sickle Cell Disease: A Biopsychosocial Model

Kermit B. Nash and Joseph Telfair

THE BIOPSYCHOSOCIAL MODEL

A biopsychosocial model for understanding and working with a chronic genetic condition such as sickle cell anemia is imperative for a holistic approach toward services. As the individual moves through the life cycle, he or she encounters frequently increasing physical, psychological, and social problems that can affect quality of life.

A biopsychosocial model, as seen in Figure 9.1, visualizes the individual in continuous interaction with internal (physical and psychological) and external (social) influences (Schwartz, 1982). The impact of any one influence can support the overall response of the individual to the chronic condition either positively or negatively. Outside influences, such as the provision of services, can help offset the deleterious impact. The negative interaction of these systems can depress, demoralize, and offset the individual's and his or her family's sense of purpose and direction.

The transaction among the elements that affect the functional status of individuals with sickle cell disease is viewed as a spinning top (Figure 9.1). The elements are the physical (molecular, genetic, cellular, and organ systems) and psychological (cognitive, affective, and behavioral). The conceptual framework offers a broader perspective than the physical and psychological by incorporating an ecological perspective. Ecology's concern is with the relationship between organisms and their environment (Germain, 1979; Bronfenbrenner, 1979). Attention is focused on the influence of social and physical environments on the adaptation and coping behaviors of people (Garbarino, 1985).

Lack of fit between individual and environment can negatively affect a person's physical and mental health (Werthiem, 1975). Likewise, ill health can negatively

Figure 9.1
Biopsychosocial Model of Health and Illness

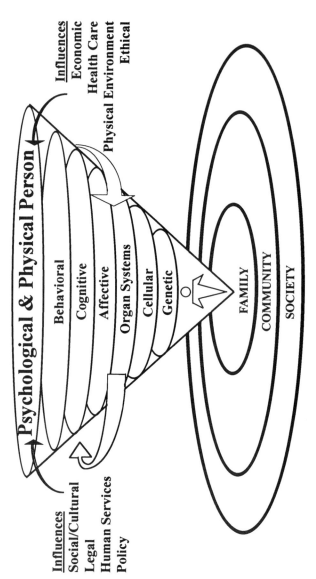

Source: Dillworth-Anderson, P., Harris, L. H., Holbrook, C. T., Konrad, R., Kramer, K. D., Nash, K. B., Phillips, G. (1993). Graphical Representation of Biopsychosocial Model of Health and Illness. *Journal of Health and Social Policy.* (In Press).

affect the degree of congruence between the individual and the environment. Therefore, understanding a condition such as sickle cell disease from a biopsychosocial perspective allows one to formulate a holistic approach vital to competent comprehensive care (Schwartz, 1982).

African Americans experience complex health disadvantages that are compounded by a combination of poverty, racial bias, ignorance, and lack of access to quality health care. Having sickle cell disease only exacerbates these conditions.

This chapter will focus on the utilization of the biopsychosocial model, not only in understanding sickle cell disease and its various current and future treatments but also in the delivery of services to those with the condition.

OVERVIEW OF SICKLE CELL ANEMIA

Understanding the impact that sickle cell disease has on the lives of those with the condition must begin with a basic understanding of the condition itself. This section will provide an overview of the geographic, historical, and bioclinical aspects of the condition.

Sickle cell disease (SCD) refers to a group of genetic disorders in which the sickling of red blood cells caused by a loss of oxygen gives the cell a sickle-like shape and results in chronic anemia and the obstruction of the body's smaller circulatory system (Vichinsky, Hurst & Lubin, 1983). In the United States, the disease occurs mostly (but not exclusively) in African Americans. It is the most common genetic disorder within a specific population, having an incidence of 1 in every 500 live Black births (Rooks & Pack, 1983). To date there are about 65,000 individuals with the disorder (Charache, Lubin & Reid, 1984).

Unexpected, intermittent, and at times life-threatening complications characterize the course of the disease (Vichinsky, Hurst, & Lubin, 1983). Like individuals with similar chronic conditions, these variations are reported to have a profound impact on the biological, psychological, and social development of these individuals, as well as implications for their overall management (Hurtig, 1986).

The disease's inheritance type is autosomal recessive. As Figure 9.2 illustrates, individuals must inherit a sickle cell gene from both parents in order to have sickle cell disease (symptomatic), but if they inherit both a normal and a sickle cell gene, they have only sickle cell trait and are asymptomatic.

Prognostic expectations for morbidity, mortality, and life expectancy of patients with the disease have improved significantly over the past 20 years with improvements and wider availability of medical care to infants and young children with the condition (Vichinsky & Lubin, 1980; Scott, 1985; Thomas & Holbrook, 1987).

Figure 9.2
Inheritance Patterns of Sickle Cell Trait and Anemia

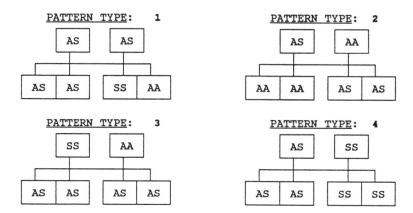

PATTERN SUMMARY:

PATTERN TYPE: 1.

Each parent carries a sickle (S) gene (trait). With each pregnancy, there is 50% chance the child will inherit a sickle (S) gene and a 25% chance that the child will inherit a normal hemoglobin pattern (AA) and a 25% chance the child will have sickle cell anemia (SS).

PATTERN TYPE: 2.

One parent carries a sickle (S) gene. With each pregnancy, there is 50% chance the child will have a normal hemoglobin pattern (AA), and a 50% chance the child will inherit a sickle (S) gene. There is no chance of having sickle cell anemia.

PATTERN TYPE: 3.

One parent has sickle cell anemia and the other has normal hemoglobin (AA). All children will inherit a sickle (S) gene. None will have sickle cell anemia.

Figure 9.2—Continued

PATTERN TYPE: 4.

One parent has a sickle (S) gene and the other sickle cell
anemia (SS). With each pregnancy there is 50% chance the
child will inherit a sickle gene (S) and a 50% chance the
child will have sickle cell anemia (SS).

Source: Pattern and text developed specifically for this chapter by Joseph Telfair, Dr.P.H., MSW-
MPH, School of Public Health, University of North Carolina at Chapel Hill, 1993.

Note: If both parents have sickle cell anemia (SS) or any combination of sickle cell disease (i.e.,
SC, Sβ⁺ thalassemia, etc.) the child will inherit sickle cell disease. Likewise if both parents
have normal hemoglobin (AA), the chance of the child inheriting sickle cell disease is zero.

Geographic Distribution

It is unclear whether or not the sickle cell gene (Hgb S) arose as a single
mutation that spread through migration or from identical mutations in different
areas throughout the world (Serjeant, 1985). It is recognized that the gene is
widespread and not racially linked. The common factor in its spread is falciparum
malaria; the sickle gene existed in high concentrations in the equatorial regions
of Africa and several Mediterranean regions, areas where malaria is endemic
(Serjeant, 1985).

In these areas the heterozygote (the individual with a single Hgb S gene or
sickle cell trait) has a natural resistance to malaria. Consequently, these individuals had a greater chance to transmit the gene. Serjeant (1985) suggests that
migration from and exploration of equatorial and West Africa were key in spread-
ing the gene to India, Saudi Arabia, Spain, Southern Italy, and other Mediterranean regions (p. 380). Gaston (1987) notes that the slave trade was a primary
catalyst in bringing the gene to the New World. This explains the high incidence
of the various sickle hemoglobinopathies among African Americans and peoples
of the Caribbean.

Clinical and Treatment Aspects of the Disease

Clinical Aspects

The most common types of sickle cell disease are Hemoglobin SS (homozygous sickle cell disease), SC, Sβ°, and Sβ⁺ Thalassemia (heterozygous types)
(Vichinsky, Hurst & Lubin, 1983; Richardson & Milner, 1983). The inheritance
pattern for all forms of sickle cell disease is autosomal recessive. In Figure 9.2,
an example is provided of the homozygous form of the disease, which is referred
to as sickle cell anemia. The disease results from an abnormality in the structure

of the main oxygen-carrying compound in the red blood cell (hemoglobin). Under low oxygen conditions, sickle hemoglobin polymerizes, changing the red cell from the usual flexible disc shape to a hard, jagged, irregular shape. This increased rigidity, due to polymerization, results in early cell breakdown (Vichinsky, Hurst & Lubin, 1983). These cells pass through the individual's blood system with much difficulty, often collecting at the junctures in the smaller veins and capillaries, causing blockage, resulting in the disease's most common symptom, the sickle cell "pain episode" (Scott, 1985; Rooks & Pack, 1983). These pain episodes are often severe and unpredictable, lasting from several hours to several days (Vichinsky, Hurst & Lubin, 1983).

Developmentally, the ever-present sickling condition with underlying hemolysis and secondary vaso-occlusion in early life may lead to dactylitis (hand-foot syndrome), stroke, osteomyelitis, anemia, priapism, aseptic necrosis, and in older patients the potential for blindness, cardiopulmonary problems, renal failure, and other major organ damage (e.g., spleen, liver) (Wagner & Vichinsky, 1989).

Complications associated with the disease vary in severity and frequency across all individuals and disease types (Hemoglobin SS being the most common and most severe) (Vichinsky, Hurst & Lubin, 1983). With the advances in the early detection and treatment of these complications over the past 10 to 15 years, the severity of most have been reduced (Scott, 1985; Gaston, 1987).

Treatments

Current and experimental techniques of the management of sickle cell disease are directed at early prevention, early detection, and prevention before major irreparable damage is done and supportive management once damage has occurred (Thomas & Holbrook, 1987). Most are discussed below.

Before newborn screening for sickle cell disease and the initiation of prophylaxis with oral penicillin, hundreds of children died each year due to severe bacterial infections (Wagner & Vichinsky, 1989). Currently, children with sickle cell disease begin to receive prophylatic oral penicillin by four months of age to decrease the risk of mortality associated with infections.

Exchange transfusion therapy, in many cases, is the treatment of choice for reducing the concentration of sickle hemoglobin and thereby the rate of progressive organ damage or conditions such as stroke, aseptic necrosis, and chronic pain (Charache, Lubin & Reid, 1984). It is an immediate management tool of priapism, acute chest syndrome, splenic sequestration, and other conditions that require emergent intervention but not long-term management (Vichinsky, Hurst & Lubin, 1983). Because of the risk of iron overload (Charache, Lubin & Reid, 1984), concurrent chelation therapy with deferoxamine (Desferal) is used to rid the body of excess iron that could cause severe damage to vital blood-profuse organs (Lubin & Vichinsky, 1991). Relatedly, the improved preparation of blood products has reduced the incidence of secondary viral infection and alloimmunization (Charache, Lubin & Reid, 1984).

The vaso-occlusive episode and its complications is the most common symptom associated with sickle cell disease (Konotey-Ahulu, 1974; Schecther, Noguchi & Rodgers, 1987). Clinical research is currently aimed at methods that can possibly decrease the frequency of these events such as the use of "new drug therapies" aimed at decreasing the amount of hemoglobin S cells in the individual's circulatory system. Two of these experimental drugs are erythropoietin (EPO) and hydroxyurea (HU).

Erythropoietin (EPO) is a hormone that is produced by the kidney and stimulates the bone marrow to increase the production of red blood cells (Noguchi, 1988; Brunara, Goldberg, Dover & Bunn, 1990). Hydroxyurea (HU) is a medication that has been used for several years in the treatment of Polycythemia vera and other myeloproliferative disorders (Charache, Dover, Moyer & Moore, 1987). Recent experiments have shown that EPO or HU, when given in sufficient doses, will enhance the synthesis of fetal hemoglobin (Hgb F) (Noguchi, 1988). Fetal hemoglobin is a normal hemoglobin present at birth and is gradually replaced by adult hemoglobins at between 6 and 18 months of age (Noguchi, 1988). It is argued that, by using agents that stimulate Hgb F synthesis, this "hemoglobin switch" can be reversed, therefore increasing the percentage of cells in the individual's circulatory system containing normal fetal hemoglobin and decreasing the percentage of hemoglobin S (sickle hemoglobin) (Brunara et al., 1990; Rodgers, 1990). The hypothesized end result is the improvement in general health by reduction of the rate of organ damage from vaso-occlusion and other complications related to hemolysis (Dover, 1986).

HU's use over long years, however, has not been studied in children. Concerns regarding the potential risk of carcinogenesis and other chronic long-term complications are raised by clinical investigators and social scientists alike (Vichinsky, 1992). Because of these concerns, the drug is currently recommended only for individuals who have had a severe disease course (Charache, Dover, Moyer & Moore, 1987; Vichinsky, 1992). Also, research is under way to evaluate the combined use of HU and EPO to increase and maintain the level of Hgb F (Brunara et al., 1990). Preliminary studies have shown the potential for EPO to augment the increase in Hgb F obtained by HU alone (Noguchi, 1988; Brunara et al., 1990). Further studies are necessary, but this combined therapy could be extremely beneficial to some individuals with sickle cell disease (Lubin & Vichinsky, 1991).

Lastly, an early study by Perrine et al. (1989) suggests that butyric acid (Butyrate) is another drug that could alter the levels of fetal hemoglobin production by blocking the switch from fetal to adult hemoglobin. Although this drug does not have the toxic side effects associated with HU, studies are still very preliminary.

Another alternative therapy, bone marrow transplantation, has recently been reported as the "cure" for sickle cell disease (Vermylen, Ninano, Robles & Cornu, 1988). Johnson et al. (1984) reported on the first such transplant, successfully performed on an 8-year-old child with sickle cell anemia and acute myeloblastic leukemia. Few bone marrow transplants have been used for persons with sickle cell disease, but several transplants have been performed in patients with thalassemia (Lucarelli et al., 1987).

Bone marrow transplant can cure children with sickle cell disease, but at what cost? Bone marrow transplantation has an inherent 10 to 50 percent risk of death from complications associated with the procedure and immediate side effects such as infection and graft-versus-host disease (Kodish et al., 1991). Cost-benefit decisions also must consider the psychological, legal, ethical, and nonmedical cost (i.e., out-of-pocket cost borne by parents) issues (Williams, 1984; Vaughan, Purtilo, Butter & Armitage, 1986; Durbin, 1988; Billings, 1989).

Young children who have experienced few complications secondary to their condition are considered ideal candidates for the procedure (Kodish et al., 1990; Billings, 1989). It is also recommended that children suffering from a major complication, such as stroke, who demonstrate full recovery would be suitable candidates for an attempt at cure with bone marrow transplantation because of the inevitable risk of another stroke with debilitating results (Kodish et al., 1991). Yet, knowing that many children with sickle cell anemia survive into adulthood with limited problems and become productive citizens and parents makes this a difficult choice for parents and professionals alike (Billings, 1989; Kodish, Lantos, Siegler, Kohrman & Johnson, 1990).

Future research includes the development of genetic therapy that can be effectively administered without complication. Gene therapy involves the transfer of normal genes into certain marrow cells. Unlike bone marrow transplantation, gene therapy does not require chemotherapy to destroy marrow. It only adds the normal gene in place of the defective gene. The question is, ''Can the gene be altered to maintain the production of fetal hemoglobin instead of increasing synthesis of sickle hemoglobin and reduce the overall clinical severity based on persistence of fetal hemoglobin?'' If effective, this therapy would prove less complicated and cheaper than bone marrow transplantation. The use of genetic therapy in young children before the onset of organ failure is also conceptually possible (Ryan et al., 1990). Although the technology for gene therapy is not yet available, much progress is being made in the area, and such therapy could possibly be available within the next 10 years (Holbrook, 1992). Despite its potential, genetic therapy implies the treatment of a fetus in utero as one means of altering the genetic outcome. Use of this therapy raises ethical issues that must be addressed before the therapy can be sanctioned as an option for expectant parents.

PSYCHOSOCIAL SICKLE CELL DISEASE LITERATURE

Clinical reports (narratives) suggest that psychosocial issues can significantly affect the overall well-being of the sickle cell patient (Whitten & Fischoff, 1974; Vavasseur, 1987; Whitten & Nishiura, 1985; Lemanek, Moore, Gresham, Williamson & Kelly, 1986; Hurtig & White, 1986). Compared to the biomedical and bioclinical areas, very few empirical studies exist that address the question of how these issues may contribute to the life course of these individuals (Hurtig & White, 1986; Briscoe, 1986). Briscoe notes, "As the physical aspects of sickle cell anemia (SCA) become progressively more manageable, the psychosocial problems associated with this chronic illness assume greater importance. Unfortunately, research on this aspect of SCA has been scarce and fragmented" (pp. 8–9). Thus, what is known about the impact of these issues on the child or adult have come from clinical reports (two types) and empirical studies.

Clinical Reports

Bioclinical and Allied Medical Reports

The first type of clinical reports are those based on clinical experiences of biomedical and adjunct medical personnel that reflect both psychological and community concerns (Whitten & Fischoff, 1974; Williams, Earles & Pack, 1983; Barrett et al., 1988). For example, Whitten and Fischoff (1974) were among the first to discuss the possible psychological impact of the disease on children and families (p. 681).

A study by Barrett et al. (1988) used the Chronic Illness Problem Inventory (CIPI) to assess the level of psychosocial functioning of 89 adults with sickle cell disease. Their findings indicated that patients were having difficulties in a number of areas indicative of underlying depression. However, these difficulties were found in only a small number of individuals, and the number of psychosocial problems found was lower than had been expected by the Sickle Cell Program's staff. This was the case in similar studies of adults with sickle cell disease (Damlouji, Keves-Cohen, Charache, Georgopoulos & Folstein, 1982; Leavell & Ford, 1983; Morgan & Jackson, 1986). The authors concluded that the staffs' attitudes may reflect their contact with a few patients who are high service utilizers and that further research is needed to distinguish between staff and patient adjustment perceptions (Barrett et al., 1988).

Psychological and Psychiatric Reports

The second type of clinical report came from psychological and psychiatric personnel who recognized that persons with the disease were at risk for adverse psychological consequences (commonly called "effects of the disease") (Lemanek et al., 1986; Fischoff & Jenkins, 1987). Their discussions reflect assumptions based on their own theoretical frameworks and professional experiences. For example, based on the psychoanalytic model that views the sickle cell individual as pathological, McElroy (1980) describes how neurotic disorders may be linked with recurring symptoms of a chronic condition. He discusses each disorder as it relates to persons with sickle cell disease, specifically as they relate to the experience of pain (the "pain personality") (McElroy, 1980, pp. 20, 25). Throughout his book, McElroy suggests that practitioners should assume that sickle cell patients have varying degrees of disturbance in their personalities due to their physiological pain experiences and that this should be the focus of any psychological intervention; this assumption is also shared by Morin & Waring (1981), Damlouji et al. (1982), and Leavell & Ford (1983).

A second example is that of Fischhoff and Jenkins (1987), who take a developmental or maturational approach and view the child as adaptable and the influence of the parent as fundamental for ego development in the child with sickle cell disease. They discuss the important role parents have in influencing children's psychological adaptation to their conditions.

Empirical Studies

Most of the psychosocial research on individuals with sickle cell disease focuses on the psychological outcomes or adverse psychosocial "consequences" of individuals with the disease (Morin & Waring, 1981; Damlouji et al., 1982; Morgan & Jackson, 1986; Dillworth-Anderson and Slaughter, 1986). For example, Damlouji et al. (1982) measured the psychosocial "adjustment" of 30 adults with diabetes and 30 with sickle cell disease. The subjects' adjustments were assessed adjustment using both the Social Functioning Schedule (SFS) and the Emotional Well-Being subscale of the General Health Questionnaire (GHQ). The results showed that almost three-quarters of the sickle cell disease group and more than half of the diabetes group were "psychosocially disabled," indicating "conspicuous psychiatric morbidity" (73% and 63% vs. 57% and 50%, respectively) and that the sickle cell group had more areas of difficulty (12) on the SFS than the diabetes group. Contrary to their expectations, the researchers did not find a correlation between the scale results and the medical complications experienced by these patients.

Past Problems and Recent Progress in the Psychosocial Sickle Cell Disease Literature

These psychosocial sickle cell disease studies focus on the struggle individuals have with their condition and the impact the condition has on their psychological well-being (e.g., anxiety, depression, body image, and self-esteem) (Vavasseur, 1987; Briscoe, 1986; Evans, Burlew & Oler, 1988). However, a number of problems have been associated with this body of work.

The first major problem is the many conceptual and methodological difficulties, including the assumption of psychopathology because of severe disease, the misapplication of standardized measures, the use of small convenient samples, and the use of samples that were not carefully selected. Consequently, the generalizability of these findings is often limited. Recent studies like those of Hurtig & White (1986), Lemanek, Moore, Gresham, Williamson & Kelly (1986) and Morgan & Jackson (1986) have attempted to address some of these problems.

A second major problem is that, while much of the literature focuses on the psychological consequences of sickle cell disease (Williams, Earles & Pack, 1983; Hurtig & White, 1986), very few investigators (Battle, 1984; Dillworth-Anderson & Slaughter, 1986; Burlew, Evans & Oler, 1989) have attempted to examine directly or concurrently the social variables that might influence how children and adults cope with their condition. Thus, for the clinical practitioner who relies on the literature for enlightenment, the understanding of how psychological and social variables influence, interact with, and are influenced by the child's condition remains incomplete.

A notable exception is the recent literature looking at the relationship between children's conditions and their families. The primary focus of these studies has been on the effects of the disease on overall family dynamics that include family social support, coping style, parental self-esteem, kinship network, parental relations, and parent-child relations. Dillworth-Anderson and Slaughter (1986), in their study of the impact of the child with sickle cell disease on extended family functioning, examined variables of family social support and coping style. This was one of the first studies to explore the relationship between children's extended family environments and their condition.

In the recent past, Evans, Burlew and Oler (1988) explored how the presence of a child with sickle cell disease affects parental relations, parent-child relations, and parent's perceptions of the child's behavior (p. 127). These authors concluded that the child's illness may cause interpersonal difficulties for the parent, particularly in single female-headed households, who the researchers postulate are at risk for family dysfunction (p. 130). Evans and his colleagues advocate an aggressive outreach program that includes a parent education support group that emphasizes understanding of the cognitive and psychological development of the child, parenting a child with sickle cell disease, and effective family communication (p. 130).

BIOPSYCHOSOCIAL SERVICES

Sickle cell anemia is a lifelong stressor that influences an individual and his or her family's medical and psychosocial functioning. Different periods of the life cycle are vulnerable to specific medical and psychosocial problems. For example, the young adult may experience infections, fevers, and difficulties with social relationships and vocational development. The adolescent may experience strokes and some school and peer-related problems. Families of individuals with sickle cell disease must continuously contend with modification of their activities, increased financial burdens, and overall intrafamily tension and conflict. Institutional stresses such as fragmented services, racism, and inadequately trained and insensitive health care providers further compound the situation for the individual and his or her family.

Biopsychosocial services are divided into four categories: medical, educational, counseling (psychotherapy), and support services. Such services enable the individual (and family) to better manage the physical condition and mediate stressful situations that promote a higher level of coping. It is anticipated that this will facilitate the better adaptation of the individual to his or her chronic condition. Such adaptation allows individuals to define their limitations and to achieve goals they set for themselves.

The array of services may include:

1. Medical services: comprehensive health maintenance, nutrition counseling, genetic counseling, psychosocial support, symptomatic treatment, treatment of complications, avoidance or elimination of factors that enhance sickling, prevention (clinical and educational), and availability of new therapies (Davis, Vichinsky & Lubin, 1980; Lubin & Vichinsky, 1991).

2. Psychosocial services that may or may not include the following: education, counseling (psychotherapy) and an array of support services (Nash, 1986; Vavasseur, 1987). These services are designed to complement the medical services for a holistic approach to patient care (see Figure 9.1).

As with the medical diagnosis, there must also be a psychosocial diagnosis to determine what services will be needed by the individual and family. A psychosocial paradigm for assessment is the impact of the condition in four areas: reaction, roles, relationship, and resources. The reaction focuses on how individuals feel and view their conditions. Role explores the impact of their conditions on the function they may not be able to fulfill with regards to their relationships with significant others. Resource determines what the individual or family has to work with, instrumental resources (food, shelter, transportation), and affective services such as education, counseling (psychotherapy), and support system.

The range and number of services that are required to help the individual and family cope may be multiple services offered by several different providers. Kinney and Nash (1989) examined the utilization of multipsychosocial resources by children and adolescents with sickle cell disease. The most frequently requested services that cross socioeconomic class included the educational, mental health, vocational rehabilitation, and financial. For those families whose income was under $20 thousand, the most frequently requested services were transportation, financial assistance, and employment. Other requested services included housing, medical services, recreation, and legal services. It becomes clear that when multiple resources are required, coordination, communication, and collaboration are needed among multiple institutions who may provide these services.

Barriers to Psychological Care

Barriers to biopsychosocial care have been systematically scrutinized in the past. These barriers can be examined through the dimensions of the individual, institution, and society. Many believe that it is easier to change the personal barrier (meaning client barriers) and institutional barriers (meaning staff and agency policy) than societal barriers.

Minimizing these disparities and the delivery of services require multiple strategies that will affect the individual and family, the institution that provides the services, and the societal context in which the population lives. Considerations necessary to deliver services to this population include recognition of cultural factors, economic factors, problems of access to services, a generalized suspicion and fear of government controls, and language differences (Murray, 1980). The provider should make an effort to minimize these differences through (a) reexamination of the nature of the relationship between practitioner and patient; (b) exploration of mutual role expectations; (c) exploration of the nature of the power in the relationship in terms of gender, class, and racial differences; (d) development of a capacity to cope with cultural value differences; (e) development of a capacity to work with patients' perception of services; and (f) response to the patients' needs, both physical and psychosocial.

SUMMARY

Sickle cell anemia is a varied and complicated disorder. Insights into its history, biology, pathophysiology, and treatment serve to emphasize this complexity. Although its origins remain a point of much debate, advances in the detection and treatment of many of its symptoms (Scott, 1985; Wagner, Vichinsky, 1989) have highlighted the variability of the disease across individuals and groups. Until a cure is found, further research on biomedical and bioclinical aspects of sickle cell disease and the promotion of effective treatment must be done. Finally, because of treatment advances, research that gives some insights into how individuals who suffer from sickle cell disease can and do learn to cope with the condition must be conducted. Therefore, critical attention to psychosocial interventions and research are also important.

NOTES

This work was supported in part by NIH Grants #P60 HL28391-06, #5P60 HL28391-08-303-6638 and #P60 HL28391-04.

The authors would like to thank Michelle Hughes for her editorial suggestions.

Please address all correspondence to Kermit B. Nash, Ph.D., School of Social Work, CB #3550, 223 East Franklin Street, University of North Carolina at Chapel Hill, Chapel Hill, NC 27599-3550.

REFERENCES

Barrett, D. H., Wisotzek, I. E., Abel, G. G., Rouleau, J. L., Plait, A. F., Plooand, W. E., & Eckman, J. R. (1988). Assessment of psychosocial functioning of patients with sickle cell disease. *Southern Medical Journal, 81*, 745–750.
Battle, S. (1984). Chronically ill children with sickle cell anemia. In Blum, R. W. (Ed.),

Chronic illness and disabilities in childhood and adolescence (pp. 265–276). Orlando: Grum and Spraton.

Billings, F. T. (1989). Treatment of sickle cell anemia with bone marrow transplantation: Pros and cons. *Trans-Am-Clin-Climatol-Assoc, 10*, 8–20.

Briscoe, G. (1986). The psychosocial impact of sickle cell anemia: A review. Unpublished paper, Comprehensive Sickle Cell Center, Children's Hospital Research Center Foundation, Cincinnati, Ohio, 1986.

Bronfrenbrenner, U. (1979). *The ecology of human development: Experiments by nature and design.* Cambridge: Harvard University Press.

Brunara, C., Goldberg, M. A., Dover, G. J., & Bunn, H. F. (1990). Evaluation of hydroxyurea and erythropoietin therapy in sickle cell disease. Paper presented at the 15th Annual Meeting of the National Sickle Cell Disease Centers, Berkeley, California.

Burlew, A. K., Evans, R., & Oler, C. (1989). The impact of a child with sickle cell disease on family dynamics. *Annals of New York Academy of Sciences, 565,* 161–171.

Charache, S., Lubin, B. H., & Reid, C. D. (Eds.). (1984). *Management and Therapy of Sickle Cell Disease,* U.S. Department of Health and Human Services, USDHHS, Publication, No. (PHS) 84-21177. Washington, DC: National Institutes of Health.

Charache, S., Dover, G. J., Moyer, M. A., & Moore, J. W. (1987). Hydroxyurea-induced augmentation of fetal hemoglobin production in patients with sickle cell anemia. *Blood, 30,* 109–116.

Damlouji, N. F., Keves-Cohen, R., Charache, S., Georgopoulos, A., & Folstein, M. F. (1982). Social disability and psychiatric morbidity in sickle cell anemia and diabetic patients. *Psychosomatics, 23,* 262–265.

Davis, J. R., Vichinsky, E. P., & Lubin, B. H. (1980). Current treatment of sickle cell disease. *Current Problems in Pediatrics, 10,* 1–64.

Dillworth-Anderson, P. & Slaughter, D. T. (1986). Sickle cell anemic children and the black extended family. In A. L. Hurtig & C. T. Viera (Eds.), *Sickle cell disease: Psychological and psychosocial issues* (pp. 114–130). Urbana and Chicago: University of Illinois Press.

Dover, G. J., Humphries, R. K., Moore, J. G., Young, N. S., Charache, S., & Nienhaus, A. W. (1986). Hydroxyurea induction of hemoglobin F production in sickle cell disease: Relationship between cytoxicity and F cell production. *Blood, 67,* 735.

Durbin, M. (1988). Bone marrow transplantation: Economic, ethical and social issues. *Pediatrics, 82,* 774–783.

Evans, R. C., Burlew, A. K., & Oler, C. H. (1988). Children with sickle cell anemia: Parental relations, parent-child relations and child behavior. *Social Work, 33,* 127–130.

Fischoff, J., & Jenkins, D. S. (1987). Sickle cell anemia. In E. Noshipts (Ed.), *Basic handbook of child psychiatry* (pp. 97–102). New York: Basic Books.

Garbarino, J. (1985). Human ecology and competence in adolescence. In J. Garbarino (Ed.), *Adolescent development: An ecological perspective* (Chapter 2). Columbus: Charles E. Merrill Publishing Company.

Gaston, M. H. (1987). Sickle cell disease: An overview. *Seminars in Roentgenology, 22,* 150–159.

Germain, C. (1979). *Social work practice: People and environment.* New York: Columbia University Press.

Holbrook, C. T. (1992). Personal communication, February.

Hurtig, A. L., & White, L. S. (1986). Psychological adjustment in children and adolescents with sickle cell disease. *Journal of Pediatric Psychology, 11*, 411–427.

Hurtig, A. L. (1986). The invisible chronic illness in adolescence. In A. L. Hurtig & C. T. Viera (Eds.), *Sickle cell disease: Psychological and psychosocial issues* (pp. 42–61). Urbana and Chicago: University of Illinois Press.

Johnson, F. L., Look, A. T., Gockerman, J., Ruggiero, M. R., Dalla-Pozza, L., & Billings, F. T. (1984). Bone-marrow transplantation in a patient with sickle cell anemia. *New England Journal of Medicine, 311*, 780–783.

Kinney, T., & Nash, K. B. (1989). *Final Report: Demonstration of Impact of Multiple Psychosocial Resources on Children and Adolescents with Sickle Cell Disease.* Supported by a grant from the National Institutes of Health—Maternal and Child Health, Genetics Services Branch, 1989, Grant # MCT-371-003.

Kodish, E., Lantos, J., Siegler, M., Kohrman, A., & Johnson, F. L. (1990). Bone marrow transplantation in sickle cell disease: The trade-off between early mortality and quality of life. *Clinical Research, 38*, 694–700.

Kodish, E., Lantos, J., Stocking, C., Singer, P. A., Siegler, M., & Johnson, F. L. (1991). Bone marrow transplantation for sickle cell disease: A study of parent's decisions. *New England Journal of Medicine, 325*, 1349–1353.

Konotey-Ahulu, F. I. D. (1974). The sickle cell diseases: Clinical manifestations including the "sickle crisis." *Archives of Internal Medicine, 133*, 611–619.

Leavell, S. R., & Ford, C. V. (1983). Psychopathology in patients with sickle cell disease. *Psychosomatics, 24*, 23–25, 28–29, 32, 37.

Lemanek, K. L., Moore, S., Gresham, F., Williamson, D., & Kelly, H. (1986). Psychological adjustment of children with sickle cell anemia. *Journal of Pediatric Psychology, 11*, 397–410.

Lubin, B., & Vichinsky, E. (1991). Sickle cell disease. In R. Hoffman, E. J. Benz, S. J. Shattil, B. Furie, & H. J. Cohen (Eds.), *Hematology: Basic Principles and Practice* (pp. 450–471). New York: Churchill Livingstone.

Lucarelli, G., Galimberti, M., Polchi, P., Giardini, C., Politi, P., Baronciani, D., Angelucci, E., Manenti, F., Delfini, C., Aurelli, G., & Muretto, P. (1987). Marrow transplantation in patients with advanced thalassemia. *New England Journal of Medicine, 316*, 1050–1055.

McElroy, S. R. (1980). *Handbook on the Psychology of Hemoglobin-S: A Perspicacious View of Sickle Cell Disease.* Lanham: University Press of America.

Moise, J. R. (1986). Toward a model of competence and coping. In A. L. Hurtig & C. T. Viera (Eds.), *Sickle cell disease: Psychological and psychosocial issues* (pp. 7–23). Urbana and Chicago: University of Illinois Press.

Morgan, S. R., & Jackson, J. (1986). Psychological and social concomitants of sickle cell anemia in adolescents. *Journal of Pediatric Psychology, 11*, 429–440.

Morin, C., & Waring, E. (1981). Depression and sickle cell anemia. *Southern Medical Journal, 74*, 766–768.

Murray, R. F. (1980). Special considerations for minority participation in pre-natal diagnosis. *Journal of the American Medical Association, 243*, 1254–1256.

Nash, K. B. (1986). Ethnicity, race and the health care delivery system. In A. L. Hurtig & C. T. Viera (Eds.), *Sickle cell disease: Psychological and psychosocial issues* (pp. 131–146). Urbana and Chicago: University of Illinois Press.

Nash, K. B. (1992). Diagnosis and management of psychosocial problems in the sickle cell patient and family. In V. N. Mankad & R. B. More (Eds.), *Sickle cell disease* (pp. 389–402). Westport, CT: Praeger.

Noguchi, C. T. (1988). Levels of fetal hemoglobin necessary for effective therapy of sickle cell disease. *New England Journal of Medicine, 318,* 96–99.

Perrine, S. P., Miller, B. A., Cohen, L., Vichinsky, E. P., Hurst, D., & Lubin, B. (1989). Sodium butyrate enhances fetal hemoglobin gene expression in erythroid progenitors of patients with HbSS and beta thalassemia. *Blood, 74,* 454.

Richardson, E. A. W., & Milner, L. S. (1983). Sickle cell disease and the child-bearing family: An update. *Maternal-Child Nursing, 8,* 417–422.

Rodgers, G. P. (1990). Hydroxyurea therapy in sickle cell disease: An update on the NIH experience. Paper presented at the 15th Annual Meeting of National Sickle Cell Disease Centers, Berkeley, California.

Rooks, Y., & Pack, B. (1983). A profile of sickle cell disease. *Nursing Clinics of North America, 18,* 131–138.

Ryan, T. M., Townes, T. M., Reilly, M. P., Asakurat, T., Palmiter, R. D., Brinsted, R. L., & Behringer, R. R. (1990). Human sickle hemoglobin in transgenic mice. *Science, 247,* 566.

Schalock, R. L., & Jensen, C. M. (1986). Assessing the Goodness-of-Fit between persons and their environment. *Journal of Association of the Severely Handicapped, 11,* 103–109.

Schecther, A. N., Noguchi, C. T., & Rodgers, G. P. (1987). Sickle cell anemia. In G. Stamatoyannopoulos, A. W. Nienhaus, P. Leder, & P. W. Majerus (Eds.), *Molecular Basis of Blood Diseases* (pp. 179–218). Philadelphia: W. B. Saunders Co.

Schwartz, G. E. (1982). Testing the biopsychosocial model: The ultimate challenge facing behavioral medicine. *Journal of Consulting and Clinical Psychology, 50,* 1040–1053.

Scott, R. B. (1973). Sickle cell anemia: Problems in education and mass screening. In H. Abramson et al., (Eds.), *Sickle Cell Disease: Diagnosis, Management, Education and Research* (pp. 285–292). St. Louis: C. V. Mosby Company.

Scott, R. B. (1985). Advances in the treatment of sickle cell disease in children. *American Journal of Diseases in Children, 139,* 1219–1222.

Serjeant, G. R. (1985). *Sickle cell disease.* Oxford: Oxford University Press.

Thomas, R., & Holbrook, T. (1987). Sickle cell disease: Ways to reduce morbidity and mortality. *Postgraduate Medicine, 81,* 265–280.

Vaughan, W. P., Purtilo, R. B., Butler, B. B. A., & Armitage, J. O. (1986). Ethical and financial issues in autologous marrow transplantation: A symposium sponsored by the University of Nebraska Medical Center. *Annals of Internal Medicine, 105,* 134–135.

Vavasseur, J. W. (1987). Psychosocial aspects of chronic disease: Cultural and ethnic implications. *Birth Defects, 23,* 144–153.

Vermylen, C., Ninane, J., Robles, E. F., & Cornu, G. (1988). Bone marrow transplantation in five children with sickle cell anemia. *Lancet, 1,* 1427–1428.

Vichinsky, E. P., Hurst, D., & Lubin, B. H. (1983). Sickle cell disease: Basic concepts. *Hospital Medicine,* 128–158.

Vichinsky, E. P., & Lubin, B. H. (1980). Sickle cell anemia and related hemoglobinopathies. *Pediatric Clinics of North America, 22,* 429–447.

Vichinsky, Elliot P. (1992). Personal communication, June.

Wagner, G. M., & Vichinsky, E. P. (1989). Sickling syndromes and unstable hemoglobin diseases. In W. C. Mentzer & G. M. Wagner (Eds.), *The hereditary hemolytic anemias* (Chapter 4). New York: Churchill Livingstone.

Werthiem, E. S. (1975). Person-environment interaction: The epigenesis of autonomy and competence. I. Theoretical considerations (normal development). *British Journal of Medical Psychology, 48,* 1–8.

Whitten, C. F., & Fischoff, J. (1974). Psychosocial effects of sickle cell anemia. *Archives of Internal Medicine, 133,* 590–614.

Whitten, C. F., & Nishiura, E. N. (1985). Sickle cell anemia. In N. Hobbs & J. M. Perrin (Eds.), *Issues in the care of children with chronic illnesses* (pp. 236–260). London: Jossey-Bass Publishers.

Williams, I., Earles, A. N., & Pack, B. (1983). Psychosocial considerations in sickle cell disease. *Nursing Clinics of North America, 18,* 215–229.

Williams, T. E. (1984). Legal issues and ethical dilemmas surrounding bone marrow transplantation in children. *American Journal of Pediatric Hematology/Oncology, 6,* 83–88.

10

Ophthalmology in Blacks: A Survey of Major Entities

Stephen Dale McLeod and Maurice F. Rabb

The leading causes of visual impairment and blindness (defined by visual acuity less than 20/200) in the United States include cataract, glaucoma, age-related macular degeneration, and diabetic retinopathy. Numerous surveys have reported significantly higher rates of blindness and visual impairment in Blacks compared with Whites in almost all age groups (Kahn & Moorhead, 1973). Furthermore, marked differences in the prevalence of cataract, glaucoma, and age-related macular degeneration, the latter being found rather less frequently in Black populations (Jampol & Tielsch, 1992), have been documented. This chapter will also include a discussion of sickle cell retinopathy as a unique ophthalmologic entity of black populations.

GLAUCOMA

From data from blindness registries and prevalence surveys it is clear that Blacks are at a significantly higher risk of glaucoma than are Whites (Martin, Sommer, Gold & Diamond, 1985). The National Survey carried out in St. Lucia in the West Indies indicates a prevalence of 8.8 percent in patients over 30 years of age (Mason et al., 1989), while a survey of Barbadians indicates an overall prevalence of 6 percent and among patients over 54 years a rate of 13 percent (Leske, Connell & Kehoe, 1989). These rates are notably higher than the reported prevalence of about 1 percent in American Whites under 70 years of age (Wilensky, Ghandi & Pan, 1978). Indeed, in the United States, the prevalence of blindness registries based on glaucoma are 8 times higher in Blacks than in Whites (Cowan, Worthen, Mason & Anduze, 1988). The Baltimore Eye Survey described glaucoma rates of 1.23 percent in Blacks aged 40 through 49 to 11.26

percent in those 80 and over, compared with 0.92 percent to 2.16 percent in Whites of comparable age groups (Tielsch et al., 1991a).

Glaucoma also appears to be a more aggressive disease in Blacks as compared to Whites (Martin, Sommer, Gold & Diamond, 1985). Numerous independent studies have demonstrated an earlier age of onset in Blacks, as well as more severe visual field loss and optic nerve damage (Wilson, Richardson, Hertzmark & Grant, 1985).

The glaucomas are a heterogeneous group of diseases characterized by optic nerve head damage and visual field loss associated with intraocular pressure greater than the eye tolerates. It should be noted that no definition of glaucoma indicates a specific intraocular pressure value. It is quite common for people to have intraocular pressures significantly above the general population's mean without sustaining optic nerve head damage or demonstrating visual field defects. This is referred to variously as ocular hypertension, early glaucoma, or glaucoma without damage, while the person might be referred to as a glaucoma suspect. Such persons are considered to run a risk of developing glaucoma of 1 percent per year (Leske, 1983). Conversely, in low-tension glaucoma, eyes without documented pressure elevations demonstrate the characteristic glaucomatous optic disc and visual field changes.

The majority of glaucoma patients have chronic or primary open-angle glaucoma, that is, a diagnosis of glaucomatous damage in the absence of obvious anatomic features that explain the associated elevated intraocular pressure. Risk factors other than race for the development of primary open-angle glaucoma include a family history of glaucoma, increased age, myopia, diabetes mellitus, and cardiovascular disease (Katz & Sommer, 1988). All three parameters contributing to the diagnostic triad of elevated intraocular pressure (usually greater than 21 mmHg), increased optic nerve cupping, and visual field defects are observed in evaluating the extent of disease and the effect of therapy.

Intraocular Pressure

Because clinically it is impractical to routinely cannulate eyes to measure intraocular pressure directly, a number of methods of estimating intraocular pressure through the behavior of the cornea when applanated or indented are employed. Many factors are thought to affect intraocular pressure, including family history of open-angle glaucoma, age, refractive error, and race (Armaly, 1965). The HANES data show the mean intraocular pressure of Blacks to be about half a millimeter of mercury higher than that of Whites (Klein & Klein, 1981). Across the general population, mean intraocular pressure is in the region of 15 mmHg, but the distribution is non-Gaussian and is skewed towards higher pressures (Armaly, 1965). As two standard deviations above the mean is approximately 20.5 mmHg, 21 mmHg is generally accepted as the upper limit of normal though, as previously pointed out, many nonpathologic eyes will maintain pressures well over 21 mmHg.

Optic Nerve Cupping

Pressure-mediated damage to the optic nerve head, either through compromise of local microvascular circulation or mechanical damage perhaps through deformation of the lamina cribrosa, is thought to be a central pathophysiologic feature of glaucoma (Shields, 1992). Enlargement of the optic nerve head's cup-to-disc ratio is a cardinal sign of optic nerve damage. The cup refers to the central, depressed paler area of the nerve head, while the neural rim refers to the ring of tissue between the edge of the cup and the disc margin. Across the general population, studies using direct ophthalmoscopy report a non-Gaussian distribution of cup-to-disc ratios, with the vast majority measuring 0.0 to 0.3 and with only 1–2 percent equal to or greater than 0.7 (Schwartz, Rueling & Garrison, 1975). Beck, Messner, Musch, Martone, and Lichter (1985) found an average cup-to-disc ratio of 0.35 in Blacks that was significantly higher than the ratio of 0.24 found in Whites, while Chi et al. (1989) describe a mean cup-to-disc ratio of 0.62 in Blacks as opposed to 0.41 in Whites.

It is therefore especially important when attempting to diagnose glaucoma based on optic nerve atrophy in Blacks that one include other features of glaucomatous optic nerve atrophy such as the color and health of the neural rim, the nerve fibre layer quality, peripapillary atrophy, and asymmetry between the two eyes. A critical feature in such a diagnosis is documentation of change in the appearance of the disc, with progression of cupping or nerve fibre layer loss.

Visual Fields

Visual loss in glaucoma is marked by various changes in the visual field as measured by the automated or manual perimeter. Generalized changes such as diffuse reduction in sensitivity, concentric contraction, and enlargement of the blind spot appear to be some of the earliest changes, but none is specific enough to be useful in diagnosis (Shields, 1992). Nerve fibre bundle defects that produce abnormalities such as arcuate scotomas or nasal and vertical steps are considered more specific and useful in diagnosis.

Screening

Efforts have been made to identify patients early in the course of their disease through screening. It is of particular concern that persons might sustain quite significant glaucomatous damage to the optic nerve before visual field deficits become apparent, but it is assumed that the institution of therapy will slow the progression of the disease and help to preserve useful vision (Grant & Burke, 1982). Parameters available for examination in screening programs include intraocular pressure, the appearance of the optic disc, visual fields, and historical risk factors. A number of other psychophysical tests are under investigation at present, such as contrast sensitivity and color vision, but none has yet proved useful in diagnosis or screening.

One of the most popular forms of screening at present is that of single intra-ocular-pressure measurements. This type of screening is fraught with problems. To begin with, this process renders a single number that in isolation is often very difficult to interpret, because many glaucomatous eyes will have pressures below the standard cut-off level of 21 mmHg and many normal eyes will have elevated pressures. Furthermore, characteristically hypertensive eyes might be read as normal and normal eyes as hypertensive. In the Welsh Ferndale study (Hollows & Graham, 1966), 9.4 percent of the population had an intraocular pressure of greater than 20 mmHg; in the U.S. Framingham study, 7.6 percent of the population had an intraocular pressure of greater than 21 mmHg (Leibowitz et al., 1980). In both populations, only about 0.3 percent went on to demonstrate glaucomatous changes in the presence of first screening measurement elevated intraocular pressure. This indicates that this screening procedure will produce a great many false positives. Raising the cut-off pressure does not improve matters because at higher levels the sensitivity becomes unacceptably poor.

It might be argued that it is of greater concern that truly glaucomatous eyes are not missed. The Baltimore Eye Survey found that more than 50 percent of glaucomatous eyes in a Black population had a survey intraocular pressure of less than 21 mmHg whether receiving therapy or not (Sommer et al., 1991b). Such a group will include persons with spuriously low pressure measurements as well as those with glaucoma in spite of pressures less than 21 mmHg.

Isolated assessments of the optic nerve head have been shown to have an unacceptably low sensitivity in glaucoma detection of about 40 percent (Neumann, Eibschitz, Hyams & Friedman, 1971) and are subject to observer inconsistency and variation (Kahn et al., 1975). Both manual and automated perimetry are considered too expensive and time consuming at present to be recommended for screening programs, though the development of cheaper, quicker perimetric methods would greatly enhance present screening methods.

The most sensitive practical method of mass screening at present is probably a combination of risk-factor recognition (including a family history of glaucoma), tonometry, and optic disc evaluation by an experienced observer. In a recent Japanese study, which combined intraocular pressure measurements with an assessment of the optic disc, it was observed that intraocular pressure measurements alone would have missed one-half of the glaucoma cases, while optic nerve head evaluation alone would have missed one-third of the cases (Shiose et al., 1981). The Baltimore Eye Survey found the vertical or horizontal cup-to-disc ratio of equal to or greater than 0.5 to have a sensitivity of 52 percent and a specificity of 85 percent, while a combination of intraocular pressure greater than 21 and vertical cup-to-disc ratio greater than or equal to 0.5 had a sensitivity of 61 percent and a specificity of 84 percent. Sensitivity was increased to 66 percent by including a family history of glaucoma as a risk factor, but specificity was reduced to 79 percent (Tielsch et al., 1991a).

It is important to recognize that the results of these various surveys should not be applied directly to the Black population, as the prevalence of glaucoma is so much higher than in most of the populations described. This significantly enhances the predictive value of any screening test. Nevertheless, the combination of risk-factor assessment, tonometry, and disc evaluation remains only modestly sensitive, a fact that makes the efficiency of the screening environment critically important. Specific features of this environment include the general population's access to screening, the competence of screeners (especially in the evaluation of the optic disc), and follow-up and treatment of glaucoma suspects and patients. Though mass screenings staffed by volunteers can reach a great many people, the staff are usually inexperienced observers, detection rates are low, and follow-up is often poor (Berwick, 1985). McPherson (1980) has demonstrated that public health departments can play a useful role in well-organized detection programs, though follow-up remains a problem.

The environment best suited for the detection and referral for treatment of glaucoma is probably the primary physician's office. Internists and family practitioners should be educated in the risk factors for glaucoma, trained in the recognition of suspicious optic discs, and encouraged to routinely check intraocular pressure (Levi & Schwartz, 1983). As they follow the general condition of the patient, they can ensure that patients with suspicious features or a diagnosis of glaucoma are indeed under the care of an ophthalmologist.

Even when glaucoma has been identified, it is suggested that Blacks might not receive adequate therapy. A recent study of Medicare clinics demonstrated that the rate of glaucoma surgery in Blacks was 45 percent lower than the expected calculated rate and that Whites were receiving proportionally higher rates of treatment (Javitt et al., 1991). It is not at all clear why a disparity in the delivery of care to identified Black and White glaucoma patients should exist, but a great deal of interest has arisen in the possible social and economic contributors to this phenomenon. It is important that ophthalmologists recognize the aggressive nature of the disease in Blacks and that primary physicians concern themselves with timely referrals and follow-up.

The psychology of the disease is in some respects comparable with that of systemic hypertension: both tend to be asymptomatic for much of the course, therapy is inconvenient to irritating, if not frankly noxious, and successful treatment as perceived by the patient is undramatic. It is therefore tremendously important that patients understand the nature of the disease, its natural history and its potentially devastating consequences. Therefore, patient and physician education is paramount.

CATARACT

According to the Department of Health and Human Services and the National Center for Health Studies, cataract extraction is one of the most frequently performed adult operations (National Center for Health Statistics, 1982). Though the Model Reporting Area for Blindness Statistics (1962 to 1970) found cataracts to be the third leading cause of blindness in the United States (Kahn & Moorhead, 1973), the National Health Interview Survey found cataracts to be the first cause of visual impairment (National Society to Prevent Blindness, 1980). The more recently conducted Baltimore Eye Survey found cataracts to be the leading cause of bilateral blindness (Sommer et al., 1991a).

The crystalline lens, which lies behind the iris, is the final refracting medium that light must traverse on its way to the retina. It is composed of a central nucleus and an enveloping cortex within a clear capsule. A cataract is an opacity of any element of this crystalline lens that impedes the normal passage of light. At present, no standard definition specifies the degree of reduction in visual acuity. This results in various estimates of frequency and incidence of cataract in the United States based on various definitions of cataract.

The most common type and therefore the most important to examine in terms of public health issues is the senile cataract. This can be defined as the presence of lens opacity in a person over 45 years of age in the absence of other causes for cataract. The HANES study required a visual acuity of 20/30 or worse (Hiller, Sperduto & Ederer, 1983), while the Framingham study required a visual acuity of 20/25 or worse (Leibowitz et al., 1980). Based on these definitions, the HANES study reported a cataract prevalence of 10 percent for people aged 55 to 64 and of 28 percent for those aged 65 to 74, while the Framingham study reported a prevalence of 4.5 percent for those aged 52 to 64 and of 46 percent for those 75 to 85 (Kahn, Leibowitz, Ganley, Kini & Colton, 1977).

Recent epidemiologic study has attempted to define demographic, environmental, and other risk factors for senile cataracts. Under demographic factors, age is the most obvious. Both the Framingham and the HANES studies have demonstrated an increasing prevalence of senile cataracts with advancing age. Numerous studies have also suggested that women over 60 years of age are at a slightly higher risk of cataracts than are men (Kahn & Moorhead, 1973).

Geographic variations in the age-adjusted prevalence of cataracts have suggested that environmental factors might contribute to cataract formation. The frequently cited Punjab study found an age-adjusted cataract prevalence almost three times higher than that of the Framingham study (Chatterjee, Milton & Thyle, 1982). Closer to home, the HANES data showed cataracts to be more common in rural than in urban dwellers, though it should be noted that this assessment was based on current residence rather than history. Ultraviolet light has been shown to be a risk factor for cataract formation in numerous studies in different parts of the world (Hollows & Moran, 1981).

A number of host factors are considered risks at present. Various studies have indicated that diabetes is such a factor (Phillips, Bartholomew & Clayton, 1980), but it is of interest that Sommer has suggested that diabetics are merely at a higher risk of diagnosis and cataract extraction (Sommer, 1977). Elevated systemic blood pressure has been identified as a risk factor by some (Phillips, Bartholomew & Clayton, 1980), but this was not supported by the HANES study. Current research addresses the contribution of poor nutrition to cataract formation and the role of supplements in retarding cataract formation.

There is general consensus in the current literature that Blacks are at an increased risk of cataract formation and subsequent visual debilitation. The HANES study found that blacks had an age-adjusted relative risk of 1.50 compared to Whites. Hiller, Sperduto, and Ederer (1983) point out that previous studies that failed to demonstrate an association of cataract formation and race were too small to detect a relative risk of that magnitude. A later analysis of the same data set revealed more specifically that Blacks had three times the risk of cortical cataracts and twice the risk of nuclear cataracts than that of Whites. Within Blacks, cortical cataracts were far more common than posterior subcapsular cataracts, though far fewer subcapsular cataracts were available for analysis (Hiller, Sperduto & Ederer, 1986).

The Baltimore Eye Survey found unoperated cataract to be the leading cause of blindness in Blacks (nearly one-third of the total) as opposed to age-related macular degeneration, the leading cause in Whites. The age-adjusted risk of cataract blindness in Blacks was 5.25 times that of Whites. The study also noted that the White subjects rendered blind by cataract were all at least 80 years old, while the Black subjects included much younger people (Sommer et al., 1991a).

The relative prevalence of cataract and consequent blindness is a particularly interesting public health concern because it depends not only upon the relative risk of cataract development but also upon the risk of curative cataract extraction. The latter risk, as suggested by the authors of the Baltimore Eye Survey, is to a great extent dictated by access to surgery. If we accept the relatively small increased risk of cataract development based on race, then we must conclude that a substantially greater risk of blindness due to unoperated cataract in Blacks indicates a marked disparity of interest in or access to cataract surgery. The fact that the disparity in blindness due to cataract between Whites and Blacks was reduced from an age-adjusted risk of 5.25 to 2.5 in patients over 80 might be explained by proposing that older patients may be comparatively reluctant to undergo surgery, but younger black patients might have more difficulty in gaining access to surgery. The Baltimore Eye Survey also reported greater percentages of White patients with a history of cataract surgery in one or both eyes in all age groups. The overall age-adjusted rate was 4.98 percent for Whites and 3.71 percent for Blacks (Sommer et al., 1991a). However, one must entertain the possibility that not only might the rates of surgery in Blacks be depressed, but that rates in Whites might be elevated by unnecessary procedures. Furthermore, as the timing of cataract surgery is based upon the patient's level of function and degree of debilitation, there may be different thresholds of patient demand for surgery in the two groups.

Analysis of the Baltimore Eye Survey data with regard to socioeconomic status indicated that in this population, where approximately 40 percent of blindness was potentially correctable, visual impairment was associated with lower socioeconomic status (Tielsch et al., 1991b). More specifically, both the HANES and the Framingham studies found poor education to be a risk factor for cataract. It is not clear what environmental or personal features marked by education and socioeconomic factors contribute to risk of cataract formation, but one might postulate that poorer or less-educated people might be less informed about health care issues in general including cataract and available treatment centers.

Though cataract surgery should not be regarded as an entirely benign procedure (a number of complications are themselves causes of ocular morbidity, visual impairment, and indeed blindness), it is in general highly successful in restoring useful and, in many cases, excellent vision. In recent years the procedure has become quite streamlined, and the vast majority of cataract extractions are performed under local anesthesia on an outpatient basis. The identification, diagnosis, and treatment of visual impairment due to cataract is comparatively straightforward in individual cases. The pressing issue is that of providing service to communities as a whole. A person who sits at home blinded by potentially curable cataracts either does not know about the cure, does not want it, or cannot get it. If primary physicians have blind or visually impaired patients, they and the patient should both know the cause. If indeed it is cataract, the physician who makes the diagnosis should be able to inform the patient of the risks and benefits of cataract surgery. Finally, we must ensure that communities have the resources to provide this essential service.

The question of why people with reversible disease go untreated, even in urban areas where people are aware of the disease entity and treatment centers are available, is a difficult one. It is significant that the Baltimore Eye Survey, with 40 percent potentially reversible blindness in its study population, found no association between use of general health care or eye care services and blindness or visual impairment (Tielsch et al., 1991b). This particular sociologic and epidemiologic question demands further investigation.

DIABETES

Though data exist that describe the relative incidence of diabetes in Black and White populations, very little data exist that describe the incidence, prevalence, and relative severity of diabetic retinopathy in the Black population. Kahn and Hiller (1974) describe an age-adjusted risk of blindness for non-Whites that is twice that of Whites, but this is not specific for the Black population.

In general, legal blindness is 25 times more common in the diabetic population. Diabetes is associated with a number of ocular manifestations, including cataract and glaucoma. The most common and clinically significant manifestation is retinopathy, which in its proliferative form causes 85 percent of all blindness in diabetics (Garcia & Ruiz, 1992). Severe retinal disease has been associated with age, duration of diabetic disease, degree of blood sugar control, hypertension, and renal disease (Klein, Klein, Moss, Davis & DeMets, 1988). Before the introduction of insulin in 1922, most diabetics died before the retinopathy became severe enough to cause blindness. However, now that treated patients live longer, proliferative retinopathy has become a far more common problem. Retinopathy develops more quickly in type II than in type I diabetes. In type II diabetes, retinopathy is evident in 20 percent of patients after two years of diagnosis; but in type I disease, only 2 percent to 7 percent have evidence of retinopathy after 2 years. However, 10 to 12 years after diagnosis, the prevalence of retinopathy in the two groups is similar (Garcia & Ruiz, 1992).

The pathology of diabetic retinopathy is primarily vascular. Changes are caused by loss of vascular competence leading to microaneurysms, dot and blot hemorrhages, hard exudates (the precipitated residue of clearing hemorrhage), and edema and by capillary occlusion leading to ischemia and cotton wool spots or soft exudates (retinal nerve fiber layer infarcts). The ischemia is believed to lead to the proliferation of new and abnormal blood vessels (neovascularization), which themselves cause vitreous hemorrhage, and to fibrous proliferation, which can cause vitreo-retinal traction and detachment.

Diabetic retinopathy can be divided into three stages, background, pre-proliferative and proliferative disease. In background and pre-proliferative disease, all pathology remains intraretinal, whereas in proliferative disease the vascular pathology extends to the pre-retinal space and the vitreous. Background diabetic retinopathy is characterized by cotton wool spots, dot-blot hemorrhages, microaneurysms, and hard exudates. Pre-proliferative retinopathy is an intermediate stage characterized by corkscrew-like intraretinal microvascular abnormalities (IRMA), venous beading, and arteriolar abnormalities. Proliferative diabetic retinopathy is the most visually threatening stage and is characterized by the development of neovascularization, either of the optic disc (NVD) or elsewhere in the retina (NVE), vitreous hemorrhage, fibrous proliferation, and tractional retinal detachment. Macular edema, caused by incompetent vessels, can exist at any one of these stages as a contributor to or cause of decreased vision.

At present, no medical therapy beyond the control of blood sugar has been demonstrated to alter the course of diabetic retinopathy. Indeed, the data demonstrating the effect of glycemic control remain somewhat controversial. Chase et al. (1989) have found that poor long-term glucose control is associated with a 2.5 times greater prevalence of severe retinopathy, while Klein, Klein, Moss, Davis, and DeMets (1988) have demonstrated in a prospective manner that higher levels of glycosylated hemoglobin (which indicates poorer glucose control) are related to a higher incidence and more severe progression of retinopathy.

The mainstay of treatment for both clinically significant macular edema (CSME) and proliferative diabetic retinopathy (PDR) with high risk characteristics as defined by the Early Treatment Diabetic Retinopathy Study (ETDRS) and the Diabetic Retinopathy Study (DRS), respectively, remains laser photocoagulation (Garcia & Ruiz, 1992). Surgery, which may involve vitrectomy, membranectomy, release of fibrous traction bands, retinal detachment repair, and retinotomy, is reserved for cases of nonclearing vitreous hemorrhage and tractional retinal detachment.

The primary epidemiologic and public health considerations of diabetic retinopathy include the identification of patients at risk and patients with disease, the minimization of risk factors for the development and progression of disease, and treatment when necessary. All patients with diabetes are patients at risk. Therefore, all diabetic patients must be referred for examination by an ophthalmologist regularly. A recent study of Black and Hispanic diabetic patients referred for initial ophthalmologic evaluation found that 37.3 percent of Black patients had severe retinopathy (either pre-proliferative or proliferative disease) at the time of initial evaluation. Indeed, many of these patients had not been referred in a timely fashion by their internists, but had sought care because of decreased visual acuity (Appiah, Ganthier & Watkins, 1991).

The most obvious exacerbating metabolic and physiologic factors that should be monitored closely by the internist are the degree of blood sugar control and blood pressure. Current data indicate that elevated systemic blood pressure is associated with more severe diabetic retinopathy (Chase et al., 1990) and that there is a higher incidence of retinopathy in patients with uncontrolled hypertension compared to treated hypertensives or normotensives (Teuscher, Schnell & Wilson, 1988). Furthermore, diabetes-related capillary nonperfusion and ischemia, severe CSME, chronic foveal hard exudates, and diffuse retinal edema are thought to be exacerbated by hypertension. It has been suggested that blood pressure control might improve the results of focal laser treatment in CSME (Rabb, Gagliano & Sweeney, 1990). It is therefore extremely important that ophthalmologists follow the blood pressure of their diabetic patients and that internists make every effort to establish both blood sugar and blood pressure control. Comprehensive studies have yet to be performed to examine the relationship between the increased risk of hypertension in the Black population and the risk and severity of diabetic retinopathy and visual impairment, as well as the more fundamental questions of the risk, severity, and course of diabetic eye disease.

SICKLE CELL

Ocular manifestations of sickle cell disease are the consequences of vascular occlusions and ischemia. They include the conjunctival sickle sign of linear dilation of conjunctival vessels (which has been shown to correlate with the irreversibly sickled cell count, the hemoglobin S concentration, and the intraerythrocytic hemoglobin concentration), segmental iris atrophy and iris neovascularization, disc vascular abnormalities, and retinal vascular occlusions with attendant ischemic complications including the black sunburst of retinal pigment epithelium hypertrophy, macular ischemia with vision loss, neovascularization, vitreous hemorrhage, and retinal detachment.

Proliferative sickle retinopathy can be divided into five stages of severity, which presumably occur sequentially. In stage I, there are peripheral arteriolar occlusions; in stage II, peripheral arterovenular anastomoses; in stage III, peripheral neovascularization; in stage IV, vitreous hemorrhage; and in stage V, retinal detachment. Proliferative sickle retinopathy (PSR) is observed primarily during the third and fourth decades of life, and its severity varies by hemoglobin type.

The sickle hemoglobinopathies result from the substitution of various amino acids in the beta hemoglobin chain. In sickle S, there is a substitution of valine for glutamic acid; and in sickle C, a substitution of lysine for glutamic acid at the same location. Though accurate data are not available, 8–10 percent of the U.S Black population are estimated to be heterozygous for the sickle S gene (AS) and 0.3–1.3 percent are estimated to be homozygous (SS). Two percent of Blacks living in the United States are estimated to be heterozygous for the sickle C gene (AC), 1 in 6,000 to be homozygous (CC), and 1 in 1,500 to carry both the S and C genes (SC). Ocular complications are noted to occur more commonly in SC and SThal disease than in SS disease. The prevalence of PSR is 60–70 percent in SC disease and 10 percent in SS disease (Bernhart, Henry & Lusher, 1974).

The risk of developing PSR varies with age in both types. In SC disease, it is greatest for males between 15 and 24 years and for females between 20 and 39 years. In SS disease, the greatest risk is between 25 and 39 years for both sexes (Fox, Dunn, Morris & Serjeant, 1990). Central visual loss occurs in approximately 12 percent of eyes with PSR (Condon & Serjeant, 1980). In a non-U.S. population (Curacao), 50 percent of patients with SC disease had PSR, 18 percent had vitreous hemmorhage, and 8 percent had gone on to retinal detachment. Four percent of the total population had a blind eye, which included 6 percent of the SC population (Van Meurs, 1991). According to data presented by Fox, Dunn, Morris, and Serjeant (1990), 50 percent of patients with SS disease will have bilateral PSR, while 70 percent of SC patients will have bilateral disease. They also note that risk factors for PSR in SS disease include high hemoglobin in males and a low fetal hemoglobin in both sexes, while risk factors in SC disease include a high mean cell volume and low fetal hemoglobin in females.

Treatment of PSR aims to induce regression of neovascularization to prevent vitreous hemorrhage and retinal detachment. This is achieved through laser photocoagulation by various techniques including feeder vessel photocoagulation, focal scatter photocoagulation, and peripheral circumferential photocoagulation. If nonclearing vitreous hemorrhage or retinal detachment has occurred, then vitreo-retinal surgery including vitrectomy and scleral buckling procedures may be indicated.

In order to minimize the number of people who go on to sustain vision loss because of proliferative disease, early treatment of PSR is essential. Internists should be aware that their sickle cell patients must be closely followed by ophthalmologists, who should regularly perform dilated funduscopic examinations. Internists should also be aware that even though the systemic manifestations of the heterozygous forms of sickle cell disease (SC and SThal) tend to be less severe than those of the homozygous form (SS), the opposite is true of the ocular complications. Further investigation of various approaches to reducing the propensity of sickle hemoglobin-containing cells to polymerize, such as the administration of calcium channel blockers or the elevation of fetal hemoglobin, could greatly reduce the incidence of systemic and ophthalmic sickle cell disease.

SUMMARY

Epidemiologic evidence available to date indicates the prevalence of visual impairment is greater among Blacks than Whites in the United States, and that there are significant differences in the prevalence of the most common conditions. As opposed to Whites, for whom the leading cause of blindness is the largely untreatable age-related macular degeneration, the leading causes in Blacks are the generally treatable cataract and glaucoma. Obviously, the approach to the problem of preventable and treatable blindness involves both diagnosis and treatment. In the way of diagnosis, general primary care physicians should be able to identify visual impairment, be aware of its most common causes, and direct appropriate referral to ophthalmologists. However, as previously discussed, even when a diagnosis has been made, lower than expected rates of treatment for Blacks have been described. These and other factors suggest that general access to ophthalmologic care remains a very important issue that demands attention.

REFERENCES

Appiah, A. P., Ganthier, R., & Watkins, N. (1991). Delayed diagnosis of diabetic retinopathy in black and Hispanic patients with diabetes mellitus. *Annals of Ophthalmology, 23,* 156–158.

Armaly, M. F. (1965). On the distribution of applanation pressure. I. Statistical features and the effect of age, sex and family history of glaucoma. *Archives of Ophthalmology, 73,* 11.

Beck, R. W., Messner, D. K., Musch, D. C., Martone, C. L., & Lichter, P. R. (1985). Is there a racial difference in physiologic cup size? *Ophthalmology, 92,* 873–876.

Bernhart, M. I., Henry, R. I., & Lusher, J. M. (1974). *Sickle cell.* Kalamazoo, MI: Scope Publication, Upjohn.

Berwick, D. M. (1985). Screening in health fairs. A critical review of benefits, risks and costs. *Journal of the American Medical Association, 254,* 1492.

Chase, H. P., Garg, S. K., Jackson, W. E., Thomas, M. A., Harris, S., Marshall, G., & Crews, M. J. (1990). Blood pressure and retinopathy in type I diabetes. *Ophthalmology, 97,* 155–159.

Chase, H. P., Jackson, W. E., Hoops, S. L., Cockerham, R. S., Archer, P. G., & O'Brien, D. (1989). Glucose control and the renal and retinal complications of insulin-dependent diabetes. *Journal of the American Medical Association, 261,* 1155–1160.

Chatterjee, A., Milton, R. C., and Thyle, S. (1982). Cataract prevalence and aetiology in Punjab. *British Journal of Ophthalmology, 66,* 35–42.

Chi, T., Ritch, R., Stickler, D., Pitman, B., Tsai, C., & Hsish, F. Y. (1989). Racial differences in optic nerve head parameters. *Archives of Ophthalmology, 107*, 836–839.

Condon, P. I., & Serjeant, G. R. (1980). Behavior of untreated proliferative sickle retinopathy. *British Journal of Ophthalmology, 64*, 404–411.

Cowan, C. L., Jr., Worthen, D. M., Mason, R. P., & Anduze, A. L. (1988). Glaucoma in blacks (Editorial). *Archives of Ophthalmology, 106*, 738–739.

Fox, P. D., Dunn, D. T., Morris, J. S., & Serjeant, G. R. (1990). Risk factors for proliferative sickle retinopathy. *British Journal of Ophthalmology, 74*, 172–176.

Garcia, C. A., & Ruiz, R. S. (1992). Ocular complications of diabetes. *Clinical Symposia, 44*, 7–34.

Grant, W. M., & Burke, J. F., Jr. (1982). Why do some people go blind from glaucoma? *Ophthalmology, 89*, 991.

Hiller, R., Sperduto, R. D., & Ederer, F. (1983). Epidemiologic associations with cataract in the 1971–1972 National Health and Nutrition Examination Survey. *American Journal of Epidemiology, 118*, 239–249.

Hiller, R., Sperduto, R. D., & Ederer, F. (1986). Epidemiologic associations with nuclear, cortical and posterior subcapsular cataracts. *American Journal of Epidemiology, 124*, 916–925.

Hollows, F., & Moran, D. (1981). Cataract: The ultraviolet risk factor. *Lancet, 2*, 1249–1250.

Hollows, F. C., & Graham, P. A. (1966). Intraocular pressure, glaucoma and glaucoma suspects in a defined population. *British Journal of Ophthalmology, 50*, 570–586.

Jampol, L. M., & Tielsch, J. (1992). Race, macular degeneration, and the Macular Photocoagulation Study. *Archives of Ophthalmology, 110*, 1699–1700.

Javitt, J. C., McBean, A. M., Nicholson, G. A., Babish, J. D., Warren, J. L., & Krakauer, H. (1991). Undertreatment of glaucoma among black Americans. *New England Journal of Medicine, 325*, 1418–1422.

Kahn, H. A., & Hiller, R. (1974). Blindness caused by diabetic retinopathy. *American Journal of Ophthalmology, 78*, 58–67.

Kahn, H. A., Leibowitz, H., Ganley, J. P., Kini, M., Colton, T., Nickerson, M. A., & Darber, T. R. (1975). Standardizing diagnostic procedures. *American Journal of Ophthalmology, 79*, 768.

Kahn, H. A., Leibowitz, H. M., Ganley, J. P., Kini, M. M., & Colton, T. (1977). The Framingham Eye Study. I. Outline and major prevalence findings. *American Journal of Epidemiology, 106*, 33–41.

Kahn, H. A., & Moorhead, H. B. (1973). Statistics on Blindness in the Model Reporting Area 1969–1970. Office of Biometry and Epidemiology, National Eye Institute. Department of Health, Education and Welfare, Publication NIH 73–427, Washington, DC.

Katz, J., & Sommer, A. (1988). Risk factors for primary open-angle glaucoma. *American Journal of Preventive Medicine, 4*, 110–114.

Klein, B. E., & Klein, R. (1981). Intraocular pressure and cardiovascular risk variables. *Archives of Ophthalmology, 99*, 837–839.

Klein, R., Klein, B. E. K., Moss, S. E., Davis, M. D., & DeMets, D. C. (1988). Glycosylated hemoglobin predicts the incidence and progression of diabetic retinopathy. *Journal of the American Medical Association, 260*, 2864–2871.

Klein, R., Moss, S. E., Klein, B. E. K., Davis, M. A., & DeMets, D. C. (1989). The

Wisconsin Epidemiologic Study of Diabetic Retinopathy. XI. The incidence of macular edema. *Ophthalmology, 96,* 1501–1510.

Leibowitz, H. M., Krueger, D. E., Maunder, L. R., Milton, R. C., Kini, M. M., Kahn, H. A., Nickerson, R. J., Pool, J., Colton, T. L., Ganley, J. P., Lowenstein, J. I., & Darber, J. R. (1980). The Framingham eye study monograph. *Survey of Ophthalmology, 24,* (supp.), 335–707.

Leske, M. C., Connell, A. M. S., & Kehoe, R. (1989). A pilot project of glaucoma in Barbados. *British Journal of Ophthalmology, 73,* 365–369.

Leske, M. C. (1983). The epidemiology of open-angle glaucoma—a review. *American Journal of Epidemiology, 118,* 166.

Levi, L., & Schwartz, B. (1983). Glaucoma screening in the health care setting. *Survey of Ophthalmology, 28,* 64.

Martin, M. J., Sommer, A., Gold, E. B., & Diamond, E. L. (1985). Race and primary open-angle glaucoma. *American Journal of Ophthalmology, 99,* 383–387.

Mason, R. P., Kosoko, O., Wilson, M. R., Martone, J. P., Cowan, C. L., Gear, J. C., & Ross-Degnan, D. (1989). National survey of the prevalence and risk factors of glaucoma in St. Lucia, West Indies, I: Prevalence findings. *Ophthalmology, 96,* 1363–1368.

McPherson, S. D., Jr. (1980). The challenge and responsibility of a community approach to glaucoma control. *Sightsaving Review, 50,* 15.

National Center for Health Statistics. (1982). Utilization of short-stay hospitals: Annual summary for the United States, 1980. National Center for Health Statistics. *Vital and health statistics,* Series 13: Data from the National Health Survey, No. 64, DHHS publication No. (PHS) 82–1725. Hyattsville, MD: Author.

National Society to Prevent Blindness. Vision problems in the U.S. (1980). New York: Author.

Neumann, N., Eibschitz, N., Hyams, S., & Friedman, Z. (1971). Ophthalmic screening in child welfare clinics in Israel with particular reference to strabismus and amblyopia. *Journal of Pediatric Ophthalmology, 8,* 257–260.

Phillips, C. I., Bartholomew, R. S., & Clayton, R. (1980). Cataracts: A search for associations or causative factors. In F. Regnault (Ed.), *Symposium on the lens* (pp. 19–25). *Amsterdam Excerpta Medica.*

Rabb, M. F., Gagliano, D. A., & Sweeney, H. E. (1990). Diabetic retinopathy in blacks. *Diabetes Care, 13* (supp. 4), 1202–1206.

Schwartz, J. T., Rueling, F. H., & Garrison, R. J. (1975). Acquired cupping of the optic nerve head in normotensive eyes. *British Journal of Ophthalmology, 59,* 216.

Shields, M. B. (1992). *Textbook of Glaucoma* (3rd ed.). Baltimore: Williams & Wilkins.

Shiose, Y., Komuro, K., Iioh, T., Amano, M., & Kawase, Y. (1981). New system for mass screening of glaucoma, as part of automated multiphasic health testing services. *Japanese Journal of Ophthalmology, 25,* 160.

Sommer, A. (1977). Cataracts as an epidemiologic problem. *American Journal of Ophthalmology, 83,* 334–339.

Sommer, A., Tielsch, J. M., Katz, J., Quigley, H. A., Gottsch, J. D., Javitt, J. C., Martone, J. F., Royall, R. M., Witt, K. A., & Ezrine, S. (1991a). Racial differences in the cause-specific prevalence of blindness in East Baltimore. *New England Journal of Medicine, 325,* 1412–1417.

Sommer, A., Tielsch, J. M., Katz, J., Quigley, H. A., Gottsch, J. D., Javitt, J., &

Singh, R. (1991b). Relationship between intraocular pressure and primary open-angle glaucoma among white and black Americans. The Baltimore Eye Survey. *Archives of Ophthalmology, 109,* 1090–1095.

Teuscher, A., Schnell, H., & Wilson, P. W. F. (1988). Incidence of diabetic retinopathy and relationship to plasma glucose and blood pressure. *Diabetes Care, 11,* 246–251.

Tielsch, J. M., Sommer, A., Katz, J., Royall, R. M., Quigley, H. A., & Javitt, J. (1991a). Racial variations in the prevalence of open-angle glaucoma. The Baltimore Eye Survey. *Journal of the American Medical Association, 266,* 369–374.

Tielsch, J. M., Sommer, A., Katz, J., Quigley, H., & Ezrine, S. (1991b). Socioeconomic status and visual impairment among urban Americans. *Archives of Ophthalmology, 109,* 637–641.

Van Meurs, J. C. (1991). Ocular findings in sickle patients on Curacao. *International Ophthalmology, 15,* 53–59.

Wilensky, J. T., Ghandi, N., and Pan, T. (1978). Racial influences in open-angle glaucoma. *Annals of Ophthalmology, 10,* 1398–1402.

Wilson, R., Richardson, T. M., Hertzmark, E., & Grant, W. M. (1985). Race as a risk factor for progressive glaucomatous damage. *Annals of Ophthalmology, 17,* 653–659.

III

Mental and Behavior-Related Conditions

11

AIDS and Sexually Transmitted Diseases

Wayne L. Greaves

AIDS is primarily a sexually transmitted disease, although it can be transmitted in nonsexual ways. People who contract HIV often have a history of repeated infections with other sexually transmitted diseases. These diseases have had a disproportionate impact on the Black community. In particular, AIDS has aggravated existing health-care problems within the Black community and underscored the racial inequalities and injustices of American society. The economic consequences of the disease have been staggering, especially for poor Blacks, who often have no medical or disability insurance. The church, historically an important cultural institution in the Black community, as well as other professional groups and organizations have only slowly begun to respond to the problem of AIDS. As a result, the epidemic of AIDS and other sexually transmitted diseases threatens to decimate the Black community.

EPIDEMIOLOGY

Almost 300,000 cases of AIDS have been reported to the Centers for Disease Control (CDC) since 1981 when the first cases were recognized; almost one-half of these persons have died (CDC, 1993). It is estimated that one million people are infected with HIV in the United States and that approximately 40,000 to 80,000 adults and adolescents become infected each year.

The first 100,000 cases of AIDS were reported in 8 years and 6 months; the second 100,000 in 2 years and 2 months; and it is projected that in slightly less than 2 years another 100,000 cases will be reported (CDC, 1992). Sixty-one percent of the first 100,000 reported cases occurred among homosexual/bisexual men with no history of injection drug use (IDU) and 20 percent among female or heterosexual male injection drug users, while 5 percent were attributed to heterosexual transmission (CDC, 1992). In comparison, 55 percent of the second 100,000 reported cases occurred among homosexual/bisexual men with no history of IDU, 24 percent among female or heterosexual male injection drug users, while 7 percent were attributed to heterosexual transmission. The second 100,000 cases reflect an increase in the proportion of Blacks with AIDS from 27 percent to 31 percent (CDC, 1992).

AIDS is now one of the major causes of death in the United States. As early as 1988, AIDS was the leading cause of death among Black women aged 15–44 in New York and New Jersey (CDC, 1991; Chu, Buehler, Oxtoby & Kilbourne, 1991a). By 1990, AIDS had become the leading cause of death nationwide for Black men between the ages of 35 and 44, and the second leading cause of death for Black children between the ages of 1 and 4 (Chu et al., 1991a). The epidemiologic pattern of transmission for AIDS among adult Blacks differs from that of the White population, with a greater proportion of cases caused by heterosexual transmission (Selik, Castro & Papaionnou, 1988).

Injection Drug Use (IDU) and transmission of HIV by injection drug users is the driving force behind the epidemic of HIV among Blacks in the United States, especially among women and children. Factors other than IDU associated with heterosexual transmission include number of sex partners, frequency of unprotected sexual contact, prostitution, sex with a prostitute, history of STDs, lack of circumcision, and ulcerative as well as non-ulcerative genital disease. Of all AIDS cases among Blacks, 78 percent have been in adult men, 19 percent in adult women, and 3 percent in children younger than 13 years (National Commission on AIDS, 1992). Among Black men, who account for 26 percent of all AIDS cases in adult men, homosexual contact accounts for 43 percent of the cases and IDU use accounts for 36 percent, and homosexual men who inject drugs account for another 7 percent of cases (National Commission on AIDS, 1992).

SEROPREVALENCE

Serosurveys in various population groups emphasize the higher HIV infection rates among Blacks. HIV seropositivity rates of 3.9 per 1,000 have been reported among Black military recruits versus 0.9 percent per 1,000 among White recruits (CDC, 1987). Among clients attending STD clinics in Baltimore, HIV seropositivity rates were 5.2 percent among Blacks compared to 1.2 percent among Whites (Quinn et al., 1988). Among patients presenting to an inner-city emergency department, Kelen et al. (1988) found a 6.0 percent HIV seropositivity rate among Blacks compared to a 2.6 percent rate among Whites. Job Corps screens disadvantaged youth between the ages of 16 and 21, approximately two-thirds of whom are Black and Hispanic and one-third White. Among Black applicants, the seroprevalence rate was found to be 5.3 per 1,000 (Louis et al., 1991).

WOMEN AND AIDS

Cases in women are increasing faster than they are in men. In 1991, the proportional increase in AIDS cases among women was 33 percent (CDC, 1991). The majority of women acquire AIDS heterosexually through injection drug use or by being a sexual partner of an injection drug user. Black women are approximately 13.2 times more likely to contract AIDS than are White women and account for approximately 52 percent of all cases of AIDS among women (National Commission on AIDS, 1992). AIDS grew from not being a known cause of death to being the eighth leading cause of death among women ages 15 to 44 in the United States in 1987; it now is the fifth leading cause of death (Chu, Buehler & Berkelman, 1991b). For the last 5 years, AIDS has been the leading cause of death in young women in New York City (Friedland et al., 1991).

As a cause of death, AIDS is 9 times higher among Black women than it is among White women. The increasing numbers of cases of AIDS among Black women is of concern because of the impact on pediatric cases of AIDS. Currently, 58 percent of all pediatric AIDS cases are Black children (CDC, 1992). Ninety-four percent of these cases have been due to perinatal transmission from mothers infected with HIV. Only 4 percent have been due to contaminated blood products. Data from surveys of infants suggest that one out of every 625 women who gave birth in the United States in 1991 was infected with the AIDS virus; and the rate is almost 1 percent in metropolitan Washington, D.C., and other areas in the Northeast.

In recent years attention has focused on women with AIDS largely because of concerns and pressure from women's groups. One important consequence has been the recognition that some clinical manifestations of HIV disease may be different in women. Chronic, persistent, or recurrent vaginal candidiasis and invasive cervical cancer may be the initial manifestations of AIDS in women, and oesophageal candidiasis may be a more common AIDS-indicator disease than pneumocystis pneumonia.

INJECTION DRUG USE

The significant historical morbidity and mortality among injection drug users complicates assessment of the direct impact of HIV in the Black community. Among injection drug users the frequency of sharing contaminated paraphernalia is a major risk factor, as is the type of exposure. Risk may be enhanced by the practice of "booting," in which blood is drawn back into the syringe in order to extract any remaining blood in the needle or syringe. The National Institute of Drug Abuse estimates that there are 1.2 million injection drug users in the United States today. The smallest proportion of these are in drug treatment; a slightly larger group are in jail or prison; and the largest number are on the streets injecting drugs. These groups are unlikely to be medically insured, unlikely to have regular medical providers, and typically use the health care system only for acute interventions and only as a last resort. They are often victims of the prejudice against substance abusers that permeates the health care system.

One controversial approach to the problem of HIV among injection drug users is the provision of sterile needles and syringes. This is viewed with disdain by those who argue that such a program simply reinforces the problem and encourages illicit trading in needles. Many are skeptical about "the establishment's" interest in helping injection drug users now; other serious problems have existed all along but have been ignored (Dalton, 1989). The injection drug user has learned to live on the edge, to accept pain and suffering as a way of life, and is not readily impressed by messages that promise freedom from infection and good health. Still others are uncomfortable with the emphasis on sterilizing "works" and exchanging needles rather than promoting abstinence. Even strict advocates of needle exchange admit that, if this approach is to work, needle exchange programs must function in tandem with drug treatment programs. Unfortunately, in most urban areas, the long wait to enter drug treatment programs adds to the frustration of the drug user and perpetuates the vicious cycle of drug use.

SEXUALLY TRANSMITTED DISEASES

The incidence of sexually transmitted diseases in the Black community is very high (Aral & Holmes, 1991; Moran, Aral, Jenkins, Peterman & Alexander, 1989). To the extent that certain sexually transmitted diseases (STDs) are risk factors for HIV transmission, the higher incidence of STDs in Blacks may contribute to the disproportionate numbers of AIDS cases in Blacks. Both the increase and distribution of heterosexual AIDS cases in the U.S. population closely parallel those of other sexually transmitted infections (Moss & Kreiss, 1990).

While overall rates of gonorrhea and syphilis have decreased in the United States, one discouraging note is the extraordinarily rapid increase of infectious primary and secondary syphilis among Black men and women since 1985. This increase in syphilis has predominantly occurred in heterosexual Black men and women, despite major declines in gay White men. In 1987, incidence rates for early syphilis in the United States were 25 times higher among Black men than among White men and 31 times higher among Black women than among White women (Aral & Holmes, 1991; Moran et al., 1989). The increase in the number of women with syphilis has led to a big increase in congenital syphilis, fatal to newborns. Syphilis and other genital ulcer diseases are of concern because they may facilitate acquisition and transmission of HIV infection. The increase in syphilis has been associated with sex for drugs and cocaine use and has been concentrated in areas of poverty and urban depression among persons who are the hardest to reach and at the greatest risk for HIV infection.

Chancroid, another ulcerative genital disease, has been increasingly reported in the United States since 1985. In patients with HIV infection, the response of chancroid to standard drug therapy appears to be decreased (Aral & Holmes, 1991). Overall, the incidence of gonorrhea has decreased in the United States, but this has been associated with an increase in the proportion of antibiotic-resistant strains and an increase in disease incidence among Blacks (Rice, Roberts, Handsfield & Holmes, 1991).

While genital ulcer disease is recognized as a risk factor for AIDS, there is now speculation that any inflammatory sexually transmitted disease may increase the risk of HIV transmission once exposure to the virus has occurred. Studies in African women suggest that the risk of heterosexual transmission of HIV is increased in women with gonococcal or chlamydia cervicitis and vaginal trichomoniasis (Plummer et al., 1991). HIV may also alter the clinical manifestations and course of some STDs. Syphilis may be difficult to diagnose by traditional serologic tests and may not respond to the usual dose of benzathine penicillin; clinical manifestations may be unusual, and the course of the disease may be accelerated. Genital herpes ulcers may be slow to heal and persist for months even with therapy. The prevalence of antibody to Herpes simplex virus type 2 is higher in the Black community than in any other group (National Commission on AIDS, 1992).

Finally, although use of condoms during sexual intercourse is promoted as a way to make sex safer, irritation of the vaginal mucosa by nonoxynol-9 coated condoms may lead to increased risk because of the associated inflammatory reaction and by causing some patients to abandon condom use altogether. Further, many Black men still refuse to use condoms; for many reasons some Black women are afraid to assert themselves in sexual relationships and therefore allow their partners not to use condoms during sexual intercourse.

HOMOSEXUALITY AND BISEXUALITY

Of all AIDS cases Blacks account for 13 percent of cases related to homosexual transmission and 28 percent of bisexual cases (Chu, Peterman, Doll, Buehler & Curran, 1992). Even here, Blacks are disproportionately represented. Black males over age 12 make up only 10.6 percent of the population, compared to 85 percent of White males over age 12, yet the latter account for only 77 percent of AIDS cases in homosexual men (Mays, 1989). Black homosexual and bisexual men account for 46 percent of all cases in Blacks and heterosexual IDUs account for 35 percent in Blacks, compared to 89 percent and 5 percent, respectively, among Whites. Homosexuality is still largely taboo in the Black community, and the attitudes and responses to alternative sexual life-styles are complex (Dalton, 1989; Mays, 1989).

SIGNS AND SYMPTOMS

AIDS is the end of the spectrum of HIV infection. The common clinical manifestation in Blacks and others are generally similar (Greaves, 1987). It appears, however, that opportunistic infections occur more frequently in Blacks and that HIV-related renal disease is more severe (Cantor, Kimmel & Bosch, 1991). Opportunistic infections are also common in injection drug users; the greater frequency of these infections in Black patients may simply reflect the high proportion of Black patients who are injection drug users. In contrast, there is a relatively lower incidence of Kaposi's sarcoma among Black patients with AIDS. It is of interest that despite the high prevalence of Kaposi's sarcoma among Blacks in equatorial Africa, the disease is relatively uncommon among Blacks with AIDS in the United States.

The course of HIV disease appears to be more rapid in Black patients. This may reflect the underlying nutritional or other health status of these individuals or presentation at a later stage of illness and destruction of the immune system. Prior to the availability of AZT, the median survival for Black patients, that is, the time from an AIDS-defining diagnosis to death, was approximately 7 months in contrast to 12 months for White patients (Greaves, 1987). Some have suggested that wasting disease (slim disease) may be more frequent and pronounced in Black patients, but there are no carefully controlled studies to support this view. Like syphilis, tuberculosis occurs with increased frequency among Blacks with AIDS (Barnes, Bloch, Davidson & Snider, 1991).

ISSUES IN THERAPY

The availability of AZT and similar agents combined with prophylaxis for opportunistic infections has prolonged life and transformed HIV disease into a chronic illness for many persons, particularly White gay men with good access to health care and to research centers. In contrast, therapeutic advances have had far less impact on Black persons with AIDS. This may be due to the lack of easy access to medical care, to postponing medical care until serious complications occur, or to a fatalistic attitude by some toward the disease.

Access to health care is a major obstacle in terms of both geographic location and ability to pay for medical care. Blacks tend primarily to use public health clinics and hospital emergency rooms for their health care and to be less likely than their White counterparts to have a private physician (Weissman, Stern, Fielding & Epstenin, 1991; Hayward, Bernard, Freeman & Corey, 1991). Consequently, care is often fragmented. Blacks also tend to seek medical care late in the course of their disease. This is reflected in the low CD_4 counts of many patients when first seen for medical care. In many cases the first reason for seeking medical care is the onset of an opportunistic infection or other serious complications associated with HIV disease. The long incubation period of AIDS and the fact that most individuals remain and feel healthy until there is a significant decrease in their CD_4 count may contribute to postponing medical care.

Another factor affecting the impact of therapy is the strong interest in and lobby for use of low-dose oral alpha interferon as an alternative to currently recommended agents such as AZT. Despite the paucity of available scientific data, there is a vocal minority within the Black community who strenuously promote the use of low-dose oral alpha interferon (Kemron). They argue that the currently used therapeutic agents are toxic and of little efficacy. Nevertheless, the current consensus of scientific opinion is that the advantages of the approved therapeutic agents outweigh the disadvantages of their adverse effects.

CLINICAL RESEARCH

The White gay community was the first to participate in clinical trials and benefit from approved drugs for AIDS. In contrast to the Black community, the White gay community is well-organized, generally better educated, and better off economically. The White gay community tends to be aware of current research findings, is more assertive, and often aggressive in seeking medical care. As a result, gay White men have been the ones to benefit most from advances in therapy.

Despite the efforts made by some sectors of the government to improve care and access to the newer therapeutic agents, these avenues have been relatively limited to Blacks, in many cases, some agents have been limited to research centers and protocols. Only recently have such protocols become available at minority institutions. Three minority medical centers are currently funded for AIDS research by the National Institutes of Health. Of these three centers, only Howard University is focusing on AIDS research among Blacks. On the other hand, more than 30 other research centers are conducting AIDS research through-out the United States. However, the general distrust of the medical and health care establishment, particularly where researchers are White and from traditional institutions, has deterred Blacks from fully utilizing these resources. The legacy of Tuskegee is so deeply rooted in the minds of many Black patients that new therapeutic agents, even when effective, are often viewed with suspicion before they are accepted by the Black community (Dalton, 1989; Thomas & Quinn, 1992); and Blacks are reluctant to participate in AIDS clinical trials (El-Sadr & Capps, 1992). This general distrust of clinical trials and new research findings can be detrimental to Blacks if the result is failure to use an effective drug or other therapy.

AZT and Kemron

Research has shown AZT can slow the course of HIV disease and contribute to the quality of life in persons with AIDS (Fischl et al., 1987). Though AZT has been embraced by the White community, it has not enjoyed such rapport in the Black community, partly because of the emphasis on its toxicity but partic-ularly because of the strong interest in Kemron, a drug reported to be effective by Kenyan researchers (Koech, Obel, Minowadge, Hutchinson & Cummings, 1990). The attitude of many in the Black community, at least in some geographic areas in the United States, is that Kemron is deliberately being withheld from clinical study and use because of institutional racism in the U.S. government in general and the National Institutes of Health (NIH) in particular. Scientists at NIH and other academic centers counter that there are few published data to support the original claims of the Kenyan researchers. Hence, there is controversy in the Black community, even among Black health professionals, about the efficacy of Kemron and other low-dose oral alpha interferon preparations.

Another controversy is the interpretation of the findings of a multicenter Veterans Administration cooperative study, which concluded that starting AZT therapy early, prior to a CD_4 count of 200, compared to starting later when the CD_4 count is below 200, was not beneficial to Blacks and Hispanics compared to Whites (Hamilton, Hartigan and Simberkoff et al., 1991). The study further suggests that early AZT may be harmful to Blacks, as the risk of dying was greater in the early AZT group. In addition, the drug showed little efficacy among persons who were injection drug users. The study has been severely criticized by some researchers, and others remain skeptical about the efficacy of AZT in Blacks and Hispanics (Smith, 1991).

An important criticism about the Veterans Administration cooperative study is that it was not designed to look specifically at the efficacy of AZT therapy by race. Also, to compensate for the small sample size, Blacks and Hispanics were combined into a single group. The controversy continues, despite evidence from retrospective reviews of earlier AIDS research studies which show no differential efficacy or outcome in Blacks given AZT compared to Whites (Lagakos, Fischl, Stein, Lim & Volberding, 1991). Within the scientific community, therefore, one can find those who are confident that AZT prolongs survival for Blacks when started early and others who are not sure AZT therapy should be initiated early.

ORIGIN OF AIDS

Other than low-dose alpha interferon, no single issue about AIDS is more controversial and engenders as much hostility in the Black community than the question of the origin of the HIV virus. Several theories have been promulgated, most of them by White researchers. In response to such theories, the Black community has come up with its own theories.

The common theory in White scientific circles is that AIDS began in Africa, because of a virus that occurred naturally in the wild, in animals like the African green monkey (Essex & Kanki, 1988). Some in the White community suggest that the virus, initially present in animals, was transmitted to man through sexual union with animals or by drinking the blood and eating the flesh of monkeys killed for food. These theories are vehemently rejected by the Black community and dismissed as racist interpretations of available scientific data. White researchers counter that there is virologic evidence to support some similarity between a virus that occurs in African green monkeys (Simian Immunodeficiency Virus or SIV) and the human immunodeficiency virus (HIV). Black researchers report that similarity does not prove causality and that the differences in the genetic sequences between SIV and HIV-1 and HIV-2 do not necessarily imply that the virus in animals was the precursor to HIV-1 as we know it today.

There are many other theories, including some that border on the ridiculous. However, one important theory espoused by many in the Black community is that the AIDS virus is man-made and represents the results of genetic engineering or research designed to eliminate Black people. While there is no hard evidence to support this view, the proponents of this theory quickly add that if such a research venture were undertaken by a government it would be classified and thus little proof would be available to scientists or laypersons. In defense, they allude to other research experiments conducted in the past by the U.S. government where the goal of research was placed above the interest and welfare of the participant. When viewed in the context of the historical data on race relations in the United States and the Tuskeegee experiments, the Black community remains extremely skeptical. Blacks consider theories that point to Africa as simply another excuse to blame them for this disease.

It is unlikely there will be any resolution of these different theories about the origin of AIDS in the near future. What is more relevant than knowing the origin of the disease is finding ways to address the serious problems we presently face. Knowledge of the origin of the AIDS virus is unlikely to contribute significantly to advances either in prevention or control of the disease.

FUTURE IMPERATIVES

For a long time, the media led the Black community to believe that AIDS was a disease of White gay men while social scientists and epidemiologists ignored the racial aspects of the AIDS epidemic. The color and face of the epidemic have now changed as well as the attitude of society to the epidemic. The danger of accepting AIDS as a chronic disease contributes to the loss of attention to AIDS-related issues. Several issues are of concern to the Black community. A prerequisite is the recognition that race is an important factor in the current AIDS epidemic and the need to address historically racist attitudes and policies in American society.

A major obstacle to controlling the epidemic among Blacks is poor access to health care and institutional racism in the health care system of the United States. The current health insurance system must change drastically so that the poorest patient, Black or White, has equal access to the same medical care as those who are wealthy. The health care system needs to provide better social services along with medical care for AIDS patients. Financially strapped urban hospitals and physicians and other health providers caring for poor Black patients must be better remunerated. Health education and AIDS prevention messages need to be more relevant and culturally appropriate, and greater attention must be given to the medium of the message.

The false dichotomy between AIDS and other sexually transmitted diseases must be avoided. All sexually transmitted diseases are behaviorally related. Although basic science has dominated AIDS research thus far, urgent attention should now be given to behavioral research. We know the genetic structure of the virus and how the disease is spread; however, we remain powerless to persuade people to change the very behaviors that place them at risk for AIDS.

Finally, everyone in the Black community, not only health professionals but corporate organizations, the clergy, and laypersons as well, must become involved in the struggle against AIDS. Without such collective involvement, the medical, social, and economic consequences of AIDS will destroy us, our families, our community, and perhaps our very existence.

REFERENCES

Aral, S. O., and Holmes, K. K. (1991). Sexually transmitted diseases in the AIDS era. *Scientific American, 264,* 62–69.

Barnes, P. F., Bloch, A. B., Davidson, P. T., and Snider, D. E. (1991). Tuberculosis in patients with human immunodeficiency virus infection. *New England Journal of Medicine, 324,* 1644–1649.

Cantor, E. S., Kimmel, P. L., & Bosch, J. P. (1991). Effect of race on expression of acquired immunodeficiency syndrome-associated nephropathy. *Archives of Internal Medicine, 151,* 125–128.

Centers for Disease Control (CDC). (1993). U.S. AIDS cases reported through December 1992. *HIV/AIDS Surveillance. Report, Year-End Edition,* issued January.

Centers for Disease Control. (1992). The second 100,000 cases of acquired immunodeficiency syndrome—United States, June 1982–December 1991. *Morbidity and Mortality Weekly Report, 41,* 218–229.

Centers for Disease Control. (1991). Mortality attributable to HIV infection/AIDS-United States, 1981–1990. *Morbidity and Mortality Weekly Report, 40,* 41–44.

Centers for Disease Control. (1987). Trends in human immunodeficiency virus infection among civilian applicants for military service—United States, October 1985–December 1986. (1987). *Morbidity and Mortality Weekly Report, 36,* 273–276.

Chu, S. Y., Peterman, T. A., Doll, L. S., Buehler, J. W., & Curran, J. W. (1992). AIDS in bisexual men in the United States: Epidemiology and transmission to women. *American Journal of Public Health, 82,* 220–224.

Chu, S. Y, Buehler, J., Oxtoby, M. J., & Kilbourne, B. W. (1991a). Impact of the HIV epidemic on mortality in children, United States. *Pediatrics, 87,* 806–810.

Chu, S. Y., Buehler, J. W., & Berkelman, R. L. (1991b). Impact of the human immunodeficiency virus epidemic on mortality in women of reproductive age, United States (1991). *Journal of the American Medical Association, 264,* 225–229.

Dalton, H. L. (1989). AIDS in black face. *Daedalus, 118,* 205–227.

El-Sadr, W., & Capps, L. (1992). The challenge of minority recruitment in clinical trials for AIDS. *Journal of the American Medical Association, 267,* 954–958.

Essex, M., & Kanki, P. J. (1988). The origins of the AIDS virus. *Scientific American, 259,* 64–71.

Fischl, M. A., Richman, D. D., Grieco, M. H., Gottlieb, M. S., Volberding, P. A., Laskin, O. L., Leedom, J. M., Groopman, J. E., Mildvan, D., Schooley, R. T., Jackson, G. G., Durack, D. T., & King, D., and the AZT Collaborative Working

Group. (1987). The efficacy of Azidothymidine (AZT) in the treatment of patients with AIDS and AIDS-related Complex. *New England Journal of Medicine, 317,* 185–191.

Friedland, G. H., Saltzman, B., Vileno, J., Freeman, K., Schrager, L., & Klein, R. (1991). Survival differences in patients with AIDS. *Journal of Acquired Immune Deficiency Syndromes, 4,* 144–153.

Greaves, W. L. (1987). The black community. In H. L. Dalton and S. Burris (Eds.), *AIDS and the Law: A Guide for the Public* (pp. 281–289). New Haven: Yale University Press.

Hamilton, J. D., Hartigan, P. M., Simberkoff, M. S., & the Veterans Cooperative Study Group, Department of Veterans Affairs. (1991). Early vs. later zidovudine treatment of symptomatic HIV infection. *Clinical Research, 39,* 216a.

Hayward, R. A., Bernard, A. M., Freeman, H. E., & Corey, R. C. (1991). Regular sources of ambulatory care and access to health services. *American Journal of Public Health, 81,* 434–438.

Kelen, G. D., Fritz, S., Qaqish, B., Brookmeyer, R., Baker, J. L., Kline, R. L., Cuddy, R. M., Goessel, T. K., Floccare, D., Williams, K. A., Sivertson, K. T., Altman, S., & Quinn, T. C. (1988). Unrecognized human immunodeficiency virus infection in emergency department patients. *New England Journal of Medicine, 318,* 1645–1650.

Koech, D. K., Obel, A. O., Minowadge, J., Hutchinson, V. A., & Cummings, J. M. (1990). Low dose oral alpha-interferon for patients seropositive for human immunodeficiency virus type-1 (HIV-1). *Molecular Biotherapy, 2,* 91–94.

Lagakos, S., Fischl, M. A., Stein, D. S., Lim, L., & Volberding, P. (1991). Effects of Zidovudine therapy in minority and other subpopulations with early HIV infection. *Journal of the American Medical Association, 266,* 2709–2712.

Louis, M. E., Conway, G. A., Hayman, C. R., Miller, C., Petersen, L. R., & Dondero, T. J. (1991). Human immunodeficiency virus infection in disadvantaged adolescents: Findings from the U.S. Job Corps. *Journal of the American Medical Association, 266,* 2387–2391.

Mays, V. M. (1989). AIDS prevention in black populations: Methods of a safer kind. In V. M. Mays, G. W. Albee, J. Jones, & S. F. Schneider (Eds.), *Primary prevention of AIDS: Psychological approaches* (pp. 264–278). Newbury Park: Sage.

Moran, J. S., Aral, S. O., Jenkins, W. C., Peterman, T. A., & Alexander, E. R. (1989). The impact of sexually transmitted diseases on minority populations. *Public Health Reports, 104,* 560–565.

Moss, G. B., & Kreiss, J. K. (1990). The inter-relationship between human immunodeficiency virus infection and other sexually transmitted diseases. *Medical Clinics of North America, 74,* 1647–1660.

National Commission on AIDS. (1992). *Special Report: The challenge of HIV/AIDS in communities of color,* pp. 3–6, 27–30.

Plummer, F. A., Simonsen, N., Cameron, D. W., Netinya-Achola, J. O., Kreiss, J. K., Gakinya, M. N., Waiyaki, P., Cheang, M., Piot, P., Ronald, A. R., & Ngugi, E. N. (1991). Co-factors in male-female sexual transmission of human immunodeficiency virus type 1. *Journal of Infectious Disease, 163,* 233–239.

Quinn, T. C., Glasser, D., Cannon, R. O., Matuszak, D. L., Dunning, R. W., Klone, R. L., Campbell, C. H., Israel, E., Fauci, A. S., & Hook, E. W. (1988). Human immunodeficiency virus infection among patients attending clinics for sexually transmitted diseases. *New England Journal of Medicine, 318,* 197–203.

Rice, R. J., Roberts, P. L., Handsfield, H. H., & Holmes, K. K. (1991). Sociodemographic distribution of gonorrhea incidence: Implications for prevention and behavioral research. *American Journal of Public Health, 81,* 1252–1258.

Selik, R. M., Castro, K. G., & Papaionnou, M. (1988). Racial/ethnic differences in the risk of AIDS in the United States. *American Journal of Public Health, 789,* 1539–1546.

Smith, M. D. (1991). Zidovudine: Does it work for everyone? *Journal of the American Medical Association, 266,* 2750–2751.

Thomas, S. B., & Quinn, S. C. (1992). The Tuskeegee syphilis study, 1932 to 1972: Implications for HIV education and AIDS risk education programs in the black community. *American Journal of Public Health, 81,* 1498–1505.

Weissman, J. S., Stern, R., Fielding, S. L., & Epstenin, A. M. (1991). Delayed access to health care: Risk factors, reasons and consequences. *Annals of Internal Medicine, 114,* 325–331.

12

Homicide, Suicide, and Assaultive Violence: The Impact of Intentional Injury on the Health of African Americans

Darnell F. Hawkins, Alexander E. Crosby, and
Marcella Hammett

The study of the incidence and correlates of nonfatal assaultive violence, homicide, and suicide has long been of interest to social and behavioral scientists. Many disciplines, including anthropology, criminology, law, psychology, psychiatry, and sociology, have contributed to the analysis of these forms of aggression and violence. Recently, the injury that results from self-directed and interpersonal aggression has come to be viewed as a public health concern (National Research Council and the Institute of Medicine, 1985; Rosenberg & Fenley, 1991).

The application of public health and medical models to the study of assault, homicide, and suicide has been heralded by many. It has been argued that the trend toward thinking of these behaviors and their consequences as public health concerns rather than as deviant/criminal conduct will lead to changed perceptions regarding the extent to which they can be predicted and prevented. As opposed to being seen as inevitable by-products of the social order or abnormal psyches, it is argued that the rate of injury and death resulting from intentional actions can be reduced through the use of traditional public health modes of intervention.

In this vein, our chapter provides data on recent rates of homicide, suicide, and assaultive injury in the United States to illustrate their impact on the health and life expectancies of African Americans. We conclude with a discussion of intervention and prevention strategies currently being considered to attempt to reduce the rates of these forms of injury.

AFRICAN AMERICANS AND HOMICIDES

Analysts have long noted the disproportionate rate of homicide among African Americans as compared to Whites. Brearley (1932) reported that the Black homicide rate in the United States during the decades following the turn of the century was nearly 6 times the White rate. Follow-up studies at both the national and the local levels have reported a similar racial disparity (Wolfgang, 1958; Farley, 1980; Hawkins, 1986; Harries, 1990; Rose & McClain, 1990). In recent years the rate of homicide among Blacks has exceeded that for all other racial groups in the United States and may rank among the highest in the world (Fingerhut & Kleinman, 1990).[1]

According to the National Center for Health Statistics, there were 217,578 homicides in the United States from 1979 through 1988, an average of more than 21,000 per year. In 1988 there were about 22,000 victims of homicide, and more than 10,000 of these were African Americans. For every year of this period and in every region of the country, the rate of death for Blacks greatly exceeded that for Whites and persons of other races. This racial gap was also evident for both sexes and for all age groups (Hammett, Powell & Clanton, 1992).

Age and Gender Differences

Between 1979 and 1988, 56 percent of all homicide victims were 15 to 34 years of age. Homicide was the second most common cause of death among all Americans in this age group, exceeded only by unintentional injuries. It was the fourth most common cause of death among White females and the third most common cause among White males in this same age range. Among 15- to 34-year-old Black males and females, it was the most common cause of death. It was the second most common cause of death among 10- to 14-year-old Black males and females (Tables 12.1 and 12.2).

Most of the increase in the rate of homicide among all Black males from 1984 to 1988 (Figure 12.1) was due to an increase in rates among those 15 to 34 years old. Within this age range, the rate increased from 61.5 to 101.8 per 100,000 during this five-year period, while the rate among those 25 to 34 years old increased from 96.3 to 108.9 per 100,000 (Table 12.3). Although the rate of death was higher in the 25–34 age group than among the younger age group, the increase was more significant among those 15 to 24 years old (56%), with the most dramatic rise occurring among those 15 to 19 years old.

The media have recently highlighted the extremely high rates of homicide found among young Black males. As we indicated above, these rates are alarmingly high. But attentiveness to the plight of young males has often meant a disregard for the extremely high rates of homicide found among other segments of the Black population. These include adolescent and young adult females, older males, and infants of both sexes. Figure 12.2 shows that the Black-White homicide gap, although most pronounced at the young adult age range, extends throughout the life span. Black children under 1 year of age and Black adults in their 40s or older become victims of homicide at rates 5 to 6 times those of their White counterparts.

Table 12.1
Ten Leading Causes of Death for Black Males, by Age Group, United States, 1988*

Rank	<1	1-4	5-9	10-14	15-24	25-34	35-44	45-54	55-64	65+	Total
1	Perinatal Period 3,660	Unintentional Injuries 400	Unintentional Injuries 316	Unintentional Injuries 263	Homicide 2,762	Homicide 2,827	Heart Disease 1,961	Heart Disease 4,041	Heart Disease 8,072	Heart Disease 24,331	Heart Disease 39,584
2	Congenital Anomalies 747	Homicide 84	Malignant Neoplasms 46	Homicide 78	Unintentional Injuries 1,592	Unintentional Injuries 1,920	HIV 1,592	Malignant Neoplasms 3,460	Malignant Neoplasms 7,266	Malignant Neoplasms 17,749	Malignant Neoplasms 30,321
3	Unintentional Injuries 160	Congenital Anomalies 73	Homicide 38	Malignant Neoplasms 38	Suicide 394	HIV 1,632	Unintentional Injuries 1,551	Unintentional Injuries 991	Cerebro-vascular 1,419	Cerebro-vascular 5,228	Unintentional Injuries 9,608
4	Heart Disease 128	Heart Disease 61	Congenital Anomalies 35	Heart Disease 26	Heart Disease 214	Heart Disease 716	Homicide 1,375	Cerebro-vascular 763	Unintentional Injuries 867	Bronchitis Emphysema Asthma 2,520	Homicide 8,314
5	Pneumonia and Influenza 123	Malignant Neoplasms 38	Heart Disease 22	(Tied) Congenital Anomalies 17	Malignant Neoplasms 169	Suicide 574	Malignant Neoplasms 1,180	Liver Disease 652	Bronchitis Emphysema Asthma 631	Pneumonia and Influenza 2,375	Cerebro-vascular 8,098
6	Homicide 58	HIV 36	Anemias 10	Suicide 17	HIV 161	Malignant Neoplasms 363	Liver Disease 640	Homicide 618	Diabetes 585	Unintentional Injuries 1,523	HIV 4,202
7	Septicemia 37	Perinatal Period 29	(Tied) HIV 8; Bronchitis, Emphysema, Asthma 8	Bronchitis Emphysema Asthma 15	Congenital Anomalies 49	Pneumonia and Influenza 201	Cerebro-vascular 449	HIV 517	Liver Disease 676	Diabetes 1,430	Pneumonia and Influenza 4,047
8	Meningitis 34	Meningitis 27	Pneumonia and Influenza 8	Pneumonia and Influenza 8	Bronchitis Emphysema Asthma 44	Liver Disease 193	Pneumonia and Influenza 327	Pneumonia and Influenza 401	Pneumonia and Influenza 538	Nephritis 1,190	Perinatal Period 3,693
9	Nephritis 28	Pneumonia and Influenza 23	Pneumonia and Influenza 8	Anemias 4	Pneumonia and Influenza 42	Cerebro-vascular 175	Suicide 285	Diabetes 315	Nephritis 297	Septicemia 1,050	Bronchitis Emphysema Asthma 3,644
10	Cerebro-vascular 28	Anemias 17	Benign Neoplasms 4	Cerebro-vascular 3	Anemias 34	Diabetes 83	Diabetes 210	Bronchitis Emphysema Asthma 226	Homicide 282	Athero-sclerosis 639	Diabetes 2,640

Source: NCHS Mortality Tapes.

*Cause and number of deaths are represented in each cell.

Table 12.2
Ten Leading Causes of Death for Black Females, by Age Group, United States, 1988*

Rank	<1	1-4	5-9	10-14	15-24	25-34	35-44	45-54	55-64	65+	Total
						Age Groups					
1	Perinatal Period 2,906	Unintentional Injuries 266	Unintentional Injuries 182	Unintentional Injuries 124	Homicide 486	Homicide 740	Malignant Neoplasms 1,476	Malignant Neoplasms 2,771	Heart Disease 6,616	Heart Disease 30,236	Heart Disease 39,882
2	Congenital Anomalies 663	Congenital Anomalies 69	Malignant Neoplasms 37	Homicide 56	Unintentional Injuries 417	Unintentional Injuries 610	Heart Disease 1,063	Heart Disease 2,369	Malignant Neoplasms 6,313	Malignant Neoplasms 13,312	Malignant Neoplasms 23,647
3	Unintentional Injuries 121	Homicide 68	Homicide 26	Malignant Neoplasms 38	Malignant Neoplasms 136	Malignant Neoplasms 509	Unintentional Injuries 470	Cerebro-vascular 607	Cerebro-vascular 1,237	Cerebro-vascular 7,924	Cerebro-vascular 10,381
4	Heart Disease 117	Heart Disease 45	Congenital Anomalies 19	Congenital Anomalies 17	Heart Disease 122	HIV 448	Cerebro-vascular 384	Diabetes 336	Diabetes 813	Diabetes 2,948	Diabetes 4,332
5	Pneumonia and Influenza 101	Malignant Neoplasms 41	(Tied) HIV 12	Bronchitis Emphysema Asthma 16	Suicide 71	Heart Disease 383	HIV 320	Liver Disease 313	Bronch. Emphysema Asthma 397	Pneumonia and Influenza 2,270	Unintentional Injuries 3,879
6	Homicide 69	HIV 30	Heart Disease 12	Heart Disease 14	Complicated Pregnancy 50	Cerebro-vascular 165	Liver Disease 317	Unintentional Injuries 292	Liver Disease 320	Nephritis 1,643	Pneumonia and Influenza 3,144
7	Septicemia 45	Pneumonia and Influenza 22	Pneumonia and Influenza 6	Suicide 12	HIV 48	Pneumonia and Influenza 131	Homicide 302	Bronchitis Emphysema Asthma 181	Nephritis 307	Septicemia 1,464	Perinatal Period 2,921
8	Nephritis 35	Anemias 17	Anemias 5	Meningitis 9	(Tied) Anemias 33	Liver Disease 114	Pneumonia and Influenza 154	Pneumonia and Influenza 147	Unintentional Injuries 304	Unintentional Injuries 1,080	Nephritis 2,249
9	Meningitis 28	Meningitis 13	(Tied) -Septicemia 4 -Benign Neoplasms	Benign Neoplasms 8	Pneumonia 33 and Influenza	Suicide 111	Diabetes 149	Nephritis 134	Pneumonia and Influenza 276	Bronchitis Emphysema Asthma 1,046	Homicide 2,089
10	Cerebro-vascular 24	(Tied) -Septicemia 10 -Bronchitis, 10 Asthma, Emphysema, -Perinatal 10 Period	-Bronchitis, Emphysema, 4 Asthma -Mencoccal 4	(Tied) -Anemias 7 -Cerebro-vascular 7	Cerebro-vascular 30	Diabetes 68	Bronchitis, Emphysema, Asthma 96	Homicide 109	Septicemia 232	Atherosclerosis 880	Septicemia 2,011

Source: NCHS Mortality Tapes.

*Cause and number of deaths are represented in each cell.

Figure 12.1
Homicide Rates* by Race** and Sex of Victim, United States, 1979–1988

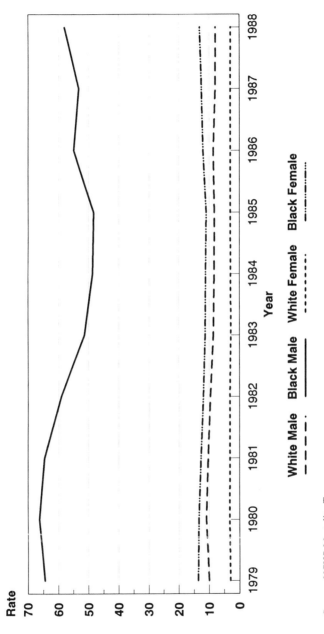

Source: NCHS Mortality Tapes.

*Homicides per 100,000 population.

**Race categories are Black and White only.

Table 12.3
Homicides and Homicide Rates for Black Males, by Age of Victim, United States, 1979–1988*

Year	<1	1-4	5-9	10-14	15-24	25-34	35-44	45-54	55-64	65+	Total
Homicide Rates - Black Males											
1979	18.0	6.2	2.3	4.1	76.9	143.1	113.9	85.5	57.6	30.0	64.5
1980	18.5	7.2	1.9	3.9	83.9	143.0	109.5	83.6	55.3	31.0	66.2
1981	12.2	8.9	2.8	5.2	78.8	136.2	106.5	82.7	52.6	34.7	64.6
1982	17.4	8.9	2.9	3.7	73.3	124.5	92.3	72.8	48.0	31.6	59.1
1983	14.1	7.2	2.1	4.0	66.7	101.3	83.1	57.8	46.6	29.2	51.4
1984	20.6	5.0	2.4	4.0	61.5	96.3	78.2	57.1	40.6	29.6	48.7
1985	16.0	6.5	2.3	4.1	66.1	94.4	76.4	51.1	37.8	25.2	48.4
1986	22.8	9.3	1.9	4.6	79.1	108.1	79.5	56.3	35.4	29.2	55.0
1987	19.4	4.8	2.0	6.8	85.5	99.0	78.5	46.0	32.8	28.5	53.3
1988	19.3	7.5	2.7	5.7	101.8	108.9	79.3	45.3	29.1	27.8	58.1
Homicides - Black Males											
1979	43	60	29	55	2,129	2,653	1,346	868	488	252	7,938
1980	50	70	24	53	2,365	2,854	1,362	858	475	264	8,385
1981	33	90	35	71	2,231	2,877	1,349	853	461	302	8,312
1982	48	92	36	51	2,066	2,739	1,223	756	429	280	7,730
1983	39	77	26	54	1,870	2,307	1,146	607	425	264	6,822
1984	56	54	31	54	1,710	2,264	1,131	607	376	273	6,563
1985	46	70	30	55	1,825	2,285	1,156	550	355	237	6,616
1986	65	102	26	60	2,184	2,688	1,265	615	337	280	7,634
1987	56	53	28	89	2,346	2,522	1,303	514	315	280	7,518
1988	58	84	38	76	2,762	2,827	1,375	518	282	278	8,314

(Age Groups)

Source: NCHS Mortality Tapes.

*Homicides per 100,000 population.

Figure 12.2
Homicide Rates* by Age, Race,** and Sex Groups, United States, 1988

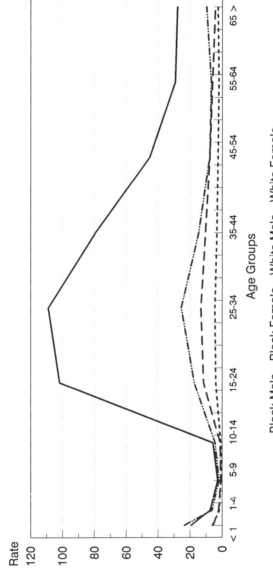

Black Male   Black Female   White Male   White Female

Source: NCHS Mortality Tapes.

*Homicides per 100,000 population.

**Race categories are black and white only.

Although most forms of violent behavior show much higher rates of both victimization and perpetration for males than females, Black females become victims of homicide at a rate greatly exceeding that of White females and also of White males (Figure 12.2). Homicide is the leading cause of death among Black females between 15 and 34 years old, and the second leading cause of death among those 10 to 14 years old. The rate among Black females of all ages increased from 11.2 to 13.2 per 100,000 from 1985 through 1988, with younger females showing the largest increases. Between 1985 and 1988, the rate for females 15 to 24 years old increased from 14.2 to 17.4 per 100,000, while the rate for those 25 to 34 years old rose from 19.8 to 25.5. The most dramatic increase was for Black female infants (less than 1 year), whose rate rose from 10.3 to 23.6 per 100,000 during this 4-year period. While the homicide rate for Black females is still substantially lower than that of Black males, it has risen faster than that of any other race-gender grouping in the United States during recent years.

Considering all types of homicide, both victims and assailants are more likely to be male than female. In 1988, 87 percent of assailants whose sex was recorded were males. In 63 percent of all homicides, both victim and assailant were male; 24 percent involved females killed by males; 11 percent were males killed by females; and in only 2 percent of all cases were both victim and assailant females (U.S. Department of Justice, 1988).

Firearms, Victim-Offender Relationships, and Other Patterns

Weapon choice plays a significant role in determining the outcome of a violent altercation. Firearms are obviously more lethal than other frequently used weapons. In 1988, 61 percent of all homicides involved the use of a firearm, and 75 percent of these were committed with a handgun. While the type of weapon involved depended more on the sex than the race of the victim, Black males continue to be more likely than any other group to be killed with a firearm. Among Black males, 70 percent of all homicides involved the use of a firearm. This compares to 63 percent of all homicides among White males, 46 percent among White females, and 45 percent among Black females (Table 12.4).

The data in Figure 12.3 are also consistent with earlier studies, which have reported that homicides are more likely to involve people who know each other and members of the same racial/ethnic group. In 1988, about half (52%) of victims were killed by family members (14%) or acquaintances (38%). The proportion of females killed by a family member (27%) was considerably higher than the proportion of males killed by a family member (10%). While females are most likely to be killed in domestic disputes, males are more likely to be killed by a nonfamily acquaintance. Females and, to a lesser extent, males are less likely to be killed by a stranger than by someone they know (Figure 12.3).

Among Blacks, 22 percent of all females are killed by family members, and an additional 40 percent are killed by other acquaintances. Their killers are most

Table 12.4
Percentage of Homicide Victims, by Type of Weapon Used, United States, 1988*

Weapon Used	Total	Total White	Total Black	Total Male	White Male	Black Male	Total Female	White Female	Black Female
Total Firearm	61.6	58.3	65.4	67.0	63.4	70.6	45.3	46.9	44.7
Handgun	46.2	41.5	51.5	50.7	45.4	55.7	32.7	31.7	34.6
Rifle	4.2	5.5	2.8	4.3	5.7	2.9	4.0	5.1	2.1
Shotgun	6.3	7.2	5.4	6.6	7.5	5.8	5.5	6.6	4.1
Other Firearm	4.9	4.1	5.7	5.4	4.8	6.2	3.1	2.5	0.1
Knife/Cutting Instrument	18.8	18.4	19.2	18.2	18.1	18.3	20.4	19.0	22.8
Undetermined	3.3	4.0	2.4	2.5	3.2	1.9	5.4	6.0	4.3
Other Weapon**	16.3	19.3	13.0	12.3	15.4	9.2	28.8	29.1	28.2
Total	100.0	100.0	100.0	100.0	100.0	100.0	100.0	100.0	100.0

Source: FBI-SHR.

*1988 FBI data does not include FL or KY

**Including bodily force

likely to be Black males who are emotionally intimate with the victim, such as husbands, boyfriends, or ex-intimates. Blacks accounted for 45.4 percent of all spouse homicide victims in the United States between 1976 and 1985. Their rate of spouse homicide was 8.4 times higher than that for Whites, with Black husbands being somewhat more likely than Black wives to be killed by a spouse (Mercy & Saltzman, 1989).

In the majority of homicides, victims and perpetrators are of the same race. In 1988, 48 percent of all homicides involved Black victims who were killed by Blacks, while 43 percent involved White victims who were killed by Whites. Less than 8 percent were interracial.

SUICIDE AMONG AFRICAN AMERICANS

Suicide in the United States has usually been viewed as a problem affecting primarily White males (Davis, 1979) and the affluent (Earls, Escobar & Manson, 1990). Among non-Whites, only the incidence of suicide among Native Americans has been widely noted (Report of the Secretary's Task Force on Black and Minority Health, Volume 5, 1986). There are several valid reasons for studying

Figure 12.3
Percentage of Homicides by Relationship of Victim to Assailant and Sex of Victim, United States, 1988

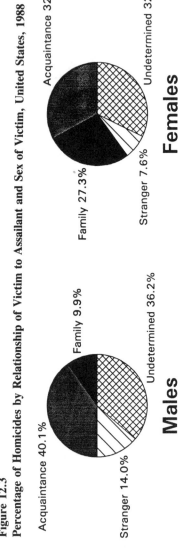

Acquaintance 40.1%

Family 9.9%

Stranger 14.0%

Undetermined 36.2%

Males

Acquaintance 32.9%

Family 27.3%

Stranger 7.6%

Undetermined 32.2%

Females

Source: FBI (SHR) Data used.

suicidal behavior among all minority populations in the United States. Although minority suicide rates are not as high as those found among Whites, it is nevertheless a leading cause of premature death and injury within these populations, including Blacks. Young Black males, who experience high rates of interpersonal violence, also have relatively high rates of suicide (Onwuachi-Saunders, 1987).

Many theories have been advanced to explain suicide among Blacks. The social, economic, and political disadvantages disproportionately associated with African Americans are often translated into the kinds of psychosocial stresses that lead to suicide. Further, as a result of their relatively lower socioeconomic status, Blacks generally experience inferior health care and are less likely to receive adequate treatment for the mental and physical disorders that contribute to the risk of suicide. Cultural beliefs, attitudes, patterns of social support, and conceptions of reality within the Black community may also differ widely from those of the majority population (Griffith & Bell, 1989). These factors may serve either to heighten or to reduce the risk of suicide among Blacks (Davis, 1980).

Rates and Trends, 1979–1988

Data for the period from 1979 to 1988 reveal both similarities and differences in trends and patterns of suicide among Blacks and Whites. During these years, 17,766 suicides occurred among Blacks of both sexes in the United States, approximately 1 suicide every 5 hours.[2] The unadjusted suicide rate for the entire Black population declined from a high of 8.5 deaths per 100,000 population in 1979 to a low of 7.1 in 1983, then rose steadily to a rate of 8.2 in 1988. Age-adjusted rates followed a similar trend. In 1988, Whites had suicide rates (12.2) almost twice the rate for Blacks (6.8), and the rate for Black males (12.2) was more than four times the rate for Black females (2.3).

From 1979 to 1988 there was only a slight change in overall suicide rates for race and gender groupings. White males consistently had the highest rates, and males of all races had higher rates than females. After 1986, Black males replaced males of other races as the group with the second-highest (after White males) rate.[3] These three male groupings were followed in 1988 by White females, females of other races, and then Black females (Figure 12.4). Of all suicides completed in the nation during that year, 72 percent involved White males, 19 percent were White females, 5 percent were Black males, and 1 percent were Black females. The remainder occurred among males and females of other races. The ratio of suicides among males as compared to females is higher for Blacks (4.9) than for Whites (3.9). For both racial groups this ratio increased between 1979 and 1988 (see Figure 12.5).

As noted earlier, from 1979 through 1988 there was an overall decrease (from 1.4 to 6.9) in the age-adjusted suicide rate for African Americans. But while this rate for Black males showed a slight, 5 percent decrease (from 12.8 to 12.2), the female rate declined by 23 percent, from 3.0 to 2.3. In addition, the overall downward trend was not evident for all age groups within the Black population.

Figure 12.4
Suicide Rates by Age Group, Race, and Sex, United States, 1988

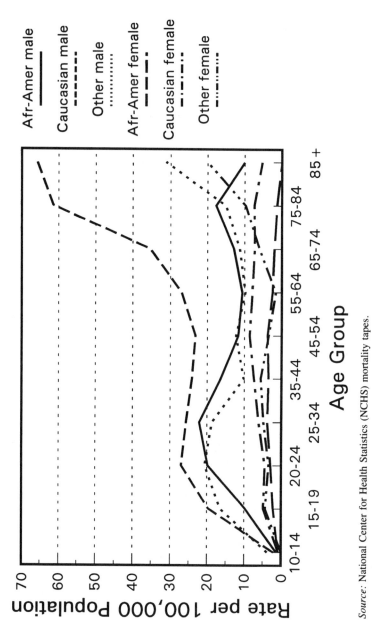

Source: National Center for Health Statistics (NCHS) mortality tapes.

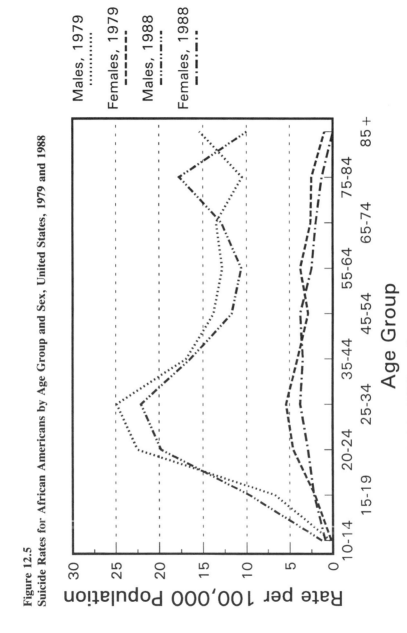

Source: National Center for Health Statistics (NCHS) mortality tapes.

During this period, there was an increase in suicide rates among both Black males and females in the 10–14 age group. The rate for males rose 333 percent from 0.3 to 1.3, while the rate for females rose from 0.2 to 0.9, a 350 percent increase. This magnitude of change reflects the variability of small numbers. On the other hand, from 1979 to 1988, suicide rates for Black males 15–19 years old increased 45 percent (from 6.7 to 9.7), while rates for females in this age group remained essentially the same. For this period, rates for Black males between 75 and 84 increased by 69 percent (from 10.5 to 17.7), while rates among Black males over 85 years of age decreased by 35 percent (from 15.4 to 10.0). The suicide rate for Black females between the ages of 20 and 24 decreased by 37 percent (from 4.6 to 2.9). The rate for Black females between 45 and 54 increased by 31 percent (from 2.9 to 3.8).

In 1988 the suicide rates for Whites and members of other races were highest among the oldest age groups, while among Blacks rates were highest for young adults. Among Black males, the highest rates and the greatest number of suicides occurred within the 20 to 44 age range. From 1979 through 1988 this age group continued to comprise the largest percentage of all Black suicides; indeed, the rates for Black males 25 to 34 years old nearly equaled that for White males of the same age range in 1988 (Figure 12.4).

Methods of Death and Regional Comparisons

The most commonly used method of suicide in the United States is firearms.[4] In 1979, 57 percent of the 27,205 suicides resulted from the use of firearms or explosives. By 1988, this had increased to 60 percent of 30,401 suicides, following a general upward trend that has continued since 1970.[5]

Among African Americans, the percentage of suicides attributed to firearms exceeded the national average in 1979, but by 1988 the national average had surpassed that for Blacks. This was due to a greater increase during the period in the overall percentage of suicides resulting from firearm or explosive use (5%) than that which occurred among Blacks (1%). The method of choice among Black males has remained fairly invariable since 1979, while that of Black females has changed substantially. In both 1979 and 1988, firearms were the leading method of suicide for Black males (60.8 percent and 61.7 percent, respectively), followed by the combined category that includes hanging and strangulation and suffocation (17.4 and 21.0 percent, respectively) (Table 12.5). For Black females, the percentage of suicides attributed to firearm use declined during this period. Though firearms remained the leading method of suicide death, the proportion who died due to poisoning by liquid or solid substances increased.

By geographical area of the country, suicide rates in 1988 among all African Americans ranged from a low of no deaths in several states to 83.8 per 100,000 persons in Montana. Due to the wide differences in the size of Black populations across states, 10-year totals were evaluated and provide the best measure of

Table 12.5

Suicides among African Americans, by Sex and Method of Suicide, United States, 1979 and 1988

Method of Suicide	Number and percent* of suicides by sex and year							
	Males				Females			
	1979		1988		1979		1988	
	Number	Percent	Number	Percent	Number	Percent	Number	Percent
Firearms and Explosives	868	60.8	1,016	61.7	185	48.2	168	44.9
Poisoning by Solids or Liquids	83	5.8	83	5.0	88	22.9	99	26.5
Jumping from height	71	5.0	53	3.2	31	8.1	20	5.4
Hanging, Suffocation and Strangulation	248	17.4	346	21.0	27	7.0	30	8.0
All other means	157	11.0	150	9.1	53	13.8	57	15.2
Total	1,427	100.0	1,648	100.0	384	100.0	374	100.0

Source: NCHS Mortality Tapes.

*Percentages may not add up to 100 due to rounding.

regional differences. Between 1979 and 1988, rates ranged from zero in South Dakota to 32.2 in Montana (see Map, Figure 12.6). Overall, Black rates were lowest in the South over the 10-year time span and were highest in the West.

ASSAULTIVE VIOLENCE AND INJURY

According to the Department of Justice's National Crime Survey (NCS), an estimated 63 million Americans were victims of rape, robbery, or assault during the period between 1979 and 1986 (U.S. Department of Justice, 1989). Of this total, 17.7 million persons suffered an injury, for an average of more than 2.2 million per year. About 1 in 6 of these victims required a hospital stay of 2 or more days for the treatment of gunshot or knife wounds, broken bones, dislodged teeth, unconsciousness, internal trauma, and so forth. Because assaultive violence, including that which leads to serious injury, often goes undetected, the figures above likely underestimate the severity of the problem in the United States.

The sociodemographic profile of the typical nonfatal assault victim mirrors that of homicide victims. Dunn (1976) suggested that many assaults may represent failed homicides, comparable to attempts at suicide for purposes of prevention. Rates of serious assault are highest among males, African Americans, persons between 19 and 24 years of age, the divorced and separated, those earning less than $10,000 annually, and residents of central cities. Of the average 2.2 million persons injured annually, just over 300,000 were Black. Their average annual rate of 14.7 per 100,000 citizens compared to rates of 11.3 for Whites and 12.9 for other races. Such rates tell only part of the story, since there were racial differences in the extent of injury. Among those injured, 23 percent of Blacks experienced a serious injury compared to 20 percent of members of other races and 15 percent of Whites.

PERSPECTIVES ON PREVENTION

The Prevention of Assaultive Injury and Homicide

In response to the high rates of assaultive violence and homicide reported in the paper, the Department of Health and Human Services has included homicide among those priority areas requiring national attention for purposes of prevention (USDHHS, 1990). Since nonfatal assaultive injury is often a precursor of later acts of homicide and itself has significant costs and consequences, it has also been targeted for preventive intervention.

While agreeing that every effort must be made to reduce the tragically high rate of homicide currently found among Blacks, researchers do not always agree as to what modes of intervention offer the best hopes for remedy. Given the diversity of types of homicide and the complex web of factors causing each

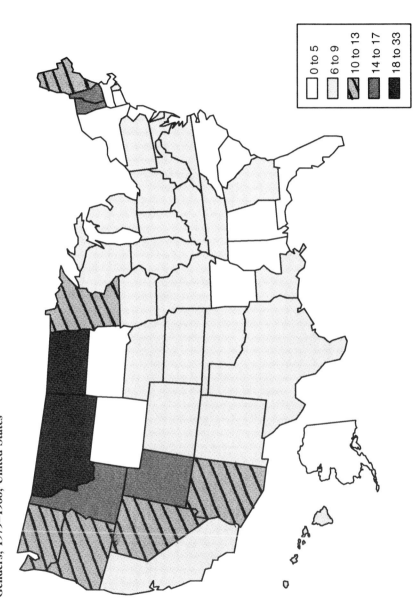

Figure 12.6

Suicide Age-adjusted Death Rate per 100,000 by State, Ages 10 to 85+ Years, African Americans, Both Genders, 1979–1988, United States

Legend:
- 0 to 5
- 6 to 9
- 10 to 13
- 14 to 17
- 18 to 33

Source: NCHS.

incident, no single solution to the prevention of violent injuries and deaths can be expected. Multiple interventions in diverse settings will be necessary.

Although the redress of certain "structural" causal and contributing factors such as poverty and racism are likely to require efforts at the national level, many interventions are most likely to succeed if originated, implemented, and controlled at the community level. Some of the possible interventions that can be incorporated into a community program are mentoring programs, school-based curricula in nonviolent conflict-resolution skills, peer-counseling programs, gun control, and special recreational programs for youth. There is also a desperate need to understand more about the psychosocial aspects of violent behavior (see Hammett et al., 1992; Prothrow-Stith & Weissman, 1991). To this end, more empirical research, especially of an "eclectic" nature, is needed to provide answers and solutions regarding psychosocial aspects of destructive behavior in African-American and other communities.

The Prevention of Suicide: The Identification of Risk Factors

Much of the injury associated with suicide involves the effects of attempts rather than completed acts. The prevention and treatment of such nonfatal injury is important in its own right. Information on unsuccessful suicidal behavior may also help prevent future fatal injury (Dorpat & Ripley, 1976). Hence, much of the research on the prevention of suicide has focused on the analysis of attempts. The Epidemiologic Catchment Area (ECA) study of the National Institute of Mental Health evaluated previous suicidal ideation (thoughts of suicide) and attempted suicides, using a broad sample of the U.S. population. The ECA study was able to measure suicidality among Blacks. Suicidality was defined using an index composed of a person's previous suicidal ideation and attempted suicide.

Using data from this survey, Moscicki et al. (1988) reported that the risk of suicide attempts for Blacks was approximately half (59%) that for non-Blacks/non-Hispanics (predominantly Whites). They also reported that, within the Black population, females and those younger than 45 were at the highest risk for suicidal ideation and attempts. However, studies have not determined what proportion of all attempters actually complete the act of suicide (Earls et al., 1990).

CONCLUSIONS

Our discussion in this chapter has illustrated the extent of injury and death that result from interpersonal aggression and self-directed violence among African Americans. No analysis of the mosaic of health within the Black community can ignore the consequences of these phenomena. Although considerable progress has been made toward treating intentional injury among Blacks as an important public health concern, significant barriers to prevention and intervention persist. These include the belief that suicide and homicide are much less amenable to remedy than are more traditional health and public health problems that affect

Americans and the idea that lower-class populations may be less affected by remedial interventions than more-advantaged groups (Hawkins, 1989).

As a result of such perceptions, the most formidable task to be confronted in the reduction of rates of intentional injury among Blacks may be that of convincing would-be interveners and those who may facilitate interventions (politicians and the larger public) that something can be done to reduce the current rates of homicide and suicide found within African-American communities. There is increasing evidence that many observers have shown a willingness to begin to think of assault, homicide, and suicide as predictable and preventable aspects of social life—yet, much skepticism remains. Through the study and delineation of risk factors and the social conditions that foster or prevent these acts of aggression, we can begin to devise strategies for the reduction of intentional injury among African Americans and others.

NOTES

1. These researchers also reported the rate of homicide among White American males to be higher than that found among males in several other industrialized countries.

2. Unless otherwise noted, suicide deaths for each year between 1979 and 1988, including tables and figures, were derived from national mortality files compiled by the National Center for Health Statistics (NCHS), of the U. S. Department of Health and Human Services.

3. Other races include all racial groups except Whites and Blacks.

4. The category for firearms in the ninth revision of the International Classification of Diseases includes firearms and explosives (E955). However, for all suicides completed in the United States, fewer than 1 percent classified in this category are due to explosives; from 1979 to 1988, none among African Americans was determined to be due to explosives.

5. The number of suicides identified in national vital statistics reflects the judgments of the physicians or coroners who certify the medical and legal cause of death on the death certificate. Suicide statistics are generally felt to underreport the actual number of suicides, but the exact extent of this underreporting is unknown. Several factors may contribute to this underreporting: variability in the criteria for classifying suicide, personal biases, incomplete information, and pressures from the community or from relatives of the dead person. We know little about the extent to which race affects these reporting practices.

REFERENCES

Brearley, H. C. (1932). *Homicide in the United States*. Chapel Hill: University of North Carolina Press.

Centers for Disease Control. (1985). *Suicide Surveillance Report, United States, 1970–1980*. Atlanta: Centers for Disease Control, April.

Davis, R. (1979). Black suicide in the seventies: Current trends. *Suicide and life-threatening behavior, 9*, 131–140.

Davis, R. (1980). Suicide and the relational system: Theoretical and empirical implications of communal and family ties. In *Research in race and ethnic relations*, Vol. 2 (pp. 43–71). Greenwich, CT: JAI Press.

Dorpat, T. L., & Ripley, H. S. (1976). The relationship between attempted suicide and completed suicide. *Comprehensive Psychiatry, 8*, 74–77.

Dunn, C. S. (1976). The patterns and distribution of assault incident characteristics among social areas. *Analytic Report 14*. Law Enforcement Assistance Administration, National Criminal Justice Information and Statistics Service, Washington, DC: Government Printing Office.

Earls, F., Escobar, J. I., & Manson, S. M. (1990). Suicide in minority groups: Epidemiologic and cultural perspectives. In S. J. Blumenthal and D. J. Kupfer (Eds.), *Suicide over the life cycle: Risk factors, assessment, and treatment of suicidal patients.* (pp. 571–598). Washington, DC: American Psychiatric Press.

Farley, R. (1980). Homicide Trends in the United States. *Demography, 17*, 177–188.

Fingerhut, L. A., & Kleinman, J. C. (1990). International and interstate comparisons of homicide among young males. *Journal of the American Medical Association, 263*, 3292–3295.

Griffith, E. E. H., & Bell, C. C. (1989). Recent trends in suicide and homicide among Blacks. *Journal of the American Medical Association, 262*, 2265–2269.

Hammett, M., Powell, K. E., & Clanton, S. T. (1992). *Homicide Surveillance Summary, United States, 1979–1988.* Atlanta: Centers for Disease Control.

Harries, K. D. (1990). *Serious violence: Patterns of homicide and assault in America.* Springfield, IL: C. C. Thomas.

Hawkins, D. F. (1986). *Homicide among Black Americans.* Lanham, MD: University Press of America.

Hawkins, D. F. (1989). Intentional injury: Are there no solutions? *Law, Medicine and Health Care, 17*, 32–41.

Mercy, J. A., & Saltzman, L. E. (1989). Fatal violence among spouses in the United States, 1976–85. *American Journal of Public Health, 79*(5), 595–599.

Moscicki, E. K., O'Carroll, P. W., Rae, D. S., Locke, B. Z., Roy, A., & Regier, D. A. (1988). Suicide attempts in the epidemiologic catchment area study. *Yale Journal of Biology and Medicine, 61*, 259–268.

National Center for Health Statistics. (1990). *Monthly Vital Statistics Report, Advance Report of Final Mortality Statistics, 1988.* DHHS publication number (PHS) 91-1120, Vol. 39, No. 7, Supplement, November. Hyattsville, MD: National for Health Statistics.

National Center for Health Statistics. (1991). Standardized micro-data transcripts—data on vital events, detailed mortality data tapes. Hyattsville, MD: Health Resources Administration.

National Research Council and the Institute of Medicine. (1985). *Injury in America: A continuing public health problem*, Committee on Trauma Research, Commission on Life Sciences, Washington, DC: National Academy Press.

Onwuachi-Saunders, E. C. (1987). The epidemiology of suicide in minorities. In P. Muehrer (Ed.), *Research perspectives on depression and suicide in minorities* (pp. 21–29). Proceedings of workshop sponsored by the National Institute of Mental Health.

Prothrow-Stith, D., & Weissman, M. (1991). *Deadly consequences: How violence is destroying our teenage population and a plan to begin solving the problem.* New York: Harper Collins.

Report of the Secretary's Task Force on Black and Minority Health. (1986). Volume 5: Homicide, suicide and unintentional injuries. U.S. Department of Health and Human Services. Washington, DC: Government Printing Office.

Rose, H. M., & McClain, P. D. (1990). *Race, Place and Risk; Black Homicide in Urban America.* Albany: State University of New York Press.

Rosenberg, M. L., & Fenley, M. A. (1991). *Violence in America: A public health approach.* New York: Oxford University Press.

U.S. Department of Health and Human Services (USDHHS). (1990). Public Health Service. *Year 2000 Health Objectives.* Washington, DC: Government printing Office.

U.S. Department of Justice, Bureau of Justice Statistics. (1989). *Injuries from Crime: Special Report.* May (NCJ-118811).

U.S. Department of Justice, Federal Bureau of Investigation. (1988). *Crime in the United States: Uniform Crime Reports, 1988.* Washington, DC: Government Printing Office.

Wolfgang, M. E. (1958). *Patterns in criminal homicide.* New York: Wiley.

13

Unintentional Injuries: The Problems and Some Preventive Strategies

Christine M. Branche-Dorsey, Julie C. Russell,
Arlene I. Greenspan, and Terence L. Chorba

WHY ARE INJURIES IMPORTANT?

Injury is one of the most serious public health problems facing the United States, claiming over 150,000 lives each year (Baker, O'Neill, Ginsburg & Li, 1992). It is the third leading cause of death nationwide, after heart disease and cancer (Baker et al., 1992) and is the leading cause of death for Americans aged 1 to 44 years. The estimated total lifetime cost of all injuries to society in 1985 was $158 billion (Rice, MacKenzie, et al., 1989).

Among Black Americans, injuries are responsible for more deaths than any other cause (13,487 deaths in 1989) (National Committee for Injury Prevention and Control, 1989). White Americans report more injuries than Black Americans (Ries, 1990) but are less likely to die of injuries than Black Americans (Gulaid, Onwuachi-Saunders, Sacks & Roberts, 1987).

Leading causes of unintentional injury death vary by race. From 1980 through 1986, the three leading causes of unintentional injury death among Black Americans were, in order: motor vehicle crashes (16.88 per 100,000 population), fires and burns (5.52), and drowning (4.22) (Baker et al., 1992). Among White Americans, however, the causes in order were motor vehicle crashes (20.42 per 100,000 population), falls (5.52), and drowning (2.34). The injury burden disproportionately affects the poor, and poor people are disproportionately represented in racial minority groups. In 1984, 33.3 percent of older Black Americans had incomes below the poverty level compared to 5.5 percent of their White American counterparts (U.S. Department of Commerce, 1986). Reliable race and ethnicity data will continue to be essential for identifying injury disparities and teasing out how poverty and race differ as risk factors.

This chapter focuses on unintentional causes of injury and injury death among

Table 13.1
Leading Causes of Unintentional Injury Death, by Race, 1988

Cause	Black American	White American	Total
Motor vehicle crashes-traffic	5,623 (18.6)[‡]	41,974 (20.2)	49,078 (20.0)
Fires and burns	1,682 (5.6)	4,222 (2.0)	5,994 (2.4)
Drowning	945 (3.1)	3,795 (1.8)	4,966 (2.0)
Unintentional firearm	266 (0.9)	1,188 (0.6)	1,501 (0.6)
Occupational[*]	704	5,696	6,400

Source: National Center for Health Statistics, Centers for Disease Control unpublished data, 1991.

*National Traumatic Occupational Fatality System, National Institute for Occupational Safety and Research, Centers for Disease Control, 1985.

‡Rates per 100,000 population in parentheses.

γRates not available.

Black Americans. We have selected motor vehicle crashes, fires and burns, drowning, unintentional use of firearms, and occupational sources for discussion here (see Table 13.1). Other causes of unintentional injury such as poisoning, bicycle crash injuries, and sports-related injuries are important, but they are not the leading causes of injury death among Black Americans. In order to address the identified problem areas more fully, discussions on risk factors and prevention are presented for each injury topic just after the basic epidemiologic data on the problem. Injuries due to violence are described in another chapter under the heading "Intentional Injuries."

MOTOR VEHICLE INJURIES

In the United States, motor vehicle crashes are the leading cause of death among people between 1 and 34 years of age (National Center for Health Statistics, 1991). For persons between 1 and 75 years of age, motor vehicle crashes are the leading cause of fatal injury and are the leading cause of work-related injury deaths (Baker et al., 1992). Crash-related death rates are similar for Black and White Americans (17 per 100,000 population versus 20 per 100,000) (NCHS, 1992). Among Black Americans, motor vehicle fatalities are highest for males ages 20 to 24 years and for females ages 20 to 29 years. Death rates, however, are about three times higher for Black American males (31 per 100,000 population) compared to Black American females (9 per 100,000 population). In the 1980s, some 40,000 to 50,000 persons were killed each year in motor vehicle crashes, and approximately 80 times that number were injured (National Highway Traffic Safety Administration, 1991).

Beyond vital statistics data, collected through death certificates, little is known about the distribution of motor vehicle-related deaths by race. The National Highway Traffic Safety Administration's Fatal Accident Reporting System (FARS), the most prominent of national surveillance systems concerned with vehicular injury, contains detailed information on motor vehicle crashes, but race and ethnicity data are not collected.

From vital statistics data, we know that in 1988 Black American males had nearly twice the pedestrian death rate of White American males, more than three times the death rate of Black American females, and over four times the rate of White American females; these ratios have remained virtually constant over many years (Gulaid et al., 1987). These data may reflect the racial mix of pedestrians, the relative frequency of walking in high-risk environments, as well as the well-known gender differences in risk-taking behaviors.

Risk Factors

Deaths due to motor vehicle injury are not randomly distributed in the population. Patterns and contributing causes of death from crashes vary by race and income. Racial differences in injury rates have often been attributed partially to different patterns of alcohol use. In Wayne County, California, examination of 10 years of medical examiner data revealed that White Americans who were killed in motor vehicle crashes were far more likely to have been drinking than Black Americans so killed (Hain, Ryan & Spitz, 1989).

Other than alcohol, factors influencing racial differences in crash-related morbidity and mortality have not been clearly defined. Motor vehicle death rates have tended to vary inversely with the per capita income of the area of residence (Baker et al., 1992), with the low-income areas experiencing inadequately designed and maintained roads, older vehicles, different driving practices, less adequate emergency and medical care, lower safety-belt use rates (Baker et al., 1992), and lower child-restraint use rates (Wagenaar, Molnar & Margolis, 1988; Baker et al., 1992). Mortality from injuries to child occupants of motor vehicles was directly related to income (Wise, Kotelchuck, Wilson & Mills, 1985), despite comparable access to emergency and tertiary medical services among all racial and income groups in a 1985 Boston study.

Preventive Strategies

Several preventive strategies are important and apply equally to Black and White Americans. Numerous studies indicate that, when used, lap and shoulder safety belts reduce the risk of both fatalities and serious injury to front-seat passenger car occupants by 45 to 50 percent. Research studies have found consistently, however, that safety-belt use is lower among persons in lower socioeconomic or educational categories, where many Black Americans are overrepresented. In a North Carolina study, however, safety-belt use rates among minority drivers have been higher than those among White American drivers in every survey conducted since implementation of that state's mandatory safety-belt legislation (Reinfurt, Campbell, Stewart & Stutts, 1988). The reasons for this differential increase in response to such legislation remain unknown. Safety-belt use, therefore, is one of the most important preventive strategies for Black Americans at this time (Graham et al., 1992).

FIRE AND BURN INJURIES

In 1988, fires and burns caused 5,994 deaths, 28 percent (1,682) of which occurred among Black Americans (NCHS unpublished data, 1991). House fires cause three-fourths of all fire and burn deaths, with smoke inhalation and resulting carbon monoxide poisoning causing two-thirds of these deaths (NCIPC, 1989). Each year, about 54,000 persons are hospitalized due to burns, and 1.4 million people experience less severe burn injuries that do not require hospitalization (Rice et al., 1989). A severe nonfatal burn may result in permanent scarring and disability. While scalds are the most common burn injury, flame burns are the most severe (McLoughlin & McGuire, 1990).

Minority populations, the very young, and the elderly are groups at increased risk for fire or burn death. The house-fire death rate among Black Americans is more than double that for White Americans (Baker et al., 1992). Males are at higher risk of both fatal and nonfatal injuries resulting from fire and burns, although the risk differences between the sexes are not as great as for other injuries (Burn Foundation, 1988).

Findings from Gulaid, Sacks, and Sattin (1989) show that elderly Black Americans had a nearly five-fold higher residential fire death rate than White Americans. Among persons older than 65 years, fire death rates increase with increasing age. Elderly Black American males are at highest risk of all age-race groups for death from residential fires, and elderly Black American females are at a higher risk than White Americans of either sex (McLoughlin & McGuire, 1990).

Risk Factors

The most common ignition source in house fires is a lighted cigarette dropped on furniture or bedding (Robertson et al., 1992), which appears to be true for

Black American homes as well (Gulaid, Sacks & Sattin, 1989). Cigarette smoking has been associated with about half of all U.S. residential fire deaths; among older people, smoking was implicated in 9 percent of burn injuries (Rossignol, Locke, Boyle & Burke, 1985; Baker et al., 1992). Fires ignited by cigarettes, furthermore, are more likely to involve the use of alcohol than fires due to other causes (Baker et al., 1992). Other sources are scalds, electrical sources, chemicals, and radiation.

Among older persons, burns are often due to clothing ignition associated with cooking; one-third occur in the kitchen. Many older persons are at increased risk for dying in residential fires because they have physical or medical conditions (Gulaid, Sacks & Sattin, 1989) that diminish their chances of escape from a fire (NCIPC, 1989). These factors include lack of mobility and decreased physical coordination, the effect of sleeping medication, impaired sense of smell, arthritic hands, and slower reaction time (Beverly, 1976; Gulaid, Sacks & Sattin, 1989). These limitations accentuate the difficulty of escaping fires in multistory buildings. In fact, older persons living in 3- to 4-story buildings have a death rate 3 to 6 times higher than people in single-story buildings (Ducic & Ghezzo, 1980).

The increased risk of fire-related death among older Black Americans may be related, in part, to poverty also; racial differences in death rates due to house fires diminish in higher-income areas (Baker et al., 1992). Many studies have shown a relationship between residential fire deaths and poverty. Poverty, in turn, is associated with substandard housing, lack of smoke detector use, and faulty heating and lighting systems (Baker et al., 1992).

Among Black Americans, house-fire death rates are twice as high in rural areas compared to other areas, whereas little variation by place of residence is evident among White Americans (Baker et al., 1992). Fire- and burn-related deaths, however, also tend to cluster in city neighborhoods (Robertson et al., 1992).

Preventive Strategies

Given the implications of cigarettes, clothing, and housing construction in fire-related injury and death, satisfactory approaches for prevention are possible. To reduce the potential for cigarettes to ignite upholstery or bedding, the manufacture of self-extinguishing cigarettes is a reasonable and technically feasible solution. The standards governing flammability in fabrics for children's clothing may be appropriate to apply also to clothing for older persons. Physicians should counsel their adult patients about the benefits of smoke detectors as a primary prevention strategy. Finally, the enforcement of effective residential building codes, which include requirements for smoke detectors and antiscald devices, is in order (Robertson et al., 1992).

DROWNINGS

About 5,000 people drown in this country each year, making drowning the fourth leading cause of unintentional injury death. According to 1985 figures, drowning and near-drowning costs $2.5 billion dollars (NCIPC, 1989), including rescue, hospitalization, and rehabilitation costs.

Drowning rates are highest mainly for two age groups: children under 5 years and persons 15 through 24 years (Gulaid & Sattin, 1988). Drowning rates were almost 4 times greater for males than for females during the years 1978 through 1984 (Gulaid & Sattin, 1988). This male-female difference is evident in every year from childhood through older age (Wintemute, Kraus, Teret & Wright, 1988).

Overall, the U.S. rates for Black Americans are twice those of White Americans (Gulaid & Sattin, 1988; Wintemute et al., 1987); however, this is not true for all age groups. For example, White American children from ages 1 to 4 years have twice the drowning rate of Black American children of these ages, largely because of drownings in residential swimming pools, but for children aged 5–19 years, Black Americans drown 2 to 4 times more often than White Americans (Rodriguez & Brown, 1990). According to data for which racial information is available, Black Americans drown in a variety of settings, but more data on specific risk factors are needed to fully understand their role in drownings among Black Americans.

Risk Factors

There are several known and suspected risk factors for drowning, which differ by age group. Overall, between one-half and three-quarters of drownings occur in lakes, ponds, rivers, and the ocean (Dietz & Baker, 1974; Centers for Disease Control [CDC], 1986), but drownings among young children usually occur in water sources around the household including bathtubs, buckets, toilets, large puddles, and swimming pools (Robertson et al., 1992), even in urban settings. Lapses in adult supervision caused by chores, socializing, or phone calls are implicated in most drowning incidents among children under 5 years of age. The danger of drowning in this age group also increases with the number of children present because of the difficulty of supervising several children at once (Robertson et al., 1992), and a lapse in adult supervision does not have to be long—in one study, young pool-drowning victims were out of sight for 5 or fewer minutes (Present, 1987).

Among adolescents and adults, drowning occurs during swimming, wading, and boating in natural bodies of water, particularly when alcohol is used in these settings (Patetta & Biddinger, 1988; Wintemute, Kraus, Teret & Wright, 1988). Forty to forty-five percent of drownings in these age groups occur during swimming (Dietz & Baker, 1974; CDC, 1986), while 12–29 percent are associated with boating (Gulaid & Sattin, 1988; Dietz & Baker, 1974). More than 50 million persons engage in various recreational (noncommercial) boating activities on at least 8 days per year (CDC, 1987), and more White Americans than Black Americans drown in boat-related incidents; but little data exist on Black Americans, their boating habits, and their drowning risks while boating.

Preventive Strategies

Black American parents need to constantly supervise their young children around all household and outdoor water sources to prevent drownings in this age group. Here is another area where physician counseling may be appropriate to warn parents of how quickly their children can drown.

For adolescent and adult Black Americans there remain many gaps in our complete understanding of risk factors for drowning. Recently federal health agencies have called for more research in drowning among Black Americans and other minority populations (Robertson et al., 1992), especially the circumstances of drowning. Some of the questions raised include these: (a) Are Black Americans who drown less likely to know how to swim? If so, are the waters in which they drown appropriate for swimming only or for boating and other activities only? (b) What is the clear relationship between alcohol use and water recreation injuries, including drowning?

UNINTENTIONAL FIREARM INJURIES

Firearms are the second leading cause of fatal injury (Baker et al., 1992). Unintentional firearm deaths account for about 5 percent of all fatal shootings, resulting in approximately 1,500 deaths annually. Unintentional shootings disproportionately affect youth nationwide. From 1982 through 1988, 32 percent of all unintentional firearm-related deaths occurred to children and teenagers below the age of 20. Of those, 81 percent occurred among those 10–19 years old (CDC, 1992), making unintentional shootings the third leading cause of unintentional injury death in this age group (Baker et al., 1992). Little is known about the incidence of nonfatal unintentional firearm-related injuries. In one study, the U.S. General Accounting Office (USGAO, 1991) estimated the ratio of nonfatal to fatal unintentional firearm-related injuries as 105 to 1, but this was based on data from only 10 U.S. cities.

Males are far more likely to die from an unintentional shooting than females. For Black Americans, the death rate for males is six times the rate for females. Males aged 15–19 are at higher risk (2.41 per 100,000) than are males in any other age group (CDC, 1992). While unintentional firearm-related fatalities peak for Black and White American males at 15–19 years, Black American males demonstrate a much more gradual decline with increasing age than their White American counterparts. In fact, the death rates for Black American males do not approach those of White American males until ages 55–59. For boys aged

1–4 years and 5–9 years, death rates for Black American males were twice those of White American males during 1988 (Fingerhut, Kleinman, Godfrey & Rosenberg, 1991). Despite these differences in age-specific rates, race differences for unintentional firearm-related fatalities are less than those for homicide (Fingerhut et al., 1991), with the unintentional firearm death rate for Black American males 1.3 times that of White American males for 1982–1988.

In contrast to males, White American females are at highest risk for an unintentional firearm-related death at ages 20–24 (0.25 per 100,000), while death rates for Black American females do not peak until 30–34 years (0.40 per 100,000) (CDC, unpublished data). Overall, Black American females were 1.5 times more likely to die from an unintentional shooting than were White American females during 1982–1988.

Although rates for unintentional firearm-related fatalities are somewhat higher for Black Americans when compared with White Americans, they are almost identical for Black and White Americans living in low-income areas (Baker et al., 1992). Furthermore, Baker et al. (1992) found an inverse relationship between per capita income of the area of residence and unintentional firearm-related mortality.

Overall, males living in the South and the West and those living in nonmetropolitan or rural areas are at greatest risk (Baker et al., 1992; CDC, 1992). White American males, however, are at greatest risk in the South (1.8 per 100,000), while Black American males are at greatest risk in the West (2.4 per 100,000) (CDC, unpublished data). Comparing metropolitan and nonmetropolitan areas, White American male children and teenagers aged 15–19 are more than twice as likely to die from an unintentional shooting if they live in a nonmetropolitan area, while there is essentially no difference in risk for Black American males aged 15–19 (CDC, 1992).

Despite differing patterns of mortality by geographic region, most fatalities occur at a residence and usually occur at the victim's home (Beaver et al., 1990; Morrow & Hudson, 1986; Wintemute et al., 1989). This is especially true for children. In a Maryland study, Beaver et al. (1990) found that 75 percent of unintentional fatal gunshot wounds in children below the age of 17 occurred at a residence; in those cases in which information existed about location of the weapon, 98 percent were unsecured. Even in predominantly rural areas most fatalities appear to be associated with shootings that occur in a residence (Morrow & Hudson, 1986).

Risk Factors

Specific factors that place Black Americans at risk for unintentional firearm-related injuries are not entirely clear. Mortality due to unintentional shootings may have less to do with race than with socioeconomic status (Klein, Reizen, Van Amburg & Walker, 1977). More studies are needed to identify race-specific factors that place Black Americans at risk for unintentional firearm-related injuries.

Preventive Strategies

Strategies to reduce morbidity and mortality should be aimed at limiting access to loaded weapons. This is especially true for children and adolescents who are at high risk for an unintentional firearm-related injury. Firearms should be stored unloaded and in a locked cabinet, with ammunition stored separately.

Modifying firearms and ammunition to render them less lethal has also been advocated as a preventive strategy (Baker et al., 1992; Christoffel, 1991). Findings from a recent study conducted by the GAO (1991) have demonstrated that the addition of childproof safety devices would prevent children below the age of 6 from discharging a firearm, while the use of loading indicators could prevent an estimated 23 percent of all unintentional firearm-related deaths. Regulation to control the amount of gunpowder and the shape and jacketing of ammunition has also been advocated as a means of reducing the severity of nonfatal firearm-related injuries (Christoffel, 1991; Robertson et al., 1992).

OCCUPATIONAL INJURIES

In 1989 Black Americans accounted for 11 percent of the civilian labor force (13.5 million workers) (Bureau of the Census, 1991) and 12.2 percent of the population in general. Recent studies indicate, however, that work-related fatal injury rates for Black Americans are higher than those for White Americans (7.7 versus 6.5 injury deaths per 100,000 workers) (Bell et al., 1990). For nonfatal work-related injuries, which account for 36 percent of all injuries requiring medical attention or restriction of activities, rates are similar for Black and White Americans (9.2 versus 9.9 per 100 persons per year) (Wagener & Winn, 1991).

Risk Factors

Historically, Black American workers have often been hired to work in jobs with the highest exposures to disease and injury-producing agents. According to 1987 data, Black American workers were still overrepresented in blue-collar jobs, where they are more likely to be exposed to work-related hazards, and were underrepresented in most white-collar occupations (15.2% of blue-collar jobs are held by Black Americans versus 8.8% of white-collar jobs) (Rubenstein, 1992). Excess fatalities and disabilities due to occupational illnesses, such as cancers and respiratory diseases, among Black American workers are well documented (Davis, 1980). A study based on data from the 1970s showed that Black American workers were more likely to be in a hazardous occupation than White American workers, and this relationship remained after controlling for differences in education and job experience (Robinson, 1984). A 1972 Social Security survey, furthermore, indicated that Black American workers are less likely to report occupational diseases than White American workers even though they are more likely to be severely disabled (Krute & Burdette, 1978). Underreporting probably occurs for work-related injuries too.

No data sources currently exist that include information both on job-specific health and safety hazards and exposures and on the racial and ethnic composition of the workers in those jobs (Rubenstein, 1992). National statistics on fatal work-related injuries by race are not available for years prior to 1980 (Bell et al., 1990). The U.S. Bureau of Labor Statistics (BLS) has not collected injury information by race in the past. This information, however, will be included in the BLS annual survey of employers in the private sector beginning in 1993.

The lack of historical data documenting the incidence of occupational injuries by race hinders efforts to understand the impact of discriminatory employment practices on occupational injuries among Black American workers. Davis (1980) describes some practices that place minority workers in high-risk jobs such as hiring certain categories of workers for the more dangerous jobs, exploiting low-income workers who are seasonally employed or dependent on small and marginal businesses (i.e. farm-workers and elderly and younger workers), and limiting access of minority workers to on-the-job training.

Robinson (1984, 1989) asserts that Black American workers may receive inadequate protection from work-related hazards because government programs, which are in place to protect against discrimination in terms of wages (Equal Employment Opportunity Commission), do not take into account unequal exposure to health and safety hazards. If discrimination exists against Black American workers in terms of wages, then it is likely there is also discrimination with respect to the allocation of workers between jobs with different levels of hazard, thus placing Black American workers at greater risk for work-related injuries. For example, a Black American worker can receive the same pay as a White American worker for a job with the same title but still be assigned to a more hazardous working environment. This problem is not addressed by the Federal Occupational Safety and Health Administration, created to promulgate and enforce standards limiting hazardous workplace exposures, which does not specifically target high-risk racial or ethnic groups of workers. Another problem facing Black American workers is employment practices that prevent them from moving out of unskilled into skilled jobs by limiting access to education and on-the-job training.

Preventive Strategies

Eliminating racial inequality in working conditions is critical to improving the health of Black Americans and other minority groups in the long run (Rubenstein, 1992). Enforcing safe working practices and supplying personal protective equipment on a large scale would be a first step toward reducing work-related morbidity and mortality. Creative and aggressive implementation and enforcement of labor laws is warranted. Employers need to ensure that Black American employees receive equal on-the-job training to assure equal opportunities to advance to higher-level jobs (Rubenstein, 1992). Workers need to be educated to recognize work-related hazards and to be protected from retribution by employers for reporting unsafe working conditions. In addition, studies are needed to establish race-specific data on workplace exposures and rates of excess morbidity (Rubenstein, 1992). These studies should provide needed data that would support appropriate intervention strategies.

CONCLUSIONS

Black Americans have higher injury rates due to pedestrian motor vehicle-related crashes, fires and burns, drowning, and unintentional use of firearms compared to their White American counterparts. Injury rates are equivocal by race for occupational injuries, and adequate injury-rate data by race are unavailable at this time to make a clear statement about the differences in risk for motor vehicle crashes.

Much of what we know about injury rates by race or ethnicity appear only as nonspecific data. We need injury research that will help us better understand the problem of injuries in Black Americans. This can be accomplished most effectively through research focused on minority groups, especially Black Americans. In such research, race as a variable needs to be used judiciously. In health research, race has long served as a proxy for powerful social inequities in the United States (Wise & Purlsey, 1992); how people live, die, and get sick or injured may depend more on socioeconomic class or income than on race (Navarro, 1990). Unfortunately, when race is reported as a variable in research, there is a tendency to assume that the results obtained manifest something about biology or genetics to explain differences in incidence or severity of outcomes, without regard to social, economic, or political factors (Osborne & Feit, 1992). Race- and cause-specific risk factors must be identified but used carefully, like any other demographic data, to guide prevention strategies to reduce the injury burden on persons of all races.

Government agencies and universities sponsor research on a variety of topics, and they must play a role in sponsoring and conducting research relevant to the Black American community. In addition, community-based prevention strategies need to be developed and evaluated to determine their efficacy and feasibility. Finally, in some cases, regulation may be necessary to ensure that preventive strategies are implemented.

Research objectives for injuries among Black Americans must:

- Provide or improve injury surveillance systems, including variables for race and ethnicity, and the circumstances and locations of injury.
- Include studies to determine specific risk factors for injury among Black Americans and other minority groups, such as (a) non-use of safety belts,

(b) drowning and near-drowning and boating injuries, (c) burns among older persons, (d) unintentional firearm-related injuries, and (e) the impact of discriminatory practices in occupational injuries.

• Develop and evaluate studies that implement preventive strategies known to have some benefit. Some of these include programs to (a) prevent pedestrian injury, fire and burn injury, and drowning; (b) routinely change batteries in smoke detectors when clocks are changed to standard time each fall; (c) encourage utility companies to check hot water temperatures when meters are read; (d) encourage owners to store firearms unloaded and in a secured and locked storage compartment with ammunition stored separately; and (e) encourage manufacturers to modify firearms and ammunition to render them less lethal.

Our regulatory or enforcement recommendations are to (a) adopt and enforce safety belt use laws and ordinances; (b) strengthen and enforce existing laws and ordinances requiring child safety seat use and extend them to cover all passenger seating positions in all motorized vehicles; (c) require cigarettes sold in the United States to have a low potential for igniting upholstered furniture; (d) apply flammable-fabrics standards to loose-fitting housecoats and bathrobes now commonly worn by older persons who are burned while cooking and smoking; and (e) develop, implement, and enforce codes to address burns in residences, including codes requiring smoke detectors and antiscald devices in hot-water systems.

REFERENCES

Baker, S. P., O'Neill, B., Ginsburg, M. J., & Li, G. (1992). *The Injury Fact Book* (2nd ed.). New York: Oxford University Press.

Beaver, B. L., Moore, V. L., Peclet, M., Haller, J. A., Jr., Smialek, J., & Hill, J. L. (1990). Characteristics of pediatric firearm fatalities. *Journal of Pediatric Surgery, 25,* 97–100.

Bell, C. A., Stout, N. A., Bender, T. R., Conroy, C. S., Crouse, W. E., & Myers, J. R. (1990). Fatal occupational injuries in the United States, 1980–1985. *Journal of the American Medical Association, 266,* 3047–3050.

Beverly, E. V. (1976). Reducing fire and burn hazards among the elderly. *Geriatrics, 31,* 106.

Burn Foundation. (1988). *Burn causes and treatment costs from 1987 Burn Center Admission Data.* Philadelphia, PA: Author.

Centers for Disease Control (CDC). (1986). North Carolina drownings, 1980–1984. *Morbidity & Mortality Weekly Report, 35,* 635–638.

Centers for Disease Control. (1987). Recreational boating fatalities—Ohio, 1983–1986. *Morbidity and Mortality Weekly Report, 36,* 321–324.

Centers for Disease Control. (1992). Unintentional firearm-related fatalities among children and teenagers—United States, 1970–1984. *Morbidity & Mortality Weekly Report, 41,* 442–445, 451.

Christoffel, K. K. (1991). Toward reducing pediatric injuries from firearms: Charting a legislative and regulatory course. *Pediatrics, 88,* 294–305.

Davis, M. E. (1980). The impact of workplace health and safety on black workers: Assessment and prognosis. *Labor Law Journal, 31,* 723–732.

Dietz, P., & Baker, S. (1974). Drowning: Epidemiology and prevention. *American Journal of Public Health, 64,* 303-312.

Ducic, S., & Ghezzo, H. R. (1980). Epidemiology of accidental home fires in Montreal. *Accident Analysis and Prevention, 12,* 67.

Fingerhut, L. A., Kleinman, J. C., Godfrey, E., & Rosenberg, H. (1991). Firearm mortality among children, youth, and young adults 1–34 years of age, trends and current status: United States, 1979–1988. *Monthly Vital Statistics Report, 39* (Supp. 11), 1–14.

Graham, J., Waller, P., Chorba, T., et al. (1992). Motor Vehicle Injury Prevention. In *Position papers from the Third National Injury Control Conference, Setting the National Agenda for Injury Control in the 1990's.* Atlanta, GA: Centers for Disease Control.

Gulaid, J. A., Onwuachi-Saunders, E. C., Sacks, J. J., & Roberts, D. R. (1987). Differences in death rates due to injury among Blacks and Whites. *Morbidity and Mortality Weekly Report, 37* (SS-3), 25–31.

Gulaid, J. A., Sacks, J. J., & Sattin, R. W. (1989). Deaths from residential fires among older people, United States, 1984. *Journal of the American Geriatrics Society, 37,* 331–334.

Gulaid, J. A., & Sattin, R. W. (1988). Drowning in the United States, 1978–1984. *Morbidity and Mortality Weekly Report, 37,* 27–33.

Hain, J. R., Ryan, D. M., & Spitz, W. U. (1989). Fatal accidents and blood ethanol levels in adolescents and adults. The Wayne County experience (1978–1988). *American Journal of Forensic Medicine and Pathology, 10,* 187–192.

Klein, D., Reizen, M. S., Van Amburg, G. H., & Walker, S. A. (1977). Some social characteristics of young gunshot fatalities. *Accident Analysis & Prevention, 9,* 177–182.

Krute, A., & Burdette, M. E. (1978). 1972 Survey of disabled and nondisabled adults: Chronic disease, injury, and work disability. *Social Security Bulletin, 11.*

McLoughlin, E., & McGuire, A. (1990). The causes, cost, and prevention of childhood burn injuries. *American Journal of Diseases in Children, 144,* 677–683.

Morrow, P. L., & Hudson, P. (1986). Accidental firearm fatalities in North Carolina, 1976–1980. *American Journal of Public Health, 76,* 1120–1123.

National Center for Health Statistics (NCHS). (1991). *Health, United States, 1990,* DHHS publication No. (PHS) 91-1232. Washington, DC: Government Printing Office.

National Center for Health Statistics. (1992). *Health, United States, 1991,* DHHS publication No. (PHS) 92-1232. Washington, DC: Government Printing Office.

National Committee for Injury Prevention and Control (NCIPC). (1989). *Injury Prevention: Meeting the challenge.* New York: Oxford University Press.

National Highway Traffic Safety Administration. (1991). *Fatal accident reporting system, 1990.* Department of Transportation publication No. HS-807-794. Washington, DC: Author.

Navarro, V. (1990). Race or class versus race and class: Mortality differentials in the United States. *Lancet, 336,* 1238–1240.

Osborne, N. G., & Feit, M. D. (1992). The use of race in medical research. *Journal of the American Medical Association, 267,* 275–279.

Patetta, M. J., & Biddinger, P. W. (1988). Characteristics of drowning deaths in North Carolina. *Public Health Report, 103,* 406–411.

Present, P. (1987). *Child drowning study: A report on the epidemiology of drownings in residential pools to children under age five.* Washington, DC: U.S. Consumer Product Safety Commission, Directorate for Epidemiology.

Reinfurt, D. W., Campbell, B. J., Stewart, J. R., & Stutts, J. C. (1988). *North Carolina's Occupant Restraint Law: A Three Year Evaluation.* Chapel Hill: University of North Carolina, Highway Safety Research Center.

Rice, D. P., MacKenzie, E. J., Jones, A. S., Kaufman, S. R., DeLissovoy, G. V., Max, W., McLoughlin, E., Miller, T. R., Robertson, L. S., Salkever, D. S., Smith, G. S. (1989). *Cost of injury in the United States: A report to Congress.* San Francisco: Johns Hopkins University, Injury Prevention Center, University of California, Institute for Health and Aging.

Ries, P. W. (1990). Health of black and white Americans. In *Vital and Health Statistics,* DHHS publication No. (PHS) 90-1599, National Center for Health Statistics. Washington, DC: Government Printing Office.

Robertson, L., Stallones, L., Branche-Dorsey, C. M., et al. (1992). Home and Leisure Injury Prevention. In *Position papers from the Third National Injury Control Conference, Setting the National Agenda for Injury Control in the 1990's.* Atlanta, GA: Centers for Disease Control.

Robinson, J. C. (1984). Racial inequality and the probability of occupation-related injury or illness. *Milbank Memorial Fund Quarterly/Health and Society, 62,* 567–590.

Robinson, J. C. (1989). Trends in racial inequality and exposure to work-related hazards, 1968–1986. *American Occupational Health Nurses Journal, 37,* 56–63.

Rodriguez, J. G., & Brown, S. T. (1990). Childhood injuries in the United States. *American Journal of Diseases in Children, 144,* 627–646.

Rossignol, A. M., Locke, J. A., Boyle, C. M., & Burke, J. F. (1985). Consumer products and hospitalized burn injuries among elderly Massachusetts residents. *Journal of the American Geriatrics Society, 33,* 768–772.

Rubenstein, H. L. (1992). Minority workers. In J. M. Last (Ed.), *Public Health and Preventive Medicine* (13th ed.). Norwalk, CT: Appleton & Lange.

U.S. Bureau of the Census. (1991). *Statistical Abstract of the United States* (111th Ed.). Washington, DC: Author.

U.S. Department of Commerce. (1986). *Bureau of the Census, Current population report.* (Series P-60 No. 152.) Characteristics of the population below the poverty level, 1984. Washington, DC: Author.

U.S. General Accounting Office. (1991). Accidental Shootings. Many Deaths and Injuries Caused by Firearms Could be Prevented. *Report to the Chairman, Subcommittee on Antitrust, Monopolies, and Business Rights, Committee on the Judiciary,* U.S. Senate (GAO/PEMD-91-9). Washington, DC: Author.

Wagenaar, A. C., Molnar, L. J., & Margolis, L. H. (1988). Characteristics of child safety seat users. *Accident Analysis and Prevention, 20,* 311–322.

Wagener, D. K., & Winn, D. W. (1991). Injuries in working populations: Black-white differences. *American Journal of Public Health, 81,* 1408–1414.

Wintemute, G. J., Kraus, J. F., Teret, S. P., & Wright, M. A. (1987). Drowning in childhood and adolescence: A population-based study. *American Journal of Public Health, 77*, 830–832.

Wintemute, G. J., Kraus, J. F., Teret, S. P., & Wright, M. A. (1988). The epidemiology of drownings in adulthood: Implications for prevention. *American Journal of Preventive Medicine, 4*, 343–348.

Wintemute, G. J., Kraus, J. F., Teret, S. P., & Wright, M. A. (1989). Unintentional firearm deaths in California. *Journal of Trauma, 29*, 457–461.

Wise, P. H., Kotelchuck, M., Wilson, M. L., & Mills, M. (1985). Racial and socio-economic disparities in childhood mortality in Boston. *New England Journal of Medicine, 313*, 360–366.

Wise, P. H., & Purlsey, D. M. (1992). Infant mortality as a social mirror. *New England Journal of Medicine, 326*, 1558–1559.

14

Chemical Use and Dependency among African Americans

Gerald Groves and Omowale Amuleru-Marshall

This chapter will review the epidemiology of alcohol, tobacco and other drug use and dependency among African Americans. This review will reveal that these are areas of significant morbidity and mortality and that African Americans suffer a higher proportion of problems associated with alcohol and other drug use/dependence than do other groups. This overall pattern exists despite anomalous findings that there are more Black than White abstainers and that Black rates of use and dependence are lower than White rates up to age 29. The authors argue that substance abuse problems are rooted in the oppressive cultural, socioeconomic, and political characteristics of Black life in the United States. Treatment efforts must acknowledge these circumstances and prevention efforts must seek to ameliorate them if problems associated with the use of psychotropic substances are to be prevented and mitigated.

EPIDEMIOLOGY

The Epidemiologic Catchment Area program (ECA) yields direct estimates of the national prevalence of alcohol and other drug abuse/dependence disorders in the United States. The ECA data were collected in the early 1980s, when substance abuse/dependence was still on the rise and before the crack epidemic became fully established. More recent data on "the use of illicit drugs, alcohol, and tobacco among members of the U.S. household population aged 12 and older" are available from the National Household Survey on Drug Abuse (NHSDA).

The ECA and the NHSDA are the major sources of the rates quoted below. Both the ECA and NHSDA 1990 and 1991 concur that alcohol and tobacco are the most used and abused substances in the United States, in general, and among African Americans, in particular.

Alcohol Consumption

If alcohol and other drug-use (AOD) disorders are combined into a single category of "substance-abuse disorders," then the national lifetime prevalence rate estimated from the ECA and undifferentiated by race is 17 percent. This lifetime rate is higher than that for any single psychiatric disorder estimated by the ECA study. Within that category, the rate for alcohol abuse/dependence was 13.8 percent and the rate for other drug abuse/dependence was 6.2 percent (Robbins, Locke & Regier, 1991).

For the country as a whole, rates of substance use appear to have been falling since peaking in the early to mid-1980s. This is supported by NHSDA 1990 and 1991 (NIDA, 1991a, 1991c). However, in 1992 the Department of Health and Human Services reported a rise in cocaine-related emergency room visits to unprecedented levels and a 15 percent increase in heroin-related emergency room visits (Treaster, 1992). Although casual use may be down, use among committed abusers of cocaine and heroin may not be.

Rates of alcohol abuse and dependence are higher than those of other drug abuse and dependence for African and other Americans. In the ECA, lifetime prevalence for alcohol abuse/dependence were surprisingly similar for Black and White persons in the aggregate, 13.8 percent and 13.6 percent, respectively, and somewhat higher for Latinos at 16.7 percent. Within each gender, lifetime prevalence was similar for African and European Americans, higher for Latino men, and lower for Latino women. In all ethnic groups, the lifetime prevalence for men was considerably higher than for women at every age level. Among both men and women, age-specific rates of lifetime, one-year, and one-month prevalence were higher for African Americans than for European Americans except for the age groups 18–29 and over 65 (Helzer, Burnam & McEvoy, 1991).

Alcohol is by far the most frequently used drug in the United States (NIDA, 1991a). According to the NHSDA, lifetime, past year, and past month prevalence figures for alcohol use among African Americans were 76.6, 55.6, and 43.7 percent, respectively. The highest lifetime and past-month prevalence in this population occurred in the 26–34 age group, and the highest past-year prevalence was in the 18–25 age group followed closely by the 26–34 age group. The 12–17 age group exhibited the lowest prevalence for all three reference periods. For all age groups and both sexes, Black rates were lower than White rates. Male rates were higher than female rates for both Black and White groups, with the exception of the 12–17 age group. Indeed, male gender is the strongest predictor of alcohol use. Only 4.2 percent of African Americans, compared to 6.9 percent of European Americans and 5.5 percent of Latino Americans, reported daily consumption of alcohol. Twenty-one percent of the total sample of the NHSDA reported one or more components of alcohol dependence in the preceding year.

Tobacco Use

The lifetime prevalence of tobacco dependence was 36 percent in the one ECA site in which it was ascertained in the early 1980s. Tobacco use continues to reflect a higher prevalence among African Americans than among European Americans. In 1987, Black Americans 20 years of age and over were more often current smokers and less often former smokers than their White counterparts. Fully 40.3 percent of Black men and 27.9 percent of Black women were current smokers in 1987, contrasted with 30.7 percent and 27.3 percent among White men and women, respectively. While trend data indicated a general decline in the proportion of light smokers (less than 15 cigarettes per day) among those who smoke, between 1965 and 1985, Black men and women who smoked were less likely to be heavy smokers (25 or more cigarettes per day) than their White counterparts (Health Resources and Services Administration, 1990).

Illicit Drug Use

Data from the ECA indicate that the lifetime prevalence rates for drug abuse/ dependence, other than alcohol, caffeine, and tobacco, were highest for European Americans and lowest for Latino Americans while African Americans displayed an intermediate rate (Anthony & Helzer, 1991). NHSDA 1990 data indicate that 14.9 percent of African Americans and 13.1 percent of European Americans reported use of illicit drugs in the previous year. Rates of illicit drug abuse/ dependence were uniformly greater for men than women, although the difference was not so marked as for alcohol abuse/dependence. Generally, lifetime prevalence rates fell with advancing age, especially after age 45. The NHSDA data for African Americans, however, indicate that the one-year prevalence rates for illicit drug use were lowest (8.3 percent) among those over 35 years of age, highest (24 percent) among the 18–34 age group, and intermediate (12.7 percent) among the 12–17 age group. Black rates were lower than White rates for those 12–25 years old but higher for those 26 years old and older.

The median age at which illicit drug use began was 16 and at which the first problem related to use developed was 18. Most individuals began drug use between ages 15 and 18 and seldom after age 20. Within each age cohort, age of onset for women was higher than for men (Anthony & Helzer, 1991). For individuals aged 30-44, 13 percent of males and 16.6 percent of females experienced their first problem associated with use after age 30.

According to the NHSDA 1990, marijuana is the illicit drug most often used. Overall use among African Americans in the previous year was 11.2 percent with the highest rates within the 18–34 year age span, the lowest rates among those 35 years and older, and intermediate rates among those 12–17 years old.

Twelve percent of the household population used psychoactive prescription drugs for nonmedical purposes, and 11 percent used cocaine sometime in their lifetimes, thereby representing the next two most frequently used illicit drugs (NIDA, 1991b).

MEDICAL CO-MORBIDITY

Alcohol, tobacco, and other drug use are risk factors for a variety of medical conditions, only some of which will be mentioned here. Despite the evidence that Black and White rates of alcohol consumption are not significantly different, there are dramatic differences in the relative rates of alcohol-related conditions. Black men had a cirrhosis death rate in 1988 that was 1.7 times greater than that of White men, while Black women had a rate that was 1.9 times that of White women (National Center for Health Statistics, 1991). Between 1969–71, the reported incidence rate of esophageal cancer among Black men was ten times greater than the rate among White men in the 35-44 age cohort (Herd, 1989). In 1988, the age-adjusted incidence rates for cancer of the esophagus and oral cavity/pharynx among Black men were 16.1 and 21.5, respectively, contrasted with 5.3 and 14.9, among White men (National Center of Health Statistics, 1991). Hypertension, which is aggravated by alcohol use, is implicated in cerebrovascular death, which occurs more frequently among Blacks than Whites.

Tobacco use is associated with coronary heart disease, chronic obstructive pulmonary disease, and cancer of the lung. In two of these three conditions, African Americans, especially males, have excessive mortality rates. Coronary heart disease is the leading cause of death among African Americans. In 1988, Black males and Black females had mortality rates of 286.2 and 181.1 as opposed to 220.5 and 114.2 for White males and White females, respectively. The mortality rate for cancer of the respiratory system was 83.4, 58.0, 24.6, and 24.8 for Black men, White men, Black women, and White women, respectively, in 1988, while White men and White women had higher death rates from chronic obstructive pulmonary disease (National Center for Health Statistics, 1991).

Acquired immunodeficiency syndrome (AIDS), for which intravenous drug use (IVDU) is a risk factor, takes a heavy toll on Blacks. Although Black men and women are merely 10.2 and 11.0 percent of U.S. men and women, they account for fully 26.1 and 55.2 percent, respectively, of gender-specific deaths due to AIDS (National Center for Health Statistics, 1991).

Perhaps the most significant behavioral cause of mortality associated with alcohol and substance abuse/dependence is homicide (Gary, 1986). The increased violence and death associated with illicit drug use and trafficking have been offered as an explanation for the recently declining life expectancy of African Americans. Homicide, the leading cause of death among young Black males in the 15–34 age range, impacts this age cohort to a degree far in excess of their White counterparts. The relevant rates are 105.3, 12.4, 21.5 and 4.2, for Black men, White men, Black women, and White women, respectively.

PSYCHIATRIC CO-MORBIDITY

The ECA indicated that 22 percent of alcoholics either abused or were dependent on other drugs. Conversely, the likelihood of lifetime co-morbid alcohol abuse/dependence among those diagnosed with other drug abuse/dependence is high, especially among cocaine (84%), sedative (71%), and opioid (67%) abusers. Alcoholism precedes substance abuse/dependence more often than the reverse (Anthony & Helzer, 1991). Although mania and schizophrenia are often present, antisocial personality disorder is the co-morbid condition most strongly associated with AOD abuse.

CAUSATION/ETIOLOGY

Traditional public health distinctions among the environment, the agent, and the host offer a useful way of structuring an etiological analysis.

The environment may be subdivided into its macro and micro dimensions. For African Americans, the former is characterized by racism, poverty, unemployment, alienated labor, cultural aggression, miseducation, dense residential clustering in inadequate housing, inadequate health services, disempowerment, and environmental pollutants, including alcohol, tobacco, and other drugs (Amuleru-Marshall, 1992).

Peer clusters, as well as other informal and formal social organizations of African Americans, join families to form micro environments that, while reflecting the larger ecology, have historically insulated and protected individuals. The capacity of black organizations, networks, and families to do this is a function of their Africentric cultural orientation. To the extent that micro environments are culturally depleted and merely mirror and express the sedimented violence of the larger ecology, they facilitate and exacerbate the vulnerability of high-risk individuals.

Among individuals sequestered in pathogenic macro and micro environments, vulnerability to substance abuse varies. While age and gender are risk indicators, other person-specific factors differentiate risk among individuals. Such factors include, for example, psychopathology, ethnocultural misorientation, academic/vocational undevelopment, and social incompetence.

Agent-specific factors, associated with the psychoactive chemicals themselves, have an impact of their own. The mechanisms permitting alcohol, tobacco, and other drugs to exist in black communities are also implicated in the onset of substance abuse among African Americans.

TREATMENT

Many former addicts have been able to stop or control their substance use without professional intervention (Jones, 1992). They have used other means such as self-help groups like Alcoholics Anonymous (AA) and Narcotics Anonymous (NA) and religious organizations. In a naturalistic study of alcohol abusers, factors other than professional treatment were found to be most important in relapse prevention (Vaillant, 1992).

Though there is little research available on substance abuse treatment with African Americans, relevant theoretical literature, which places the African experience as the centerpiece of psychological analysis, has been developing for more than 20 years (Nobles, 1991; Azibo, 1992). Among Africentric psychologists there is agreement that effective treatment interventions must not merely target black clients—cultural specificity—nor mimic popular black culture—cultural sensitivity—but must be prescriptively designed to heal the peculiar psychocultural trauma of African Americans—cultural appropriateness (Amuleru-Marshall, in press).

A review of treatment research (Woody, Groves & McLellan, 1993), revealed a significant literature on the treatment of addicts, albeit undifferentiated as to race/ethnicity. Effective treatment appears to occur in sequential stages: detoxification, rehabilitation, and continuing care. Detoxification alone, though it may be a critical first step in breaking the cycle of compulsive use, is ineffective in achieving sustained remission (Lee, Mavis, & Stoffelmayr, 1991). Typically, rehabilitation involves helping the addict evaluate his or her addiction and its consequences realistically, identify precipitants of drug use, develop alternative coping strategies, plan to enhance psychosocial stability, and initiate patterns of living that are inconsistent with addiction. Unfortunately, these programs generally fail to address critical experiential aspects of African-American life.

Even with the best of currently available treatment, substance abuse/dependence is often a chronic, relapsing disorder, and many who eventually become abstinent do so only after partial success or failure in previous treatment attempts. In general, the overwhelming majority of alcoholics and other addicts relapse during the first 5 years after treatment. The discouraging success rate of treatment, especially with Black clients, is due, in part, to the cultural inappropriateness of available treatment programs.

Aftercare seeks to stabilize the recovering addict in the community; monitor substance use by observation, breathalyzer, and urine testing; initiate strategies for relapse prevention; and modify values. Engagement in the anonymous self-help organizations of which Alcoholics Anonymous is the prototype is universally recommended. Such organizations include Narcotics Anonymous and Cocaine Anonymous. While African Americans do participate, especially in Narcotics Anonymous and Cocaine Anonymous, the philosophy that permeates the traditions and steps of these self-help groups is anchored in the cultural values of the European-American, middle-class male. It invites recovering alcoholics and other addicts, who are culturally different, to acquiesce to the historical, political, and cultural status quo, while fixated on their individual chemical health.

One effort to render treatment for African Americans that is more culturally appropriate is the Uhuru Recovery Model, which, developed for a 6-week, intensive outpatient program, includes an Africentric modification of the traditionally used 12 steps (Amuleru-Marshall, 1991a).

AOD addicts may present with a variety of concurrent problems. Among these are co-morbid psychiatric disorders. The addition of professional psychotherapy to addicts who had persistent psychiatric symptoms in a methadone maintenance program demonstrated additional benefits (Woody, O'Brien, McLellan & Luborsky, 1985). Other problem areas may include physical health, family relations, employment, social relations, and the legal system. They often overshadow AOD abuse at the time of the addict's entry into treatment (McLellan, O'Brien, Metzger, Alterman & Urschel, 1992). Although attention to them will not resolve the addiction, it will forestall relapse and support treatment gains (Amuleru-Marshall, 1991b). The fact that psychosocial services enhance treatment programs of which they are a part and contribute significantly to treatment outcomes has been convincingly demonstrated (McLellan, Arndt, Metzger, Woody & O'Brien, 1993).

The type of substance or substances that clients abuse also has implications for treatment. Detoxification from central nervous system (CNS) depressants requires medical supervision, as their withdrawal symptoms can be quite serious and even life-threatening. Opiate withdrawal symptoms, while not life-threatening without medical intervention, may actually deter abstinence because of their well-publicized unpleasantness. For these reasons, pharmacotherapeutic agents that reduce these symptoms may be especially useful in detoxification from these substances. Supplemental nicotine administered through routes other than by smoking is also being used to aid withdrawal from tobacco.

Methadone is the only drug approved for maintenance of opioid addicts, a disproportionate number of whom are Black. It has a therapeutic history of almost three decades in this country (Dole & Nyswander, 1965). A longer-acting congener of methadone, levo-alpha-acetylmethadol (LAAM), requires dosing only every 48 to 72 hours. It has been in experimental use for two decades (Savage, Karp, Curran, Hanlon & McCabe, 1976) and is expected to be approved by the FDA for clinical use shortly. Buprenorphine, another drug that is a partial agonist analgesic, is currently being evaluated in the treatment of opioid addiction (NIDA, 1992).

Methadone maintenance has been controversial in Black communities for several years, largely because it has been viewed as drug substitution rather than drug therapy. However, the exploding rates of HIV infection in these communities has made oral substitutes for heroin more acceptable. Making methadone dosing contingent on continued participation in AIDS education, designed with regard to culturally relevant themes and implemented by the methadone program, would likely enhance the impact of methadone maintenance on slowing the spread of HIV infection.

Of the one million inmates in U.S. prisons and jails, nearly 455,000 are African American (Meddis, 1991). The largest single factor behind the rise in incarceration rates over the past decade is probably the "war on drugs" (Mauer, 1991; Lusane, 1991), which is widely perceived in the Black community as a war against Black people, poor and otherwise (Lusane, 1991). More than 80 percent of inmates report drug-use histories, while over half of violent offenders reported that they had committed the offense while under the influence of alcohol, other drugs, or both (Innes & Greenfield, 1990). Although incarcerated addicts provide a spectacular opportunity for treatment and rehabilitation, this is seldom exploited. The authors advocate an end to unalloyed criminal justice solutions to health problems. It is poor public policy to warehouse addicted persons without deliberate efforts to treat their chemical dependency.

PREVENTION

Seventy percent of the resources allocated to AOD problems in the United States is spent on supply reduction or interdiction and law enforcement programs (Meddis, 1991). Almost three-quarters of the portion that is given to demand reduction is consumed at the tertiary or treatment end of the continuum. Treatment is considered to be tertiary prevention because it prevents the progressive debilitating course of a given disorder. Its failure rate, prohibitive cost and the resulting disparity between available treatment slots and addicts requiring treatment make it clear that effective treatment on demand is currently an inaccessible ideal. Treatment (tertiary prevention) continues to dwarf primary and secondary prevention because health care in the U.S. is consumer driven and primary and secondary prevention are difficult to integrate into the marketplace.

Secondary prevention, focusing on intervening early in the progression of substance abuse or targeting populations at excessive risk, such as children of alcoholic or addicted parents, is as important as treatment. Much more attention should be given to outreach and screening in settings that are not commonly associated with substance abuse programming such as churches, schools, and universities, primary care medical practices, dental clinics, community health centers, homeless shelters, prisons, and emergency rooms. Substance abusers could thereby be identified well in advance of the destruction of their relationships and normal patterns of coping.

Focusing on primary prevention is facilitated by separating the environment from the agent and the host. Primary prevention strategies can be targeted at one or more of these categories of risk. Many African Americans, and most who qualify as high risk, live in environments that inherently threaten human life and thriving. Preventing substance abuse in these high-risk environments requires that education, employment, housing, health care, and political empowerment become the intervention targets (Amuleru-Marshall, 1991b).

Mind-altering chemicals, both legal and illegal, are pathogenic agents. While the participation of Black people, especially young Black males, in illicit drug dealing is well publicized, the elaborate arrangements by which 70 percent of all the illegal drugs produced in the world get to American cities and towns is one of the country's best kept secrets. Despite all the resources diverted to interdiction and law enforcement, only 15 percent of the enormous volume of drugs imported into this country is ever interdicted. A highly disproportionate share of the 85 percent that manages to reach America's streets finds its way to urban Black American communities (Rangel, 1986).

The Black community is also a lucrative market for licit drugs, alcohol and tobacco. Many poor Black communities are inundated with outdoor advertisements for these substances as well as with bars, taverns, and other outlets that retail them. Additionally, magazines and radio stations that target these communities continuously advertise alcohol and tobacco, especially "high octane" malts and wines specifically produced and marketed for Black consumers. There is also the vulgar promotion of these toxins by their association with the live performance of Black music and sports, popular pastimes in the Black community. Special initiatives, including media advocacy for community education and action as well as local and national legislation, will be required to decrease the marketing and availability of alcohol and tobacco in the Black community. Countervailing advertisements, highlighting the risks of substance use and strategies to reduce them, must also be among the objectives of these initiatives.

Finally, primary prevention strategies targeted at the host are planned to reduce risk and increase resilience in individuals. Because alcohol, tobacco, and other drug use typically begin in the teen years, these interventions tend to be targeted at pre-teens and teenagers. It should be emphasized, however, that individuals are at risk for substance abuse disorders at other periods in the life span. Irrespective of the age of the targeted recipients of the primary prevention program, its messages, media, and place of intervention must be culturally appropriate. It is not enough, when working with Black persons, to present accurate information on abused substances and their effects on an individual's mind, body, and life. Their impact on the individual's family, community, and race must also be presented. The collective historical experiences of Africans and African Americans and the role these substances play in these experiences are also pertinent themes to be included. An emphasis on values associated with spirituality and collective responsibility is an additional indispensable feature. These messages form an appropriate platform from which resistance skills, decision making, and other conventional behavior rehearsal strategies might be more effectively mounted.

REFERENCES

Amuleru-Marshall, O. (1991a). Uhuru Recovery Model. An Africentric Treatment Program. Atlanta, GA. Unpublished manual.

Amuleru-Marshall, O. (1991b). African Americans. In J. Kinney (Ed.), *Clinical manual of substance abuse* (pp. 146–153). St. Louis: Mosby Year Book.

Amuleru-Marshall, O. (1992). Nurturing the black adolescent male: Culture, ethnicity, and race. In L. W. Abramczyk & J. W. Ross (Eds.), *Nurturing the black adolescent male in the family context: A public health responsibility* (pp. 38–48). Columbia: University of South Carolina.

Amuleru-Marshall, O. (In Press). Political and economic implications of drugs in the African-American Community. In L. L. Goddard (Ed.), *An African-centered model of prevention for high-risk African-American youth* (pp. 31–50). Rockville, MD: Center for Substance Abuse Prevention.

Anthony, J. C., & Helzer, J. E. (1991). Syndromes of drug abuse and dependence. In L. N. Robbins & D. A. Regier (Eds.), *Psychiatric Disorders in America* (pp. 116–154). New York: Free Press.

Azibo, D. A. (1992). *Liberation Psychology*. Trenton, NJ: African World Press.

Dole, V. P., & Nyswander, M. (1965). A medical treatment for diacetylmorphine (heroin) addiction: A clinical trial with methadone hydrochloride. *Journal of the American Medical Association, 193,* 80–84.

Gary, L. E. (1986). Drinking, homicide and the black male. *Journal of Black Studies, 80,* 397–410.

Health Resources and Services Administration. (1990). Health status of the disadvantaged: Chartbook 1990. *U.S. DHHS (HRSA) HRS-P-DV 90-1.* Washington, DC.

Helzer, J. E., Burnam, A., & McEvoy, L. T. (1991). Alcohol abuse and dependence. In L. N. Robbins & D. A. Regier (Eds.), *Psychiatric Disorders in America* (pp. 81–115). New York: Free Press.

Herd, D. (1989). The epidemiology of drinking patterns and alcohol-related problems among U.S. blacks. In S. Spiegler, D. Tate, S. Aitken, & C. Christian (Eds.), *Alcohol Use among U.S. Ethnic Minorities* (pp. 3–50). National Institute on Alcohol Abuse and Alcoholism (NIAAA), USDHHS. Rockville, MD: NIAAA.

Innes, C., & Greenfield, L. (1990). Violent state prisoners and their victims. *Bureau of Justice Statistics Special Report.* Washington, DC: Department of Justice.

Jones, R. T. (1992). What have we learned from nicotine, cocaine, and marijuana about addiction? In C. P. O'Brien & J. H. Jaffe (Eds.), *Addictive States* (pp. 109–122). New York: Raven Press.

Lee, J. A., Mavis, B. E., & Stoffelmayr, B. E. (1991). A comparison of problems-of-life for blacks and whites entering substance treatment programs. *Journal of Psychoactive Drugs, 23,* 233–239.

Lusane, C. (1991). *Pipe Dream Blues: Racism and the War on Drugs.* Boston: South End Press.

Mauer, M. (1991). *Americans behind Bars: A Comparison of International Rates of Incarceration,* Washington, DC: The Sentencing Project.

McLellan, A. T., O'Brien, C., Metzger, D., Alterman, A., & Urschel, H. (1992). How effective is substance abuse treatment—compared to what? In C. O'Brien & J. Jaffe (Eds.), *Addictive States* (pp. 231–252). New York: Raven Press.

McLellan, A. T., Arndt, I. O., Metzger, D. S., Woody, G. E., & O'Brien, C. P. (1993). The effects of psychosocial services. *Journal of the American Medical Association, 269,* 1953–1959.

Meddis, S. (1991). Black imprisonment highest in the USA. *USA Today.* January 7.

National Center for Health Statistics. (1991). *Health, United States, 1990.* Hyattsville, MD: Public Health Service.

NIDA. (1991a). *National Household Survey on Drug Abuse: Main Findings 1990,* DHHS Publication No. (ADM) 91-1788. U.S. Department of Health and Human Services.

NIDA. (1991b). *National Household Survey on Drug Abuse: Highlights 1990*, DHHS Publication No. (ADM) 91-1789. U.S. Department of Health and Human Services.

NIDA. (1991c). *Overview of the 1991 National Household Survey on Drug Abuse*. NIDA Capsules No. C-83-1(a). U.S. Department of Health and Human Services.

NIDA. (1992). LAATRC/VA/NIDA Study #999a: A multicenter clinical trial of buprenorphine in treatment of opiate dependence. In NIDA Medications Development Division, U.S. Department of Health and Human Services.

Nobles, W. (1991). African philosophy: Foundations for black psychology. In R. L. Jones (Ed.), *Black Psychology* (3rd ed.). Berkeley, CA: Cobb & Henry Publishers.

Rangel, C. B. (1986). *Reports on Drug Abuse*. Washington, DC: House Select Committee on Narcotic Abuse and Control.

Robbins, L. N., Locke, B. Z., & Regier, D. A. (1991). An Overview of Psychiatric Disorders in America. In L. N. Robbins & D. A. Regier (Eds.), *Psychiatric Disorders in America* (pp. 328–366). New York: Free Press.

Savage, C., Karp, E. G., Curran, S. F., Hanlon, T. E., & McCabe, O. L. (1976). Methadone/LAAM maintenance: A comparison study. *Comprehensive Psychiatry, 17*, 415–424.

Treaster, J. B. (1992). Emergency rooms' cocaine cases rise. *New York Times*, October 24, p. 6.

Vaillant, G. E. (1992). Is there a natural history of addiction? In C. O'Brien & J. Jaffe (Eds.), *Addictive States* (pp. 41–57). New York: Raven Press.

Woody, G. E., Groves, G. A., & McLellan, A. T. (1993). Treatment research: Findings and future directions. In M. G. Monteiro & J. A. Inciardi (Eds.), *Brasil-United States Binational Research*. Sao Paulo, Brasil: CEBRID.

Woody, G. E., O'Brien, C. P., McLellan, A. T., & Luborsky, L. (1985). Psychotherapy as an adjunct to methadone treatment. In R. E. Meyer (Eds.), *Psychiatric Aspects of Opiate Dependence* (pp. 169–195). New York: Guilford Press.

15

Infant Mortality and Related Issues

Feroz Ahmed

INTRODUCTION

Sociologists since Marx have viewed the level of infant mortality in a society as a sensitive indicator of the overall well-being of its members, just as they have viewed the status of women in any society as a reflection of the degree of freedom and enlightenment in that society. In the United States, the largest military and economic power in the world, the infant mortality rate (IMR), particularly for its Black citizens, has become the shame of the nation and an embarrassment worldwide. One writer titled her book on Black infant mortality "Capital Crime" (Boone, 1989). The Secretary of the Department of Health and Human Services' Task Force on Black and Minority Health, established in 1984, identified infant mortality as one of the six major health problems for minorities, accounting, by itself, for 27 percent of the excess mortality among Blacks (Report of the Secretary's Task Force on Black and Minority Health, 1986).

To get an overview of infant mortality among Black Americans and to locate it in its historic and current comparative contexts, it is useful to examine the data from the National Center for Health Statistics (NCHS) and other sources. While Blacks constitute only 12 percent of the U.S. population, they account for 30 percent of the nearly 39,000 infant deaths that occur in this country each year. The huge differences between the infant mortality rates for Blacks and other Americans are indicated in Table 15.1, which shows that, of every 1,000 Black babies born alive in 1988, nearly 18 died before their first birthday.

This rate is twice as high as that for White babies, and more than 4 times as high as that for Filipino or Japanese Americans. The same table also shows that these ratios hold true for both the neonatal (up to 27 days) and postneonatal (28

Table 15.1
Infant, Neonatal, and Postneonatal Mortality Rates by Ethnic Groups, United States, 1988 (Deaths per 1,000 Live Births)

Ethnic Group	Infant Mortality Rate	Neonatal Mortality Rate	Postneonatal Mortality Rate
White	8.5	5.4	3.1
Black	17.8	11.5	6.2
American Indian	9.0	4.1	4.8
Hispanic*	8.1	6.0	3.0
Hawaiian	6.9	5.1	1.8
Chinese	4.2	2.2	2.0
Japanese	3.8	2.6	1.3
Filipino	4.1	3.0	1.1
Other Asian	5.5	3.4	2.1
Other	5.2	3.4	1.9
Total	10.0	6.3	3.5

Source: National Center for Health Statistics (1990b).

*Not a mutually exclusive category. Coverage also limited.

days to first birthday) periods. Only the postneonatal mortality rate (PMR) of American Indians comes closest to that of Blacks. An international comparison, based on the United Nations' data for 1987, shows that while the IMR for White Americans ranks no better than fourteenth, that for Black Americans fares much worse—ranking thirty-fourth and exceeding that for Third World countries or territories of Hong Kong, Singapore, Trinidad and Tobago, Cuba, and Costa Rica (United Nations, 1991).

Neonatal and Postneonatal Mortality Rates

National data on infant mortality since 1940 show that both neonatal and postneonatal mortality declined for Blacks as well as for Whites (NCHS, 1990b). Our analysis of these data reveal that while Blacks experienced a much higher rate of decline than did Whites between 1940 and 1950, in the following decade there was no improvement for Blacks. Both neonatal and postneonatal mortality failed to decline for Blacks during the 1950s. The Black IMR again declined at a faster rate than did the White IMR during the 1960s. During the 1970s, the rate of decline for Blacks was even faster than in the preceding decade; but it was slightly slower than was the decline for Whites in the same period. During the 1980s, the rate of decline in IMR for both racial groups slowed down (Ahmed, 1992).

White Americans had already achieved major reductions in postneonatal mortality by the 1960s, and the White PMR has bottomed out in the last two decades. However, the Black PMR continued to decline at a faster rate than did the rate for Whites throughout the same three decades. The rate of decline in the PMR for Blacks also slowed down recently (Ahmed, 1992). Most of the reduction in the PMR for all races during the 1960s and 1970s was due to the drop in mortality from infectious diseases (Khoury, Erickson & Adams, 1984). Because of this, the percentage decline in the PMR for Blacks was much higher than was the percentage decline in the Black neonatal mortality rate (NMR) through the 1960s. However, the trend subsequently reversed itself. Since 1980, the Black PMR has remained within a narrow range of 6.1 to 6.8 deaths per 1,000 live births (Ahmed, 1992).

During the 1970s, both Blacks and Whites experienced a substantial decline in the NMR, the component which accounts for roughly two-thirds of all infant deaths. This decline was mainly due to the improvement in perinatal medical care (Lee, Paneth, Gartner, Pearlman & Gruss, 1980). Because of this and the slowing down of the decline in Black postneonatal mortality, the NMR for Blacks decreased at a much faster rate than did the PMR for Blacks during the 1970s and 1980s. During the 1980s, however, the NMR for Blacks declined at a slower rate than it did during the 1970s. Blacks, despite having a much higher NMR, experienced lower rates of decline than did Whites during both decades. Since 1980, the Black NMR has varied between 11.5 and 13.4 deaths per thousand live births (Ahmed, 1992). The two-fold gap between Black and White infant mortality rates persists in America.

Factors associated with high infant mortality among Black Americans can be understood not only from the data and studies on infant mortality per se, but also on its components and related pregnancy outcomes. As nearly two-thirds of the infant deaths in the United States occur during the neonatal period, i.e., within 27 days, many analyses are restricted to neonatal mortality. Given the fact that nearly two-thirds of the infant deaths in the United States occur among infants with a low birth weight (LBW), that is, under 2,500 grams or five-and-a-half pounds (USDHHS, 1980a), students of infant mortality often focus their studies on the determinants of LBW or very low birth weight (under 1,500 grams or three-and-a-quarter pounds). Most of the LBW babies are also born pre-term or "prematurely," and many of them either do not survive or suffer from physical and/or mental handicaps. As stated in the Public Health Service's "Objectives for the Nation'' for 1990, ''The greatest single problem associated with infant mortality is low birthweight'' (USDHHS, 1980a). Low birth weight is a preferred variable in research for yet another reason: it can be measured accurately, while gestational age cannot be estimated correctly in many cases.

Low Birth Weight

Much of our understanding concerning risk factors associated with infant mortality is derived from studies of low birth weight. From the standpoint of prevention of infant mortality, it is important to differentiate between the roles of birth weight distribution and birth weight-specific mortality rates, that is, death rates for each narrow birth weight category. If in a given population the latter are too high as compared to the rates in another population, there may be a deficiency in neonatal intensive care or other neonatal or pediatric care. However, if the birth weight-specific rates are fairly low and the infant or neonatal mortality rates are still high, the high IMR is due to a poor birth weight distribution. This poor distribution may be due to a variety of obstetrical, medical, health care, behavioral, cultural, environmental, socioeconomic, or even biological factors. In the United States the decline in the infant mortality rates during the last three decades has mainly been achieved by a dramatic improvement in neonatal care (Lee et al., 1980), at the heart of which lay the proliferation of neonatal intensive care units and regionalization of perinatal care. Thus, poor birth weight distribution stands out as the principal proximate determinant of the relatively high infant mortality rate in the United States.

Black American infants have the highest incidence (13% in 1988) of low birth weight among all ethnic groups, more than twice as high as the rate for White Americans (5.6%). This high incidence of low birth weight is mainly, but not entirely, responsible for the very high infant mortality rates among Black Americans. Blacks also have higher mortality rates among normal-weight neonates as well as higher postneonatal mortality rates.

Researchers such as Binkin and her colleagues (1985) and Sappenfield and his colleagues (1987) have demonstrated that, while Blacks have lower neonatal mortality rates than do Whites at lower birth weights, the pattern is reversed at higher birth weights, particularly at 3,500 grams and above. As the vast majority of the live births are of normal weight and the lower mortality rates at low birth weights for Blacks are still quite high, Blacks, owing to their poorer birth weight distribution, end up having much higher neonatal mortality rates than do Whites.

Many multivariate studies of Black-White differentials in LBW ratio have shown that even when several known risk factors are controlled simultaneously, there is still a substantial residual difference (Alexander, Tompkins, Altekruse & Hornung, 1985; Bross & Shapiro, 1982; Kleinman & Kessel, 1987). One study purported to show that when the hematocrit level (a measure of anemia) was kept constant in addition to several other control variables, Black-White differences in the incidence of prematurity disappeared (Lieberman, Ryan, Monson & Schoenbaum, 1987). However, this result was found to be a study artifact caused by faulty design (Klebanoff, Shiono, Berendes & Rhoads, 1989). Some recent studies have shown that American Blacks tend to have worse pregnancy outcomes than do foreign-born or non-American Blacks in the United States as well (Kleinman, Fingerhut & Prager, 1991).

RISK FACTORS

Sociodemographic and Related Factors

The risk of infant mortality, or other adverse pregnancy outcomes, varies by maternal age, marital status, educational attainment, socioeconomic status (SES), and other sociodemographic factors.

Maternal Age

Pregnancies occurring to women under the age of 18 or even 20 years old and over the age of 34 years old are considered to be high-risk pregnancies. Infants born to such women tend to have a higher incidence of low birth weight and remain at a higher risk of dying before their first birthday, as compared to infants born to mothers 20–34 years of age (IOM, 1985; Report of the Secretary's Task Force on Black and Minority Health, 1986).

Both neonatal and postneonatal mortality rates are highest among babies born to adolescent mothers. These babies have a risk of mortality from 1.5 to 3.5 times greater than the risk to babies born to mothers aged 25 to 29 years of age (Friede et al., 1987). The trends are quite similar for LBW as well. The rates peak among teens below the age of 15 years, reach their lowest level within the maternal age group of 25 to 29 years, and reflect a slow rise through subsequent older age groups (IOM, 1985). For example, according to national data for 1988, 13.6 percent of the births to mothers under age 15 years were low birth weight; compared to 9.3 percent of the births to mothers 15 to 19 years; 6.1 percent of the births to mothers 25 to 29 years; and 8.2 percent of the births to mothers between the ages of 40 and 44 years (NCHS, 1990a). For Blacks specifically, while the overall incidence of low birth weight was 13 percent, that for infants born to women under 20 years and over 34 years was 14.4 percent and 14.6 percent, respectively (NCHS, 1990a).

Black mothers are more likely to be teenagers than are mothers of any other ethnic group (IOM, 1985; Report of the Secretary's Task Force on Black and Minority Health, 1986). National data for 1988 show that nearly one-fourth (22.7%) of all Black births, but only 10.5 percent of White births, were to women under the age of 20 (NCHS, 1990a). This greater exposure of Black women to age-related risk, combined with high maternal age-specific LBW ratios, contributes to a high overall infant mortality rate among Blacks.

Despite the widely observed higher risk for poor pregnancy outcomes among adolescent females and the attribution by some medical authorities of such risk to biological conditions, there is growing evidence that young age, particularly above 15 years, does not constitute an independent risk factor for poor pregnancy outcomes (Baldwin & Cain, 1980; Lee, Ferguson, Corpuz & Gartner, 1988). Biological and socioeconomic factors as well as life-styles converge and potentiate the risk associated with young maternal age. There are numerous interrelated risk components. Therefore, young maternal age is not considered an independent risk factor for poor pregnancy outcomes (IOM, 1985). Further, a few studies have shown that even the observed relationship between teenage motherhood and poor pregnancy outcome is not as consistent among Blacks as it is among Whites (Collins & David, 1990; Geronimus, 1986).

Ahmed (1987), analyzing data on Black births in Washington, D.C., between 1980 and 1985, observed that, even without controlling for any other factors, infants born to mothers 17–19 years of age had a better birth weight distribution and a lower relative risk of mortality than did babies born to mothers of any other age group. Even mothers under age 17 did not have worse birth outcomes than did mothers 20–34 (Ahmed, 1987).

These anomalies and inconsistencies, however, do not provide a basis for underestimating the risks associated with teenage pregnancies. Teenage pregnancy and teenage childbearing put women at a much greater risk for many adverse health and social outcomes. Ahmed (1990), for example, has shown that even in a population where women 20–34 years have poorer pregnancy outcomes than do teenage females, the higher risk to women in their 20s and 30s is correlated with their having commenced childbearing in their teens.

Parity

Women having their first child and those having their fourth or subsequent child are generally at a higher risk of delivering a LBW infant than are women having their second or third child (Taffel, 1980). However, because of the interaction between birth order and age, as well as other factors, bivariate association between birth order and birth weight can be altered by the differences in the age patterns of reproductive behavior. For example, national data for 1976 showed that, while White women having a fourth or subsequent birth were at the highest risk for a LBW infant, among Black mothers, those having their first child were at a greater risk (Taffel, 1980). While a few studies (e.g., Ahmed, 1987; Bross & Shapiro, 1982) have shown that the association between parity and birth weight no longer remains significant when several other factors are controlled, other studies (e.g., Petitti & Coleman, 1990) have shown an independent elevated risk of LBW to infants born to women having their first or their fourth or subsequent live birth. The ratio of first births to all live births is somewhat lower among Blacks (39%) as compared to Whites (42%). The share of fourth and subsequent births is much higher among Blacks: 14 percent, as compared to 9 percent for Whites (NCHS, 1990a).

Birth Interval

A short interval between pregnancies or births is also deemed to be a risk factor for LBW and infant mortality. Analysis of national data showed that the incidence of LBW was highest among infants born within 12 months of the previous pregnancy termination, followed by infants who were born 12 to 23 months after the previous termination (Taffel, 1980). For Blacks, the incidence of LBW was 25.6 percent if the interval was less than 12 months, 12.1 percent if the interval was 12–23 months, and less than 10 percent for longer intervals (Taffel, 1980). Black women are more prone to having short birth intervals than are white women. According to recent national data for all single-delivery live births whose birth intervals were known, 1.2 percent of White and 3.2 percent of Black infants were born within 12 months of the previous live birth; 23.8 percent of White and 27.9 of Black infants were born 12 to 23 months after the previous live birth (NCHS, 1990a).

Marital Status

Research on the relationship between marital status and pregnancy outcome shows that infants born to unmarried women are at a higher risk of low birth weight and mortality than are infants born to married women (IOM, 1985; Report of the Secretary's Task Force on Black and Minority Health, 1986). The effect of marital status upon pregnancy risks has been observed both directly and indirectly through other factors such as maternal age and socioeconomic status (IOM, 1985). According to the 1985 national data, the incidence of LBW for the infants born to unmarried mothers was twice as high as that for infants born to married mothers for all racial groups combined; however, for Blacks the rate was only 39 percent higher (Taffel, 1989).

Even though most multivariate studies of LBW and infant mortality have ignored marital status as a variable, a few recent studies (e.g., Ahmed, 1990; Lee et al., 1988) have shown that even when factors such as race, age, education, parity, and prenatal care are controlled, the unmarried status of the mother remains significant as a risk factor for adverse pregnancy outcomes. However, the advantages of the married status and stable family are often offset by the conditions of social disadvantage and substance abuse (Ahmed, 1990; Boone, 1989; Collins & David, 1990). Despite these findings, the overall risk for poor pregnancy outcomes remains high for unmarried mothers, as compared with the outcomes for married mothers.

The marital status differential in pregnancy outcomes is especially significant when viewed within the context of the increasing rate of out-of-wedlock births. In 1980, 11 percent of the White and 55 percent of the Black women delivering a live infant were unmarried (IOM, 1985); by 1988, the unmarried birth ratios had risen to 17.7 percent and 63.5 percent, respectively (NCHS, 1990a). Even though the relative risk of poor pregnancy outcomes from being unmarried is somewhat lower among Blacks as compared with other groups, its absolute level is still quite high, and far too many Black mothers belong in this high-risk group. In the District of Columbia, where two-thirds of Black mothers were unmarried, 17 percent of all LBW births and neonatal deaths among Blacks were attributed to mothers being unmarried; in which case, the relative risk for delivering a LBW infant was 35 percent higher and for experiencing an infant death 38 percent higher (Ahmed, 1987). The odds for delivering a LBW baby were 18 percent higher even when age, education, and prenatal care were controlled (Ahmed, 1990).

Socioeconomic Status

Because of the limited information available on birth and death certificates and in the medical records, the most commonly cited socioeconomic status (SES) indicator in the demographic and epidemiological studies on pregnancy outcomes is maternal education. There is an inverse relationship between education and adverse pregnancy outcomes. The lower the level of education of the mother, the higher the incidence of low birth weight babies and infant mortality rate (IOM, 1985; Report of the Secretary's Task Force on Black and Minority Health, 1986). Bross and Shapiro (1982) showed that education has an indirect effect upon neonatal mortality through low birth weight but a direct effect upon post-neonatal mortality. Evidently, the level of the mother's educational attainment up to a point is a function of age. Nevertheless, a negative association between maternal education and the birth weight of an infant has been demonstrated for each age group among Black women (Kovar, 1977). Besides age, even when factors such as race, prenatal care, parity, and socioeconomic status are con-trolled, lower educational attainment remains a risk factor for poor pregnancy outcomes (Bross & Shapiro, 1982).

Although the median level of education attained by women has risen over the years, the gap between the risks of poor pregnancy outcomes associated with high versus low levels of education has not been narrowed. With regard to the incidence of low birth weight babies, comparative data for 1971, 1976, and 1981 reveal the increasing gap between women with a high level of education and those with a low level of education.

According to 1985 national data, for Black mothers the percentage of LBW live births ranged from 14.6 for mothers with nine to 11 years of education to 9.5 for mothers with 16 years or more of education (Taffel, 1989). Using 1983 national data, Kleinman and Kessel (1987) noted that Black women with low levels of education were at a 59 percent greater risk of having moderately low birth weight (1,500–2,500 grams) babies, but low education had little effect on very low birth weight (under 1,500 grams) births. Our computations on the 1985 national data (Taffel, 1989) show a similar pattern, with a maximum difference between levels of educational attainment of 39 percent for MLBW ratio, but only 17 percent for VLBW ratio for Blacks (Ahmed, 1992). Among uniformly disadvantaged inner-city Black women, having more education made little dif-ference in pregnancy outcomes (Boone, 1989).

The educational attainment of Black mothers is relatively low. The 1988 national data show that 31.3 percent of Black mothers had less than 12 years of education, while only 7.2 percent had 16 years or more. The respective figures for White mothers were 17.5 percent and 20.1 percent (NCHS, 1990a).

In some cases, birth certificate items other than maternal education, such as paternal education or mother's census tract have been analyzed, and a few supplemental natality and infant mortality surveys have provided information on other indicators such as income, occupation, and type of health insurance. In general, low SES, however measured, is associated with an increased risk of LBW and infant mortality (IOM, 1985; Report of the Secretary's Task Force on Black and Minority Health, 1986).

Some of the risk associated with low SES is attributed to related characteristics such as low maternal weight gain, short stature, hypertension, excessive smoking, and limited use of prenatal care (IOM, 1985). Low SES negatively affects maternal health and ultimately increases neonatal mortality, but low SES also results in unfavorable environmental conditions that exacerbate the problem of postneonatal mortality (Report of the Secretary's Task Force on Black and Minority Health, 1986). For example, in a study of White legitimate births, Gortmaker (1979a) found that birth into poverty status increased the risk of infant mortality by 50 percent, mainly by elevating the risk of postneonatal mortality. In general, a disproportionately high number of Blacks live near or below the poverty level. A relatively high portion of Black births are to mothers in the lower socioeconomic status groups (Ahmed, 1987). Overall, low SES patterns account for much of the high incidence of LBW and infant mortality among Blacks. For instance, low SES-related factors such as inadequate access to health care and unfavorable living conditions negatively affect pregnancy outcome, especially the postneonatal component of infant mortality (Report of the Secretary's Task Force on Black and Minority Health, 1986).

Maternal

Inadequate Health Care

A vast body of knowledge has borne out that the more adequate the prenatal care, in terms of the timing of the first prenatal visit and frequency of visits throughout pregnancy, the lower the risk of low birth weight and infant mortality (IOM, 1985; IOM, 1988; Report of the Secretary's Task Force on Black and Minority Health, 1986). The Institute of Medicine's Committee to Study the Prevention of Low Birthweight, after carefully reviewing a large number of clinical as well as population-based studies, concluded: "The overwhelming weight of the evidence is that prenatal care reduces low birthweight" (IOM, 1985).

Principal studies conducted on the subject include the one by Kessner and his colleagues (1973) for the Institute of Medicine, which developed a composite three-level index of the adequacy of prenatal care—adequate, intermediate, and inadequate. Other major studies include those by Gortmaker (1979b); Showstack, Budetti & Minkler (1984); and Taffel (1980). These studies have shown that even when factors such as race, socioeconomic status, educational attainment, maternal age, parity, birth interval, and pregnancy complications are controlled, inadequacy of prenatal care is correlated with adverse pregnancy outcomes.

More recent national data show that for mothers beginning care in the third trimester, the risk of having a LBW baby is nearly twice as high as that for those beginning care during the first two months of pregnancy (Taffel, 1989). However, while for Whites the risk of LBW among women not receiving prenatal care or receiving it during the third trimester is 2.9 and 1.8 times higher, respectively, than it is for mothers receiving prenatal care during the first two months of pregnancy, the corresponding risk for Blacks is 2.3 and 1.4 times higher, respectively (Taffel, 1989).

A number of analyses of data on Black Americans specifically have demonstrated the net adverse impact of not receiving adequate prenatal care. Gortmaker (1979b), for example, found that among Black mothers, those with inadequate prenatal care increased their risk of delivering a low birth weight infant by 78 percent. In addition, after controlling for several other risk factors, prenatal care was significantly related to the neonatal mortality of Black infants. For Black mothers in the District of Columbia, infant mortality was three times more likely among those receiving inadequate or intermediate care, as compared to those with adequate care, and the relative risk for LBW was 72 percent higher (Ahmed, 1987). Even when maternal age, marital status, educational attainment, pregnancy complications, prior fetal loss, previous child death, and birth interval were controlled in the analysis, Black mothers receiving inadequate prenatal care had a 23 percent higher risk of having a LBW infant than did mothers receiving adequate care (Ahmed, 1987).

Utilization of prenatal care by expectant mothers in the United States increased between 1969 and 1980; however, since 1980 the trends have remained stable or in some cases the use of prenatal care has declined (IOM, 1988). When compared to White women, Black women are less likely to receive early prenatal care, and proportionately more Black women receive no prenatal care at all (IOM, 1988). In 1988, 59.6 percent of Black mothers reported beginning care in the first trimester, 28.1 percent in the second trimester, 6.8 percent in the third trimester, and 4.2 percent reported receiving no prenatal care (NCHS, 1990a). The percentage of Black mothers with late or no prenatal care increased from 8.8 in 1981 to 11.1 in 1988 (NCHS, 1990a). In 1988, less than one-half of Black mothers (47.9%) both began prenatal care in the first trimester and maintained nine or more visits; the corresponding figure for Whites was 71.7 percent (NCHS, 1990a).

A recent Current Population Survey estimate showed that in 1989, 34.3 percent of Blacks aged 18–24 years and 22.5 percent aged 25–44 years did not have any health care coverage; the comparative figures for Whites—also quite high—

were 26.3 percent and 14.4 percent, respectively (Ries, 1991). Although overall more women, as compared with men, were covered by health insurance, this difference was largely due to a greater public assistance coverage for women. As pointed out by the National Commission to Prevent Infant Mortality, there are serious gaps in eligibility for and the provision of services in the publicly assisted Medicaid program and limitations and exclusions in the private health insurance plans for the pregnant women (NCPIM, 1988). Black women suffer disproportionately from this lack of adequate health care.

Nutrition

The effect of malnutrition on the fetus can be seriously limiting during the early stages and may cause malformations or even fetal death. After three months, there is no teratogenic effect, but there can be fetal growth retardation. During the last trimester, even mild nutritional restrictions may impede the growth of a fetus (Worthington-Roberts, 1985). Nutritional intake during pregnancy can be measured either directly, by calculating the nutritional value of the foods eaten by the pregnant mothers, or indirectly, by measuring the weight gained during pregnancy. The latter, being simpler, is used most often in the studies of the effects of nutrition on pregnancy outcomes. Reviews of studies on the subject have found a consistent association between maternal weight gain during pregnancy and the birth weight of the infant or the neonatal mortality rate (Brown, 1988; IOM, 1985). In the Collaborative Perinatal Study in the United States, for example, the risk of bearing a LBW infant was 4 times higher for women who gained less than 14 pounds as compared to women who gained 30–35 pounds (Singer, Westphal & Niswander, 1968). Perinatal mortality rates for women who gained less than 10 pounds during pregnancy were nearly 4 times higher than were the rates for women who gained more than 33 pounds (Brown, 1988).

Data on Blacks show an even greater impact of poor nutrition on birth outcomes. Simpson, Lawless, and Mitchell (1975) showed that, while the risk of having a LBW infant was 4.8 times higher for White women who gained less than 11 pounds during pregnancy as compared to women who gained more than 30 pounds, the relative risk for Black women was 8 times higher. National data have shown that Black women are twice as likely as White women to gain less than 16 pounds during pregnancy (Taffel & Keppel, 1984).

Despite the demonstrated effect of malnutrition on pregnancy outcomes and a greater exposure of socially disadvantaged women to malnutrition and undernutrition, some experts believe that malnutrition contributes very little to the high infant mortality rate in the United States (Graham, 1991). The Surgeon General's 1988 report on nutrition and health, while reviewing the relationship between nutrition and pregnancy outcomes and elaborating on the nutritional needs of the pregnant woman, fetus, and infant, makes no claim that malnutrition is a significant contributing factor to infant mortality in the United States (USDHHS, 1988).

Drug Abuse

Maternal use of illicit drugs is emerging as the greatest threat to the unborn. Cocaine—along with its more potent and cheaper derivative "crack"—is considered to be the most harmful of the illicit drugs currently in use in the United States and has received most attention from the researchers. Based on his extensive observations and research on women using drugs during pregnancy, Chasnoff listed the following neonatal outcomes of cocaine use: "Infants delivered to mothers who have used cocaine during pregnancy tend to be shorter and of lower birthweight and to have smaller head circumferences than infants delivered to drug-free women" (Chasnoff, 1987). Since most drug users tend to be polyusers, the individual effects of each drug are difficult to separate (Chasnoff, 1987).

Legal and other obstacles to obtaining accurate information on maternal drug use have made it exceedingly difficult to estimate correctly the prevalence of maternal drug use and the relative risk of adverse pregnancy outcomes to the drug-using mothers. Nonetheless, information from clinical studies, combined with the birth certificate data from New York City, provides useful quantified data on the extent of perinatal risk from maternal drug use. For instance, a study based upon pregnant women reporting no prenatal care and delivering at a large New York City hospital in 1986 showed that maternal cocaine use was directly related to premature birth and low birth weight, with drug-using mothers being at twice as high a risk for these outcomes as were non-drug-using mothers (Chouteau, Namerow & Leppert, 1988). Birth certificate data for New York City for 1985–1987 showed that 34 percent of infants born to mothers using illicit drugs during pregnancy were LBW, a rate almost 4 times as high as the overall incidence of LBW ("Maternal Drug Abuse," 1989). The IMR for drug-exposed babies was 2.6 times as high as that for babies not exposed to drugs: 34 per 1,000 live births, as compared to the overall IMR of 13.1 per 1,000 live births ("Maternal Drug Abuse," 1989). The General Accounting Office's (GAO) study, based upon the review of medical records of hospitals selected from across the country, found a relative risk of LBW ranging from 2.5 to 8 times higher for drug-exposed infants, as compared with the infants not identified as drug-exposed (GAO, 1990).

A case-control study in Alameda County, California, showed that, when several potential confounders were controlled, Black mothers using cocaine or crack throughout their pregnancy had a 4 times higher risk of delivering a LBW infant than did mothers who did not use drugs during their pregnancy (Petitti & Coleman, 1990).

The National Association of Perinatal Addiction Research and Education (NAPARE) randomly selected 36 hospitals across the nation, with 154,856 births, and conducted a survey to estimate the prevalence of maternal drug use of marijuana, cocaine, PCP, heroin, methadone, and amphetamines. Eleven percent of these births were found to have been affected by maternal drug use, giving an extrapolated annual estimate of 375,000 births involving maternal drug use nationally ("Innocent Addicts," 1988). The National Drug Control Strategy estimated in 1989 that 100,000 infants are exposed to cocaine annually in the United States (GAO, 1990). In the GAO's 1989 record review of 10 hospitals, the percentage of drug-exposed infants varied from 1.3 percent to 18.1 percent (GAO, 1990). The largest percentage of maternal drug use has been attributed to cocaine usage ("Innocent Addicts," 1988). In the GAO study, the percentage of drug-exposed infants who were exposed to cocaine ranged from 23.1 percent to 93.2 percent (GAO, 1990).

There are no reliable national data on the racial differences in the use of illicit drugs among pregnant women or even among women of childbearing ages. In Washington, D.C. hospitals, drug usage rates of up to 30 percent have been reported among the predominantly Black group of delivering mothers (Norris, 1991). Data from New York City indicated that maternal cocaine users were twice as likely as were non-users to be Black ("Maternal Drug Abuse," 1989).

Given the very high independent risk of an adverse pregnancy outcome associated with cocaine and other drug use, even a moderate increase in maternal drug use during pregnancy can result in a substantial increase in the incidence of LBW and infant mortality. In the Alameda County study, where the prevalence of cocaine and crack use among delivering Black women was estimated to be 3.9 percent, the adjusted relative risk of 4.0 for LBW due to cocaine/crack use throughout pregnancy made such use responsible for 10 percent of the LBW births (Petitti & Coleman, 1990). The 10 percent increase in the incidence of LBW among infants in New York City during the 1980s was attributed mainly to the 20-fold increase in cocaine use ("Maternal Drug Abuse," 1989). Cocaine use is also suspected to be the main contributing factor in the persistence of a high IMR in Washington, D.C. (Abramowitz, 1989).

Smoking

As early as 1957, Simpson reported that women who smoked during pregnancy delivered babies with birth weights lower than those of the infants of women who did not smoke. Over 50 subsequent studies involving over 500,000 births have confirmed those initial findings (IOM, 1985; USDHHS, 1980b; Report of the Secretary's Task Force on Black and Minority Health, 1986). Some of these subsequent findings have also demonstrated that smoking, rather than being a proxy of some other factors, has an independent effect on birth weight.

Despite the independent effect of smoking, it has been observed that the presence of other risk factors can compound the effect of smoking on LBW. Meyer and her associates (1976) found that the effect was more pronounced when the weight gain was less than 20 pounds. Hogue and Sappenfield (1987), noting this "multiplicatively independent" risk, showed that, while a White woman smoker with at least a high school education exposes her infant to a 7 percent greater risk of LBW, a Black woman with less than a high school education exposes her infant to a 20 percent greater risk if she smokes during pregnancy. The Surgeon General's 1980 report attributed up to 14 percent of premature births in the United States to maternal smoking (USDHHS, 1980b).

Cigarette smoking can also be a direct cause of neonatal death in otherwise normal infants. Such deaths are a result of the increased risk of early delivery and are secondarily related to early bleeding and premature rupture of the membrane (USDHHS, 1980b). A review of several studies showed that the risk of perinatal mortality among low-risk (that is White, upper-class, better-educated, and 20–34 years old) mothers was not significantly different for those who smoked during pregnancy and those who did not. However, among high-risk (that is, non-White, low-income, less-educated, and under 20 and over 34 years old) mothers, the women who smoked during pregnancy had a 1.26 to 2.16 times higher risk of perinatal mortality than did the women who did not smoke during pregnancy (USDHHS, 1980b).

According to the 1985 National Health Interview Survey (NHIS), 27.5 percent of Black women who had given birth between 1980 and 1985 smoked at some time during the 12 months prior to the birth, compared with 33.2 percent of White women (NCHS, 1988). Earlier, a study based on the data on married pregnant women from the National Natality Surveys of 1967 and 1980 showed that, while among women 20 years and over, Blacks had a lower prevalence of smoking than did Whites, they also had a lower rate of decline, which resulted in narrowing the gap from 7 percentage points to 2 percentage points (Kleinman & Kopstein, 1987). The 1988 NHIS survey of children under age 5 showed that, compared to White children, proportionately twice as many Black children were exposed prenatally and 3 times as many were exposed postnatally to cigarette smoke (Overpeck & Moss, 1991).

Alcohol Use

Even though drinking alcohol by a woman during her pregnancy is known to cause Fetal Alcohol Syndrome (FAS) in her offspring, with its attendant congenital anomalies, the results concerning the effect of maternal drinking on the infant's birth weight are contradictory (IOM, 1985). From the review of the literature conducted by Stein and his associates, it could not be established that alcohol consumption was an important determinant of IUGR (Stein & Klein, 1983). Mills and his colleagues (1984), however, showed that in comparison to the infants born to nondrinking mothers, infants of mothers who drank one drink a day were 14 grams lighter, and infants of those who had 3 to 5 drinks a day were 165 grams lighter. Even when race, age, education, marital status, weight for height, smoking, parity, reproductive history, preexisting hypertension, and preeclampsia were controlled, there was a significant association between the expectant mother's alcohol consumption during pregnancy and IUGR (Mills, Graubard, Harley, Rhoads & Berendes, 1984).

In a recent study, however, in which cocaine or crack use was also controlled in addition to age, parity, SES, prior LBW baby, pre-pregnant weight, weight gain during pregnancy, and cigarette smoking, the odds ratio of having a LBW infant for mothers who had more than 2 drinks a day was 1.7, as compared to nondrinkers, but the result was not statistically significant, because of a large standard error (Petitti & Coleman, 1990). The Secretary of Health's report on *Alcohol and Health* to Congress mentions prenatal growth retardation, but not LBW, as a possible consequence of maternal alcohol consumption (USDHHS, 1990).

Even though available evidence does not suggest that drinking alcohol during pregnancy independently contributes to the high incidence of LBW or infant mortality among Blacks in any major way, the fact that alcohol drinking is often combined with cigarette smoking and the use of illicit drugs would seem to indicate that women who drink alcohol during pregnancy remain at a high risk for infant mortality.

Other Medical Factors

A number of medical and obstetric risk factors adversely affect pregnancy outcomes. Obstetric factors include previous reproductive history as well as certain conditions associated with the current pregnancy. Other medical factors include preexisting diseases and non-obstetrical conditions associated with the current pregnancy. In addition to having a high parity and short birth intervals, discussed previously, Black women tend to be at a higher risk for other medical risk factors such as previous fetal loss (Kochanek, 1990), multiple pregnancies (Taffel, 1980), and hypertension, diabetes, anemia, and sexually transmitted diseases (Ahmed, 1987). Although AIDS/HIV infection does not contribute to a significant number of infant deaths in the United States, the trend of alarming increase in the overall incidence of HIV infections is likely to result in similar increases in pediatric AIDS and infant mortality. Already, 55 percent each of female and pediatric AIDS cases in the United States occur among Blacks (Ahmed, 1992).

CONCLUSION

A review of the research and an analysis of national data in this chapter underline what has been known to the professionals in the field, namely, that an extremely high incidence of low birth weight is mainly responsible for the high infant mortality rate among Black Americans. It is possible to increase the survival rate of both low birth weight and normal birth weight newborns. Nevertheless, the impact of such reduced birth weight-specific mortality on the overall infant mortality rate for Blacks would be quite small, compared to the reduction in the infant mortality rate which could be brought about by lowering the incidence of low-weight births in the first place.

Many of the more important risk factors do not operate among Blacks the same way as they do among Whites or other ethnic groups. There is growing evidence that the impact of teenage motherhood, of being unmarried, or of not having a high school education is not as great among Blacks, especially inner-city poor Blacks, as in other groups. Teenage mothers have been a popular target group for social concern and health care focus and have often been implicated in the high infant mortality rate for Blacks. There are numerous good reasons for the national concern about teenage pregnancies, but equating teenage pregnancy with high infant mortality is not empirically valid. Teenagers contribute a small number of all births and infant deaths. Additionally, among Blacks, the risk of a poor pregnancy outcome may only be marginally higher for teenage mothers than it is for mothers in their early and mid-20s. In some jurisdictions, however, even this is not true.

Even though the relative risk for infant death or low-weight birth is not as high for unmarried Black women as it is for unmarried White women, unmarried status remains a risk factor among Blacks and is more important than the age factor because nearly two-thirds of Black births take place outside of marriage. This trend has been on the increase for the past several decades and is reflected in the 1990 Census figures, which show the female-headed single parent household to be the major type of family in many urban centers of the United States. The unmarried mothers are more likely to be unemployed, poor, and dependent on public assistance. Substance abuse, high-risk sexual behavior, and crime are often the defining features of the environment these women inhabit. Such environment contributes to high morbidity and mortality rates among their infants and children.

The lack or inadequacy of prenatal care is another factor that produces a lesser impact on the pregnancy outcomes of Blacks than it does on the pregnancy outcomes of Whites. However, the proportion of Black women not receiving adequate prenatal care is so high that, by providing adequate prenatal care to the more than 50 percent of the Black pregnant women who do not receive it, a major dent can be made into the infant mortality rate among Blacks. The lack of adequate prenatal care, however, is only a part of the lack of adequate health care in general for a large section of the American population. Blacks suffer disproportionately from the absence of this basic human right. There is ample evidence in support of the recommendation of the National Commission to Prevent Infant Mortality that calls for providing universal access to early maternity and pediatric care for mothers and infants. Reaching out to women and providing them with adequate prenatal and postpartum care would be essential also for the prevention, treatment, and management of prenatal substance abuse, a major factor in high incidence of infant mortality among Blacks.

High birth rate, reflected in high parity and short birth intervals, in itself remains a risk factor for pregnancy outcomes among Black women. They remain more exposed to this risk of too many and too closely spaced births than do White or Asian-American women. This situation indicates the need for providing and utilizing adequate family planning services including abortion. Provision of adequate postpartum care could be a means of avoiding an unwanted next pregnancy.

Though measures of socioeconomic status used in the risk-factor analyses usually fail to capture the full impact of SES on pregnancy outcomes, the major risk factors discussed above can only operate in an environment of poverty, social disadvantage, and hopelessness. This, however, does not necessarily mean that macro-level social programs aimed at alleviating poverty and creating jobs and adequate incomes will automatically change the environment so radically as to cause a major decline in the infant mortality rate in the short run. Dependency on drugs and irresponsible sexual behavior—products of an environment of hopelessness, alienation, and loss of self-esteem—seem to have emerged as mega confounders that drastically offset the normal effect of many favorable factors. Maternal age, marital status, educational attainment, and even the adequacy of prenatal care, which often show anomalous patterns, may only be the variables through which the effects of the potent variables of substance abuse, risky behaviors, and dangerous environments are mediated. Thus, the health care focus, including prenatal care and substance abuse prevention programs, will remain an important stratagem in the fight against high infant mortality among Black Americans.

Realistically, however, no major reduction in Black infant mortality can be achieved in the short run, for the roots of the risk factors associated with a high infant mortality rate, like the roots of so many other social problems among Blacks, are deeply embedded in the long and devastating history of racism, oppression, social disadvantage, and injured psyche. Though specific regimes of prevention and treatment measures for each of the health and social problems are necessary, their impact will be limited in the absence of a national commitment to reverse the hounding legacy of racial injustice in America.

REFERENCES

Abramowitz, M. (1989). Infant mortality soars here. *Washington Post,* September 30, p. Al.
Ahmed, F. (1987). *Infant mortality in Washington, DC: A study of risk factors among black residents.* Washington, DC: Institute for Urban Affairs and Research, Howard University.
Ahmed, F. (1990). Unmarried mothers as a high-risk group for adverse pregnancy outcomes. *Journal of Community Health, 15,* 35–44.
Ahmed, F. (1992). *Infant mortality among Black Americans.* Washington, DC: Institute for Urban Affairs and Research, Howard University.
Alexander, G. R., Tompkins, M. E., Altekruse, J. M., & Hornung, C. A. (1985). Racial differences in the relationship of birthweight and gestational age to neonatal mortality. *Public Health Reports, 100,* 539–547.
Baldwin, W., & Cain, V. S. (1980). The children of teenage parents. *Family Planning Perspectives, 12,* 34–43.
Binkin, N. J., Williams, R. L., Hogue, C. J. R., & Chen, P. M. (1985). Reducing Black neonatal mortality: Will improvements in low birthweight be enough? *Journal of the American Medical Association, 253,* 372–375.

Boone, M. S. (1989). *Capital Crime: Black infant mortality in America*. Newbury Park: Sage Publications.

Bross, D., & Shapiro, S. (1982). Direct and indirect associations of five factors with infant mortality. *American Journal of Epidemiology, 115*, 78–91.

Brown, J. E. (1988). Weight gain during pregnancy: What is "Optimal"? *Clinical Nutrition, 7*, 181–190.

Chasnoff, I. J. (1987). Perinatal effects of cocaine. *Contemporary Obstetrics and Gynecology, 29*, 163–179.

Chouteau, M., Namerow, P. B., & Leppert, P. (1988). The effect of cocaine abuse on birthweight and gestational age. *Obstetrics and Gynecology, 72*, 351–354.

Collins, J. W., & David, R. J. (1990). The differential effect of traditional risk factors on infant birthweight among Blacks and Whites in Chicago. *American Journal of Public Health, 80*, 679–681.

Friede, A., Baldwin, W., Rhodes, P. H., Buehler, J. W., Strauss, L. T., Smith, J. C., & Hogue, C. J. R. (1987). Young maternal age and infant mortality: The role of low birthweight. *Public Health Reports, 102*, 192–199.

General Accounting Office (GAO). (1990, June 28). Drug exposed infants: A generation at risk. Statement of Charles A. Bowsher, Comptroller General of the United States.

Geronimus, A. T. (1986). The effects of race, residence, and prenatal care on the relationship of maternal age to mortality. *American Journal of Public Health, 76*, 1416–1421.

Gortmaker, S. L. (1979a). Poverty and infant mortality in the United States. *American Sociological Review, 44*, 280–297.

Gortmaker, S. L. (1979b). The effects of prenatal care upon the health of the newborn. *American Journal of Public Health, 69*, 653–660.

Graham, G. G. (1991). WIC: A food program that fails. *Public Interest, 103*, 66–75.

Hogue, C. J. R., & Sappenfield, W. (1987). Smoking and low birthweight: Current concept. In M. J. Rosenberg (Ed.), *Smoking and reproductive health* (pp. 97–103). Littleton, MA: PSG Publishing Company.

Innocent addicts: High rate of prenatal drug abuse found. (1988). *ADAMHA News* (October), pp. 1, 3.

Institute of Medicine (IOM). (1985). *Preventing low birthweight*. Washington, DC: National Academy Press.

Institute of Medicine (IOM). (1988). *Prenatal care: Reaching mothers, reaching infants*. Washington, DC: National Academy Press.

Kessner, D. M., Singer, J., Kalk, C., & Schlesinger, E. R. (1973). *Infant death: An analysis of maternal risk and health care*. Washington, DC: National Academy of Sciences, Institute of Medicine.

Khoury, M. J., Erickson, D. J., & Adams, M. J. (1984). Trends in postneonatal mortality in the United States 1962 through 1978. *Journal of the American Medical Association, 252*, 367–372.

Klebanoff, M. A., Shiono, P. H., Berendes, H. W., & Rhoads, G. G. (1989). Facts and artifacts about anemia and pre-term delivery. *Journal of the American Medical Association, 262*, 511–515.

Kleinman, J. C., Fingerhut, L. A., & Prager, K. (1991). Differences in infant mortality by race, nativity status, and other maternal characteristics. *American Journal of the Diseases of Childhood, 145*, 194–199.

Kleinman, J. C., & Kessel, S. S. (1987). Racial differences in low birthweight: Trends and risk factors. *New England Journal of Medicine, 317,* 749–753.

Kleinman, J. C., & Kopstein, A. (1987). Smoking during pregnancy, 1967–80. *American Journal of Public Health, 77,* 823–825.

Kochanek, K. D. (1990). *Induced terminations of pregnancy: Reporting states, 1987.* DHHS Publication No. (PHS) 90–1120. Hyattsville, MD: Public Health Service: National Center for Health Statistics.

Kovar, M. G. (1977). Mortality of Black infants in the United States. *Phylon, 38,* 370–397.

Lee, K. S., Ferguson, R. M., Corpuz, M., & Gartner, L. M. (1988). Maternal age and incidence of low birth weight at term: A population study. *American Journal of Obstetrics and Gynecology, 158,* 84–89.

Lee, K. S., Paneth, N., Gartner, L. M., Pearlman, M. R., & Gruss, L. (1980). Neonatal mortality: An analysis of the recent improvements in the United States. *American Journal of Public Health, 70,* 15–22.

Lieberman, E., Ryan, K. J., Monson, R. R., & Schoenbaum, S. C. (1987). Risk factors accounting for racial differences in the rate of premature birth. *New England Journal of Medicine, 317,* 743–748.

Maternal Drug Abuse—New York City. (1989). *City Health Information (CHI)* (September), p. 1–4.

Meyer, M. B., Jonas, B. S., & Tonascia, J. A. (1976). Perinatal events associated with maternal smoking during pregnancy. *American Journal of Epidemiology, 103,* 464–476.

Miller, M. K., & Stokes, C. S. (1985). Teenage fertility, socioeconomic status and infant mortality. *Journal of Biosocial Sciences, 17,* 147–155.

Mills, J. L., Graubard, B. I., Harley, E. E., Rhoads, G. G., & Berendes, H. W. (1984). Maternal alcohol consumption and birthweight: How much drinking during pregnancy is safe? *Journal of the American Medical Association, 252,* 1875–1879.

National Center for Health Statistics (NCHS). (1988). *Health promotion and disease prevention U.S., 1985.* DHHS Publication No. (PHS) 88–1591. Washington, DC: Government Printing Office.

National Center for Health Statistics. (1990a). *Vital Statistics of the United States 1988. Vol. I, Natality.* USDHHS Publication No. (PHS) 90-1100. Washington, DC: Government Printing Office.

National Center for Health Statistics. (1990b). *Vital Statistics of the United States 1988. Vol. II, Part A, Mortality.* USDHHS Publication No. (PHS) 90-1102. Washington, DC: Government Printing Office.

National Commission to Prevent Infant Mortality. (1988). *Death before life: The tragedy of infant mortality.* Appendix. The report of the National Commission to Prevent Infant Mortality. The Honorable Lawton Chiles, United States Senate, Chairman. Washington, DC.

Norris, M. L. (1991). Crack's children: Suffering the sins of the mothers. *Washington Post,* June 30, p. A1.

Overpeck, M. D., & Moss, A. J. (1991). Children's exposure to environmental cigarette smoke before and after birth: Health of our nation's children, United States, 1988. *Advance Data from Vital and Health Statistics,* No. 202. Hyattsville, MD: National Center for Health Statistics.

Petitti, B. D., & Coleman, C. (1990). Cocaine and the risk of low birthweight. *American Journal of Public Health, 80,* 25–32.

Report of the secretary's task force on black and minority health. (1986). Vol. VI: Infant mortality and low birthweight. DHEW, Washington, DC: Government Printing Office.

Ries, P. (1991). Characteristics of persons with or without health care coverage: United States, 1989. *Advance Data from Vital and Health Statistics,* No. 201. Hyattsville, MD: National Center for Health Statistics.

Sappenfield, W. M., Buehler, J. W., Binkin, N. J., Hogue, C. J. R., Straus, L. T., & Smith, C. J. (1987). Differences in neonatal and postneonatal mortality by race, birth weight, and gestational age. *Public Health Reports, 102,* 182–191.

Showstack, A., Budetti, P. P., & Minkler, D. (1984). Factors associated with birthweight: An exploration of the roles of prenatal care and length of gestation. *American Journal of Public Health, 74,* 1003–1008.

Simpson, J. W., Lawless, R. W., & Mitchell, A. C. (1975). Responsibility of the obstetrician to the fetus II: Influence of pregnancy weight gain on birth weight. *Obstetrics and Gynecology, 45,* 48–57.

Singer, J. E., Westphal, M., & Niswander, K. (1968). Relationship of weight gain during pregnancy to birthweight and infant growth and development in the first year of life: A report from the collaborative study of cerebral palsy. *Obstetrics and Gynecology, 31,* 417–423.

Stein, Z., & Klein, J. (1983). Smoking, alcohol and reproduction. *American Journal of Public Health, 73,* 1154–1156.

Taffel, S. M. (1980). Factors associated with low birthweight, United States—1976. *Vital and Health Statistics,* Series 21, No. 37, DHEW Publication No. (PHS) 80-1915. Hyattsville, MD: National Center for Health Statistics.

Taffel, S. M. (1989). *Trends in low birthweight: United States, 1975–85.* DHHS Publication No. (PHS) 89–1926, Series 21, No. 48. Hyattsville, MD: National Center for Health Statistics.

Taffel, S. M., & Keppel, K. G. (1984). Implications of mother's weight gain on the outcome of pregnancy. Paper presented at the meeting of the American Statistical Association, Philadelphia, PA.

United Nations. (1991). *1989 Demographic Yearbook.* New York: United Nations.

U.S. Department of Health and Human Services (USDHHS). (1980a). *Promoting health/preventing disease: Objectives for the nation.* Washington, DC: Government Printing Office.

U.S. Department of Health and Human Services. (1980b). *The health consequences of smoking for women: A report of the surgeon general.* Rockville, MD: Department of Health and Human Services, Public Health Service, Office of the Assistant Secretary of Health, Office on Smoking and Health.

U.S. Department of Health and Human Services. (1988). *The surgeon general's report on nutrition and health, 1988.* DHHS Publication No. (PHS) 88-50210. Washington, DC: Government Printing Office.

U.S. Department of Health and Human Services. (1990). *Seventh special report to the U.S. Congress on alcohol and health from the secretary of health and human services, January 1990.* DHHS Publication No. ADM 90-1656. Rockville, MD: National Institute on Alcohol Abuse and Alcoholism.

Worthington-Roberts, B. S. (1985). *Nutrition in pregnancy and lactation.* St. Louis: Times Mirror Mosby College.

16

Social Status, Stress, and Health: Black Americans at Risk

Ivor Lensworth Livingston

> People are healthier not because they receive better treatment when ill but because they tend not to become ill in the first place, thanks to healthier environments and ways of living.
>
> David S. Sobel

Good health is not only desirable but a prerequisite for most, if not all, of life's daily functioning. African Americans, or Blacks as they will be called here, have poorer health compared with their White counterparts. Recent vital statistics confirm the deplorable health crisis for Blacks, especially as reflected in the best summary rate, life expectancy. The latest mortality data show a continued reduction and leveling off in life expectancy of 64.8 and 73.5 years for Black men and women, respectively. However, these trends contrast with an extension of life of 0.4 and 0.3 years for White males (72.7) and females (79.2) (National Center for Health Statistics, 1992).

Although several factors are responsible for the current racial disparities in health, it is argued in this chapter, as well as in the past by this author (see Livingston, 1986/87; Livingston, 1985a), that stress is a major factor that must be addressed. One recent national survey that looked at age-adjusted and gender-adjusted reports of moderate experiences of stress (i.e., 2 weeks before the interview) showed that, for the most part, Whites reported more stress than Blacks across gender (see Table 16.1). Interestingly, Black females reported higher levels of stress than their Black male counterparts. When the question was asked about the belief that stress had some effect on health, a greater percentage of Black females, again across all age groups, said that it did than their male counterparts. In terms of interracial differences, however, more Black females between 45 and 64 years of age (49.9%) reported that it did versus their

Table 16.1
Percentage of Persons 18 Years and Over on Selected Stress Items by Race and Gender, United States, 1990

	Race			
	Black		White	
	Male	Female	Male	Female
Felt moderate stress in past 2 weeks				
All Ages	44.5	50.7	55.8	61.5
18-29	46.0	47.8	59.2	66.9
30-34	51.8	59.2	66.6	70.8
45-64	40.4	51.7	54.4	62.5
65+	25.6	34.0	28.1	37.9
Stress has some effect on health				
All Ages	32.0	43.8	34.4	46.8
18-29	26.1	40.4	32.9	49.1
30-34	37.5	47.2	41.0	52.4
45-64	33.0	49.9	35.1	47.5
65+	30.1	32.1	20.6	33.5

Source: A. Piani and C. Schoenborn (1993). Health promotion and disease prevention: United States, 1990. NCHS, *Vital and Health Statistics,* Series 10, No. 85, DHHS Publication No. (PHS) 93-1513. Hyattsville, MD.

White counterparts (47.5%). Black males in the age group 65 and older was the only age group in which more of the stress-health relationship was reported than in their White counterparts (20.6%) (see Table 16.1).

Though simple descriptive reports such as those mentioned above are important, they fail to address crucial issues relating to age, race, gender, and socioeconomic status (or SES) differences in the perception of stressors and subsequent reactions to and effects of stress. In short, lacking is a conceptual framework of the stress process on which to guide and interpret ongoing stress research. There is a need to move beyond simply reiterating and showing, especially through descriptive surveys, the importance of the stress-race-relationship and to begin explaining how stress can contribute to health dysfunctions in general and health dysfunctions of Blacks in particular. Also lacking are race-specific analyses involved with population-based empirical studies that examine these relationships, adjusting for potentially confounding covariates.

This chapter is, in part, an attempt to bridge the existing void of a conceptual framework that explains how and in what manner stress contributes to various health dysfunctions in Blacks. Specifically, the purpose of the chapter is to review critically and discuss available information concerning the negative relationship between stress and the health of Blacks, especially those who are vulnerable or at risk because of their low socioeconomic status. A related purpose of the chapter is to use a 3-stage sociopsychophysiological model (or SPPM) of the stress process as a conceptual framework to show the following: (a) variations of how Blacks are likely to perceive and experience stress, (b) how their bodies react to stress, and (c) the various effects or dysfunctional outcomes that are likely to occur, especially because of chronic and unmitigated stress.

A Comprehensive View of Health

In the preamble to its 1946 constitution, the World Health Organization, or W.H.O., defined health as a "state of complete physical, mental, and social well-being, and not merely the absence of disease and infirmity" (Leavell & Clark, 1965, p. 14). Based on what is implied in this view of health, the healthy end of the continuum represents an ideal toward which we are oriented rather than a precise condition that we expect to attain. According to Schaefer (1983), along the continuum, people define themselves as healthy or sick on the basis of criteria established, in part, by each individual, medical practitioners, and the wider society. This relativistic approach to health allows for viewing health in a social context and considering how it varies in different situations and cultures (Wolinsky, 1988). Therefore, this view of health represents the context in which the life experiences of Blacks in the United States are assessed.

SOCIAL STATUS AND HEALTH OF BLACKS: AN OVERVIEW

The positive relationship between social status (i.e., socioeconomic status) has been widely documented in the past (e.g., Report of the Secretary's Task Force on Black and Minority Health, 1985; Syme & Berkman, 1976). Therefore, any discussion about the health of Blacks has to include, among other things, their disproportionate representation in low socioeconomic status positions.

The Social Status of Blacks

To assess the social status of Blacks is to understand how they are ranked, perceived, and treated as a group. The legacy of racial oppression in the United States is vividly underscored by the disproportionately high representation of

Blacks in low-income or low socioeconomic status (SES) positions. Although Blacks make up approximately 12 percent of the total United States population, they make up 30 percent of the population below the poverty level (Anderson, 1989). Because of a protracted history of institutional inequality in the United States (Katz & Taylor, 1988; Comer, 1980), which in turn is mainly responsible for Blacks being disproportionately poor, a frequently made mistake is the assumption that Blacks are a monolithic group. However, Blacks are heterogenous in terms of ethnic background (e.g., initially coming from the Caribbean, South America) and racial composition (e.g., racial admixture), to mention only a few factors. Therefore, research efforts that seek to explain racial differences in health must, then, include interracial and intraracial research designs (Livingston, Levine & Moore, 1991a).

Though some progress has been made to upgrade Blacks' status, for example, through legislation (such as the Civil Rights Act of 1964), any grounds that have been gained have to be interpreted in a restrictive United States society, which remains today institutionally racist and both anti-black and anti-poor.

Empirically, the social status of Blacks can, in part, be assessed by their income or economic status. For example, in 1990, 31.9 percent of Blacks and 10.7 percent of Whites lived in poverty. For Blacks, this percentage means that in 1990 there were 6.5 million more Blacks in poverty than would have been if Blacks and Whites had equal poverty rates. The poverty rates are equally astonishing for Black children. For 1990, the rate of poverty among Black and White children was 44.8 percent (4,550,000) and 15.9 percent (8,232,000), respectively (Swinton, 1992; U.S. Bureau of the Census, 1991).

Social Status and Health

The general health status of Blacks, especially those whose social status relegates and maintains them in poverty, is dismally poor (Navarro, 1990). The health disparities between Whites and Blacks are increasingly attributed to social class or status and less to race. However, because many Blacks are classified as of a low SES, race continues to serve as a proxy for SES (Kessler & Neighbors, 1986).

The enormous increase in social inequality, as evidenced in the widening gap in income, has contributed heavily to the worsening of the social conditions that decide health in the Black community (Health Trends, 1992). Generally speaking, people with incomes above (versus those below) the poverty level experiences better health (Amler & Dull, 1987). It was reported that the all-cause mortality rate for Blacks exceeds that for Whites by 149 percent for those 35 to 44 and by 97 percent for those 45 to 54 (Otten, Teutsch, Williamson & Marks, 1990). For example, though homicide is the number-one killer of young Black males between the ages of 18 and 35, race appears not to be as important a risk factor for violent death as socioeconomic status (Healthy People 2000, 1990).

Inverse associations have been reported between low educational attainment and health. For example, activity limitations are 4 times more common among people with 8 years of education than among individuals with 16 years or more. It has also been reported that bed disability days increase as income decreases (National Institute on Disability and Rehabilitation Research, 1989). Low-income people and those who completed less than 12 years of schooling have higher-than-average rates of high blood pressure and obesity (Surgeon General's Report on Nutrition and Health, 1988); and they tend to smoke about 20 percent more than other, educated people (McCord & Freeman, 1990). All these conditions are major risk factors for heart disease and stroke, the number-one and number-two killers, respectively, of all Americans.

Black Children

In childhood, the best indicator of the relationship between poverty and health is infant mortality. Poor pregnancy outcomes, including prematurity, birth defects, low birth weight, and infant death are associated with low income, low educational level, low occupational status, and other conditions related to being socially and economically disadvantaged (Institute of Medicine, 1985). Black children, especially males, do not have the same prospects for a long and disability-free life as their White counterparts (Moore, 1990).

Disproportionate traumatic death and developmental limitations are also associated with children who are poor. For example, iron deficiency is more than twice as common in low-income children, aged 1 and 2, than among other children of similar ages in the wider population (Healthy People 2000, 1990). Growth retardation affects 16 percent of low-income children younger than 6 years of age; and in the mid-1980s, an estimated 3 million children, most of whom were from low-income families, had blood lead levels that exceeded 15 ug/dL. This lead level was sufficient to place them at risk for impaired mental and physical development (Healthy People 2000, 1990).

Social Status and Stress

Although research shows that the race-stress relationship is more concentrated among individuals with low incomes (Harburg et al., 1973; Kessler & Neighbors, 1986), there are additional factors to consider. For example, using one of the few large nationally representative samples of Blacks, the National Survey of Black Americans, it was reported that the association between SES and distress (or negative stress) varied by the type of "stressor" involved. When the stressor was associated with an economic crisis or physical illness, low-SES Blacks experienced more distress than their higher-SES counterparts. However, when the stressor involved emotional adjustment problems, high-SES Blacks reported more distress than their lower-SES counterparts (Neighbors, 1986).

Intraracial findings, as those mentioned above, underscore both the heterogeneity of the Black population and the complexity of the SES-stress(health)-race relationship. These findings also suggest the need for further research in the area, especially where greater emphasis is placed on (a) statistical "interaction" versus "main" effects in analyses, (b) income-related differences in "perceived" stressors, and (c) the use of interracial and intraracial research designs.

THE STRESS-HEALTH RELATIONSHIP: A NEEDED FRAMEWORK

How does the human body deal with the various "demands" arising from the environment? How are individual, SES, and racial and/or ethnic variations in stress addressed for individuals? What symptoms and/or outcome effects occur when the body is unable to respond in a "healthy" manner to these perceived demands? These are just a sample of the many questions that can be asked when addressing the stress-health relationship. It is reasoned in this chapter and elsewhere (e.g., Livingston 1988a) that answers to these and related questions can be more easily addressed by using a conceptual model of the stress process as a guiding framework.

A Conceptual Stress Model: The Focus on Blacks

It is posited that the generic sociopsychophysiological model (or SPPM) of the stress process seen in Figure 16.1 provides the needed conceptual framework on which to theoretically discuss and, subsequently, conduct empirical research to assess the stress-health relationship. The SPPM is especially useful when the focus is on low-SES persons, such as at-risk Blacks.

The dominant view of stress adopted in this paper is consistent with a cognitive and interactive view of stress alluded to in the past by this author (Livingston, 1988a, 1988b, 1990) and others (e.g., Lazarus, Cohen, Folkman & Schafer, 1980). A stressful situation is one perceived and appraised by individuals (e.g., Blacks) as personally significant to their well-being, but also as taxing or exceeding their resource capabilities. Put succinctly, stress is not what happens (stressor) to Blacks but how their bodies react (i.e., neurophysiologically) to what happens (stress).

An examination of the SPPM of the stress process, illustrated in Figure 16.1, shows an interactive (see bidirectional arrows) 3-stage process (onset, reaction, and effect) involving 9 basic components. (For a more in-depth discussion of the SPPM, see Livingston, 1988b, 1991b.) Of importance to the SPPM is the fact that the wider society or the outer system[#1] subsumes the individual or the inner system[#2], which in turn subsumes the remaining 7 component parts. Also, there is an ongoing interaction, over time, between both systems. For Blacks, this latter point is very important, given the dominant and institutionally racist nature of the wider U.S. society (#1). What follows is a brief discussion of Blacks and stress under each of the 3 defined stages of the SPPM.

Figure 16.1
A Sociopsychophysiological Model of the Stress Process

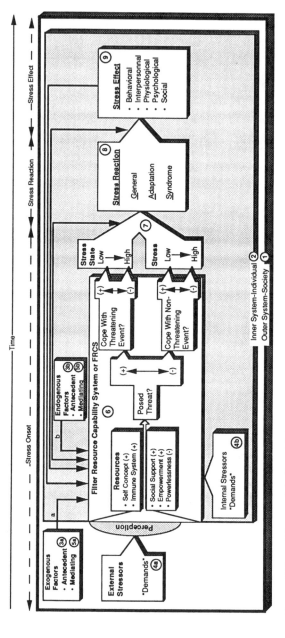

Source: This model was originally published in the *Journal of the National Medical Association*, 8 (1), 49–59, but it was specifically revised for this chapter by the author.

a External conditions in society contributing to the functioning of the FRCS.

b Internal factors within the individual contributing to the functioning of the FRCS.

↔ Bidirectional arrows reflect the reciprocal nature of designated elements in the model.

(+) Desirable qualities or *resources*.

(−) Undesirable qualities or *resources*.

Stress-Onset Stage

This first and crucial stage of the stress process [i.e., #3 thru #7] refers to the initiation of the complex series of events and processes required to be started before and including the experience of stress, that is, the stress state[#7] by Blacks. At the heart of this stage is the Filter Resource Capability system (or FRCS), which is the mind-body enduring capacity that Blacks have that filters, mediates, neutralizes, and subsequently serves to stabilize all entering noxious and other stimuli or stressors. For example, it plays an important role in (1) the perception and interpretation of external eliciting stressors[#4a], which are of primary interest in this paper for Blacks (e.g., life experiences resulting from a combination of racism and poverty). The FRCS also plays a mediating role in Blacks' experiencing internal eliciting stressors (e.g., trauma, infection)[#4b]. However, because of the focus of the chapter (i.e., less on internal and physical stressors and more on external sociopsychological stressors), these stressors are not addressed.

The strength of the FRCS, which is directly related to its ability to inhibit activation of stressful experiences or the stress state[#7] by Blacks, is in turn influenced by various other factors. First, it is related to the existence of a variety of antecedent[#3a & #3b] (i.e., precursors or possible "triggers" that exist before the stressor condition) and mediating[#5a & #5b] (i.e., factors that buffer the effects of the stressor condition) resource/competing conditions that may be exogenous or external[#1] to Blacks and/or endogenous or within[#2] (e.g., a "hardy" personality, Kobasa, 1979) Blacks. As precursors occuring outside and within Blacks, respectively, they individually and collectively lay the groundwork for the perception of external stressors as "demanding" or stressful.

In terms of exogenous antecedent conditions[#3a] affecting Blacks, institutional racism and its related factors, e.g., poverty or low socioeconomic status, are perhaps the best example. It is said that stressors related to alienation and other adverse factors resulting from discrimination make up psychological threats to Blacks (Benjamin, 1991). Therefore, if stress is used as an index of psychological threat, it should be more evident around Blacks than Whites and among the poor than among the middle and upper classes (Myers, 1982).

Two interrelated (exogenous) factors that are directly responsible for Blacks' stressful experiences have been alluded to before: (a) their disproportionate numbers in low socioeconomic positions and (b) the daily discriminatory experiences they encounter as a group living in America. Therefore, it is reasoned that these relatively unanimous experiences, especially for Blacks who are poor, put them as a group more at risk to experience stress and subsequently a variety of dysfunctional health outcomes.

Endogenous antecedent factors[#3b] that put Blacks at risk to experience stress and related conditions may relate, in part, to their developmental acquisitions. For example, developmental histories (e.g., Brown & Harris, 1978) and idiosyncratic stress (e.g., Seligman, 1975) have been associated ultimately with depression and hypertension (Livingston, 1985b). It is reported that Black children (and other minorities) are exposed to many early traumas, which are associated with race and class oppression (Dohrenwend & Dohrenwend, 1970).

In view of how stress is operationalized in the paper, some caution must be exercised by stopping short of implying that all Blacks will, because of, for example, the deleterious societal experiences associated with racism (exogenous antecedent condition), have relatively "weak" FRCSs, thereby being at risk to experience a disproportionate incidence of stress. As mentioned before, Blacks living in America exhibit commonality amid diversity. Therefore, the mere presence of predisposing racially related stressors is a necessary but not a sufficient condition to initiate the stress process (i.e., stress onset).

In terms of exogenous mediating conditions[#5a], perhaps the best example is the social support Blacks and others receive in times of need. Social support has been found to buffer the stress-health relationship (Cobb, 1976). Operationalizing social support through social integration, it was reported that Blacks who attended church more frequently had lower levels of arterial blood pressure than those who attended less frequently (Livingston, Levine & Moore, 1991a).

Of particular concern in this chapter is the contributing role of endogenous mediation factors[#5b] to increasing the strength and resiliency of Blacks' FRCSs[#6]. An additional concern is the variety of qualities and skills that Blacks must have to withstand the internal[#4b] and external[#4a] stressors, most of which relate to the "challenges" of living in America. Although there are many personal "resource" factors that can exist any time in the arsenal of Blacks' repertoire, given the inverse association between these resources (e.g., hardiness, Kobasa, 1979; experiences with comparable stressors, Livingston, 1992a; a strong immune system, Henry, 1982; Livingston, 1988b; and mastery, Pearlin et al., 1981) and stress, one empirically proven resource is the availability of requisite coping skills (Scott & Howard, 1970). See Figure 16.1 and the relationship of coping skills to posed threat or demands (e.g., [#4a]) in the context of Blacks' FRCSs and subsequent variations in stress levels (#7).

Stress Reaction Stage

Depending on the severity of the stress state[#7], the time factor involved, and the repeated failure of not having a strong and resilient FRCS[#6] to improve the situation, Blacks are likely to experience this second phase of the stress process. Essentially, this phase involves a complex series of measurable neuroendocrine reactions and changes. If activation of the sympathoadrenomedullary system lasts for any protracted period or the activation is repeated too often, the results will be functional disturbances in various organs and systems throughout the body (Green & Costain, 1981).

Cannon's (1935) research on blood hormones reported that stress that exceeded a critical threshold could strain the human system beyond its adaptive capacity. The levels of adrenocorticotrophic hormones (ACTH) from the pituitary gland

and/or corticoids in the plasma or urine are viewed as the nonspecific adaptation in the body. The presence of these (and other) substances in a (Black) person's blood is a reliable physiologic indicator of the presence of stress (i.e., the state[#7]).

A related physiologic response associated with corticosteroid hormonal secretion is the presence of a sequential syndrome—the General Adaptation Syndrome or G.A.S.[#8]—with its 3 stages: alarm, resistance, and exhaustion (Selye, 1976). The presence of the last stage, exhaustion, implies host (i.e., Black) vulnerability for illness and/or disease (Shaffer, 1983). If the stress state[#7] that contributed to it is not improved, as indicated in the SPPM by, for example, Blacks having a strong FRCS, the last stage of the stress process occurs, the stress effect.

Stress Effect Stage

This last phase of the complex stress process depicted in the SPPM is germane to explaining the disproportionate incidence of various health disorders between Blacks and Whites. Again, this stage is reached without any abatement of chronic stress experienced by Blacks.

Over 85 percent of health can be explained by life-style conditions and experiences. Therefore, because stress is reasoned to be an integral part of the lives of low-SES, at-risk Blacks, any address of racial disparities in health has then, to examine the relationship between stress and selected leading causes of morbidity and mortality among Blacks. Because of space limitations, only a brief overview follows of selected stress-related health outcomes or effects that are disproportionately shared by Blacks, e.g., infant mortality (Healthy People 2000, 1990), hypertension (Joint National Committee, 1988; Livingston, 1993), HIV/AIDS (Selik, Papaionnou & Castro, 1988), and homicide (Health United States 1991, 1992).

Infant Mortality

Although more research needs to be done, there is suggestive evidence that infants born to mothers who lived their own childhood under conditions of extreme disadvantage (or stress, as with many Black women) tend to have greater rates of low birth weight (i.e., less than 2,500 grams) and dead babies (Emanuel, Hale & Berg, 1989). Also, preterm delivery might be caused by sudden or large surges in epinephrine caused by high stress (Lobel, Dunkel-Schetter & Scrimshaw, 1992).

Hypertension

As previously discussed in this chapter, stress occurs, in part, from persons (e.g., Blacks) having a weak FRCS. Chronic stress contributes to elevated arterial blood pressure (BP) through various pathways. One likely pathway to explain the stress-BP relationship is through increased cardiac reactivity (Livingston &

Marshall, 1990) and restricted sodium excretion (brought on by the inhibitory effects of stress). These two processes are related because inhibited sodium excretion in Blacks augments reactivity (Anderson, 1989). Additionally, there are some preliminary data that suggest that greater life stress is associated with inhibited recovery from cardiovascular reactivity (Anderson, 1989).

HIV Infection and AIDS

On a physiological level, the association between stress and infectious diseases (e.g., AIDS) is very complex. Stress is reported to be responsible for the reactivation of latent viruses (e.g., HIV) (Ickovics & Rodin, 1992). Also, stress-produced corticosteriods tend to affect greatly important elements of the immunological apparatus. Therefore, it has been suggested that stress may play a role in the onset of infectious diseases (e.g., AIDS) by further suppressing the body's immune system (Livingston, 1988b) through, for example, the shrinkage of the thymus gland and reduction in the number of (T-)lymphocytes in the blood (Elliott & Eisdorfer, 1982).

Homicide

The role of chronic stress in interpersonal violence, particularly homicide, has been reported (Whaley, 1992). According to Britt and Allen (1988), poverty (i.e., an exogenous antecedent condition[#3a]) is perhaps the most common stressor associated with extreme interpersonal violence in the Black community. Chronic poverty is likely to cause anger, depression, and anxiety, to name only a few negative feelings, as Blacks struggle to survive on a daily basis (Whaley, 1992). The stresses of developmental transitions can also affect the mental health and, subsequently, the violence associated with Black youth. Relatedly, it has been said that the inability of Black adolescents to master the transition from early childhood can result in several negative outcomes, one such outcome being violent behavior (Brunswick & Merzel, 1988).

INTERVENING TO REDUCE STRESS AND IMPROVE HEALTH

Successful strategies to reduce stress and improve the health of Blacks should involve action on both the macro and micro levels. Macro-level intervention, such as addressing the all-encompassing problem of institutional racism and equity in health care, while relatively more difficult to achieve and taking a long time to rectify, is very much needed to ensure sustained success. For this chapter, however, micro-level interventions, which are more easy to achieve and, therefore, possess more immediate benefits to Blacks, are emphasized.

Micro Approaches

A pragmatic view suggests that immediate improvements in Black health are more likely to be achieved through innovative, culturally sensitive, and practical intervention strategies (see Livingston, 1992c) aimed at educating Blacks about improving their health in general and understanding and managing stress in particular. In short, although there is an intrinsic relationship between Blacks and the wider U.S. society (see Figure 16.1[#1]), to achieve faster, more stable and sustaining improvements in Black health the focus of activities must, of necessity, be on Blacks themselves. For example, through health education directives in targeted Black communities, Blacks must be provided with the needed information and skills to become more informed and empowered to recognize how and when to protect themselves from the ravages of uncontrolled stress. Blacks in local communities where the intervention is to take place must be given the opportunity beforehand to assess the cultural sensitivity of the approaches and methods to be used.

The SPPM as a Guide

Based on the discussion presented in this chapter, educators are advised about (a) understanding the important role stress plays in health and disease and (b) how this stress-health relationship is best understood in the context of a conceptual model of the stress process, as the SPPM presented in Figure 16.1. In terms of intervention approaches, it is suggested that relevant aspects of the SPPM be used as a conceptual guide in addressing practical and specific ways of reducing stress, and by that improving general health in the Black community.

More specifically, when the SPPM is used as a guide, improvements must be primarily sought in areas relating to (a) endogenous antecedent (see #3b) and mediating (see #5b) factors and (b) the FRCSs (see #6). Also, because of the central importance of the FRCS in the SPPM, the overriding concern of researchers, educators, and health care personnel must be to increase the resources (i.e., mediating and enabling) of Blacks (e.g., physical tolerance, immune functioning, self-concept, being in control, and engaging in preventive and protective behaviors. See +s next to examples of desirable resource categories and −s next to examples of undesirable resource categories in Figure 16.1). These resources (+) will, in turn, strengthen the resiliency of Blacks' FRCS.

Stress Management and Related Issues

Although the main focus of any health education appeal to the Black population is to increase the functional strength and resiliency of their FRCSs, the success of any micro-level health intervention efforts will be decided by answers to the following questions: (a) How, where, and by whom will the message be directed to at-risk Blacks as a group? (e.g., using Black media, billboards, and videos with culturally appropriate expressions and messages articulated by "known" personalities in the Black community; information presented in schools, at work environments, at community meeting places and on public transportation). (b) What are the specific messages contained in the educational directives to Blacks? (e.g., information about "enabling" and "mediating" factors that will serve to strengthen the FRCSs of Blacks) (see Livingston, 1992c; Livingston, 1993).

Given that stress has reached epidemic proportions, especially in the at-risk low-SES segments of the Black population, great care must be taken to ensure that the stress management information presented is understood, used and sustained by at-risk Blacks. Limitations associated with prior stress management approaches must be avoided. Some of these limitations include (1) the use of inappropriate esoteric stress management approaches; (2) failure first to explain the nature of stress before stress management techniques are presented; (3) failure to incorporate a holistic orientation into stress management education (see Livingston, 1992a); and (d) failure to have more interactive discussions, including information relating to life-style activities (e.g., exercise, diet, use of support systems, meditation, etc.).

Whatever stress management intervention approach is adopted, health education should be used to teach Blacks about the importance and value of relaxation (Livingston, 1993). Also, in order to make Blacks more empowered and accountable for their actions/health, they should be involved in the instructional phase and selected stress management approach. Not only should Blacks be allowed to set realistic goals for themselves regarding stress and their own health, but they should also be instructed to establish personal goals and conduct self-evaluations of their progress. In order to achieve and sustain progress, Blacks must also be educated and motivated to stay well. This can be accomplished by teaching them to build up their ''resources'' (i.e., their FRCSs) by engaging in consistent health-protective behaviors including, but not limited to, stress management.

CONCLUSION

There is no justifiable reason Blacks, especially those who are poor, should experience approximately 60,000 excess deaths a year more than their White counterparts. There is no compelling reason life expectancy for Blacks has lagged behind that of the total population throughout this century. Last, there is no compelling reason over one-third of Blacks live in poverty, which is 3 times the rate of Whites; over half live in urban areas inundated with poverty, crowded and substandard housing, poor schools, unemployment and underemployment, pervasive drug culture, excessive street violence, and generally high levels of stress.

While fully appreciating the contribution of all these (and other) factors to the health status of Blacks, the main focus of this chapter was on the detrimental nature of stress (i.e., distress) and its often unrecognized contribution to health problems in general and health outcomes of Blacks in particular.

The SPPM introduced in this chapter offers a practical and functional guide for needed change involving (a) stress management interventions, (b) theory building, and (c) research in the area of Black health. Also, as a generic and process-oriented model emphasizing (a) the ongoing *interaction* between Blacks and the wider U.S. society in which they live, (b) the *subjective* nature of the stressful experience and (c) the multiple points and ways to *intervene* (e.g., increasing the resiliency of Blacks' FRCSs) to reduce stress, the SPPM is sufficiently flexible to address *interracial* and *intraracial* variation in the stress-health relationship, especially among the truly at-risk segments of the Black community.

REFERENCES

Amler, R. W., & Dull, H. B. (1987). *Closing the gap: The burden of unnecessary illness.* New York: Oxford University Press.

Anderson, N. B. (1989). Racial differences in stress-induced cardiovascular reactivity and hypertension: Current status and substantive issues. *Psychological Bulletin, 105,* 89–105.

Benjamin, L. (1991). *The black elite.* Chicago: Nelson-Hall.

Britt, D. W., & Allen, L. (1988). Homicides and race riots. *Journal of Community Psychology, 16,* 119–131.

Brown, G. W., & Harris, T. (1978). *Social origins of depression.* New York: Free Press.

Brunswick, A. F., & Merzel, C. R. (1988). Health through three life stages: A longitudinal study of urban black adolescents. *Social Science and Medicine, 27,* 1203–1214.

Cannon, W. (1935). Stresses and the strains of homeostasis. *American Journal of Medical Science, 189,* 1–14.

Cobb, S. (1976). Social support as a moderator of life stress. *Psychosomatic Medicine, 38,* 300–314.

Comer, J. P. (1980). White racism: Its root, form, and function. In R. L. Jones (Ed.), *Black psychology* (2nd Ed.). New York: Harper and Row.

Dohrenwend, B. S., & Dohrenwend, B. P. (1970). Class and race as status-related sources of stress. In S. Levine & N. A. Scotch (Eds.), *Social stress* (pp. 111–140). Chicago: Aldine.

Elliott, G. R., & Eisdorfer, C. (Eds.). (1982). *Stress and human health.* New York: Springer Publishing Company.

Emanuel, I., Hale, C. B., & Berg, C. J. (1989). Poor birth outcomes of American black women: An alternative explanation. *Journal of Public Health Policy, 10,* 299–308.

Green, A., & Costain, D. (1981). *Pharmacology and biochemistry of psychiatric disorders.* New York: John Wiley.

Harburg, E., Erfurt, J., Hauenstein, L., Chape, C., Schull, W., & Schork, M. (1973). Socioecological stress, suppressed hostility, skin color and black-white blood pressure: Detroit. *Journal of Chronic Diseases, 26,* 595–611.

Health Trends. (1992). New vital statistics confirm worsening of black health. *Ethnicity and Disease, 2,* 192–193.

Health United States 1991. (1992). DHHS Publication No. (PHS) 92-1232, National Center for Health Statistics. Washington, DC: Government Printing Office.

Healthy People 2000. (1990). National health promotion and disease objectives. DHHS Publication No. (PHS) 91-50213. Washington, DC: Government Printing Office.

Henry, J. P. (1982). The relation of social to biological processes in disease. *Social Science and Medicine, 16,* 369–380.

Hutchinson, J. (1992). AIDS and racism in America. *Journal of the National Medical Association, 84,* 119–124.

Ickovics, J. R., & Rodin, J. (1992). Women and AIDS in the United States: Epidemiology, natural history, and mediating mechanisms. *Health Psychology, 11,* (1), 1–16.

Institute of Medicine. (1985). Preventing low birthweight. Washington, DC: National Academy Press.

Joint National Committee. (1988). The 1988 report of the Joint National Committee on Detection, Evaluation and Treatment of High Blood Pressure. *Archives of Internal Medicine, 148,* 1023–1038.

Katz, P., & Taylor, D. (Ed.). (1988). *Eliminating racism.* New York: Plenum.

Kessler, R. R., & Neighbors, H. (1986). A new perspective on the relationships among race, social class and psychological distress. *Journal of Health and Social Behavior, 27,* 107–115.

Kobasa, S. C. (1979). Stressful life events, personality, and health: An inquiry into hardiness. *Journal of Personality and Social Psychology, 37,* 1–11.

Lazarus, R. S., Cohen, J. B., Folkman, S., Kanner, A. & Schaefer, C. (1980). Psychological stress and adaptation: Some unresolved issues. In H. Selye (Ed.), *Selye's guide to stress research, Volume I* (90–117). New York: Van Nostrand Reinhold Company.

Leavell, H. R., & Clark, E. G. (1965). *Preventive medicine for the doctor in his community: An epidemiologic approach* (3rd Ed.). New York: McGraw-Hill.

Livingston, I. L. (1985a). Alcohol consumption and hypertension: A review with suggested implications. *Journal of the National Medical Association, 77,* 129–135.

Livingston, I. L. (1985b). The importance of stress in the interpretation of the race-hypertension association. *Humanity and Society, 9,* 168–181.

Livingston, I. L. (1986/7). Blacks, lifestyle and hypertension: The importance of health education. *Humboldt Journal of Social Relations, 14,* 195–213.

Livingston, I. L. (1988a). Stress and health dysfunctions: The importance of health education. *Stress and Medicine, 4,* 155–161.

Livingston, I. L. (1988b). Co-factors, host susceptibility, and AIDS: An argument for stress. *Journal of the National Medical Association, 80,* 49–59.

Livingston, I. L., & Marshall, R. J. (1990). Cardiac reactivity and elevated blood pressure levels among young African Americans. In D. J. Jones (Ed.), *Prescriptions and policies: The social well-being of African Americans in the 1980s* (pp. 77–91). New Brunswick: Transactions Publishers.

Livingston, I. L., Levine, D. M., & Moore, R. D. (1991a). Social integration and black intraracial variation in blood pressure. *Ethnicity and Disease, 1,* 135–149.

Livingston, I. L. (1991b). Stress, hypertension and renal disease: A review with implications. *National Journal of Sociology, 5,* 143–181.

Livingston, I. L. (1992a). *The ABC's of stress management: Taking control of your life.* Salt Lake City: Northwest Publishing.

Livingston, I. L., & Ackah, S. (1992b). Hypertension, end-stage renal disease and rehabilitation: A look at black Americans. *The Western Journal of Black Studies, 16,* 103–112.

Livingston, I. L. (1992c). AIDS/HIV crisis in developing countries: The need for greater understanding and innovative health prevention approaches. *Journal of the National Medical Association, 84,* 755–770.

Livingston, I. L. (1993). Stress, hypertension and young black Americans: The importance of counselling. *Journal of Multicultural Counselling, 4*, 132–142.

Livingston, I. L. (1993). Renal disease and black Americans: Selected issues. *Social Science and Medicine, 37*, 613–621.

Lobel, M., Dunkel-Schetter, C., & Scrimshaw, S. C. M. (1992). Prenatal maternal stress and prematurity: A prospective study of socioeconomically disadvantaged women. *Health Psychology, 11*, 32–40.

McCord, C., & Freeman, H. P. (1990). Excess mortality in Harlem. *New England Journal of Medicine, 322*, 173–177.

Moore, E. K. (1990). Status of African American children. Twentieth Anniversary Report 1970–1990. Washington, DC: National Black Child Development Institute.

Myers, H. (1982). Stress, ethnicity and social class: A model for research with black populations. In E. E. Jones (Ed.), *Minority mental health* (pp. 118–148). New York: Praeger.

Navarro, V. (1990). Race or class versus race and class: Mortality differentials in the United States. *The Lancet*, November 17, 1238–1240.

National Center for Health Statistics. (1992). Advance report on final mortality statistics, 1989. *Monthly Vital Statistics Report*, Vol. 40, No. 8, Supp. 2. Hyattsville, MD: Public Health Service.

National Institute on Disability and Rehabilitation. (1989). *Chartbook on disability in the United States*. Washington, DC: The Institute.

Neighbors, H. W. (1986). Socioeconomic status and psychologic distress in adult blacks. *American Journal of Epidemiology, 124*, 779–793.

Otten, M. W., Teutsch, S. M., Williamson, D. F., & Marks, J. (1990). The effect of known risk factors on the excess mortality of black adults in the United States. *Journal of the American Medical Association, 263*, 845–850.

Pearlin, L. T., Lieberman, M. A., Menaghan, E. G., & Mullan, J. T. (1981). The stress process. *Journal of Health and Social Behavior, 22*, 337–356.

Report of the Secretary's Task Force on Black and Minority Health. (1985). Volume I: Executive Summary. U.S. Department of Health and Human Services. Washington, DC: Government Printing Office.

Scott, R., & Howard, A. (1970). Models of stress. In S. Levine & N. A. Scotch (Eds.), *Social stress*. Chicago: Aldine.

Seligman, M. E. P. (1975). *Helplessness: On depression, development and death*. San Francisco: W. H. Freeman.

Selik, R. M., Castro, K. G., & Papaionnou, M. (1988). Racial/ethnic differences in the risk of AIDS in the United States. *American Journal of Public Health, 78*, 1539–1544.

Selye, H. (1976). *The stress of life*. New York: McGraw-Hill.

Shaffer, M. (1983). *Life after stress*. Chicago: Contemporary Books, Inc.

Sobel, D. S. (1979). Introduction. In D. S. Sobel (Ed.), *Ways of health* (p. 4). New York: Harcourt Brace Jovanovich.

Surgeon General's Report on Nutrition and Health. (1988). DHHS, Public Health Service. Washington, D.C.

Swinton, D. H. (1992). The economic status of African Americans: Limited ownership and persistent inequality. In B. J. Tidwell (Ed.), *The status of black America 1992* (pp. 61–117). New York: National Urban League.

Syme, S., & Berkman, J. (1976). Social class, susceptibility and sickness. *American Journal of Epidemiology, 104,* 1–8.

U.S. Bureau of the Census. (1991). The black population in the United States: March 1991. *Current Population Reports,* P20–464. Washington, DC: Government Printing Office.

Whaley, A. L. (1992). A culturally sensitive approach to the prevention of interpersonal violence among urban black youth. *Journal of the National Medical Association, 84,* 585–588.

Wolinsky, F. D. (1988). *The sociology of health* (2nd ed.). Belmont, CA: Wadsworth.

17

The Mental Health of African Americans: Findings, Questions, and Directions

David R. Williams and Brenda T. Fenton

An understanding of the distribution of mental health problems in the Black (or African American) population is a prerequisite to the development and targeting of appropriate mental health and social services. The study of African-American mental health has a long and, at times, disturbing history in the United States.

In a comprehensive and perceptive review of the study of racial differences in health during the 19th century, Krieger (1987) shows how racial comparisons in health status have been used to obscure the social origins of illness, demonstrate Black inferiority, and provide a "scientific" rationale for policies of inequality, subjugation, and exploitation of Blacks. An illustrative example was a scientific report that deliberately falsified the Black insanity rates from the 1840 U.S. Census to show that the further North Blacks lived, the higher their rates of lunacy—strong evidence, of course, that freedom drove Blacks crazy. Current research on Black mental health is no longer characterized by such blatant racism, and today we have better and more reliable estimates of the distribution of psychopathology within the African-American population. However, 150 years after the 1840 census, there are still important gaps and paradoxes in our knowledge of the mental health status of the African-American population, and much research on the health of African Americans still obscures the social origins of illness.

This chapter critically evaluates the available data on the mental health status of the African-American population. It traces the evolution of our understanding of the mental health status of the Black population and highlights important trends and developments. We consider rates of serious mental illness, as well as less severe forms of psychological impairment. In addition, we highlight a number of unresolved issues in the literature that urgently need attention and point to some emerging trends that have great promise to enhance our understanding of Black mental health.

OVERVIEW OF STUDIES OF BLACK MENTAL HEALTH

The race-comparison paradigm has been the central and dominant focus of most research on Black mental health (Neighbors, 1984). In this framework, the mental health status of the White population is used as a standard of comparison for the mental health of the African-American population. We will present a chronological overview of the major findings from the early psychiatric epidemiology studies, population-based studies of psychological distress, and the more recent studies of psychiatric disorders in community samples.

Early Studies of Mental Illness

Most of our knowledge of the mental health of the African-American population in the first half of the 20th century comes from several large studies that focused only on the severely mentally ill (hospitalized patients). These early studies examined racial differences in first-admission rates of patients in mental hospitals in the country as a whole as well as in states such as Ohio, New York, Virginia, and Illinois (Fischer, 1969). The findings of these studies with regard to race were remarkably consistent: Blacks had higher rates of mental illness than Whites.

However, these early studies had a serious methodological flaw. Only patients in certain treatment sites, predominantly state hospitals, were included in the samples. Treatment rates are not accurate estimates of the prevalence of psychiatric illness because cases in treatment tend to reflect the severe end of the illness spectrum, as well as health care access. A client's economic status, the number of available beds, health care financing options, distance, available transportation, racial discrimination, and other structural and cultural barriers affect the likelihood of both seeking and receiving medical care. Help-seeking behavior has been found to vary across race, with Blacks in need using professional services less than their White counterparts (Vernon & Roberts, 1982; Neighbors, 1985). Neighbors found that less than 10 percent of Blacks who had experienced "serious personal problems" utilized professional services. State hospitals have been and continue to be the principal inpatient care source for African Americans (Mollica, Blum & Redlich, 1980; Snowden & Cheung, 1990) and are not representative of all treatment facilities. In contrast to their Black peers, White patients could frequently avoid the stigma of a mental hospital admission by obtaining treatment outside the psychiatric specialty sector, such as admission to a general hospital ward.

As later studies expanded their study population by the inclusion of outpatients, private patients, and/or community residents, the bias inherent in the earliest studies was reduced, and the findings of racial differences in mental health status became more inconsistent (Jaco, 1960; Pasamanick, 1963). Pasamanick (1963), for example, demonstrated that Blacks had higher rates of psychiatric disorder than Whites in Baltimore only when the analyses were restricted to patients in state hospitals. The reverse was true when state hospital data were combined with data from private mental hospitals, Veterans' Administration (VA) hospitals, and a community survey of Baltimore residents. Some studies of expanded treatment populations continued to find higher rates of mental illness in Blacks. The 1960 Census Report of inmates of mental hospitals, as well as psychiatric inpatients and outpatients of general and VA hospitals and substance abuse treatment centers, found that Blacks were overrepresented in treatment and had slightly higher crude rates of mental illness (U.S. Bureau of the Census, 1960).

Studies of Psychological Distress

After World War II, a new generation of studies emerged. Community surveys using statistical methods to select a sample of residents representative of the total community were increasingly used to provide information on the social distribution of disease. However, the field of psychiatry had not reached consensus on a standardized diagnostic system for psychiatric disorders. Therefore, indicators of nonspecific emotional malaise such as psychological distress were utilized. Thus, although these studies avoided selection biases associated with treatment samples, they provided information only on psychological well-being and not on mental illness.

Although various instruments were used to measure psychological distress, higher rates of symptomatology and depressive symptoms among Blacks were fairly consistently found. However, the racial differences in distress tend to disappear when controlled for socioeconomic status (SES) (Williams, 1986; Neighbors, 1984). One exception to this trend has been Black rates of phobia, an issue to which we will return later in this chapter. Many researchers, therefore, see the higher rates of distress in Blacks as attributable to characteristics of their social situation, such as a greater number of life stressors among Blacks (Kessler, 1979) and higher levels of alienation and powerlessness (Mirowsky & Ross, 1989).

It is important to recognize that the mental health of African Americans was not a central concern for many of the major studies conducted during this period. Most of the landmark studies in psychiatric epidemiology (see review in Weissman, Myers & Ross, 1986) excluded African Americans or included them in insufficient numbers to make racial comparisons. For example, the classic study of social class and mental illness in New Haven, Connecticut, included only 96 African Americans. Similarly, the Midtown Manhattan Mental Health Study, a prime source of our early knowledge of psychiatric impairment in an urban setting, was drawn from a population that was 99 percent White, and the Sterling County Study, an important ongoing prospective study of mental illness, included only 47 Blacks.

EPIDEMIOLOGIC CATCHMENT AREA STUDY

One of the first community-based studies to utilize both standard psychiatric diagnostic criteria and a structured interview was completed in New Haven, Connecticut in the mid-1970s (Weissman & Myers, 1978). The study found no significant racial differences for any affective diagnosis, but Whites tended to have lower rates of current minor depression and higher rates of current or lifetime major depression, lifetime minor depression, grief reaction, and cyclothymic and depressive personality than non-Whites. This study was a forerunner to the National Institute of Mental Health Epidemiologic Catchment Area (ECA) Study, with Weissman and Myers serving as investigators at the first ECA site, Greater New Haven.

The ECA Study is the largest study of mental health ever conducted in the United States (Robins & Regier, 1991). Its goals were to estimate the prevalence and incidence of specific psychiatric disorders (both current and lifetime) in representative samples of institutionalized and non-institutionalized persons, to assess potential risk factors for disorders, and to examine health care utilization. Between 1980 and 1983, almost 20,000 adults were interviewed in 5 mental health catchment areas in the United States. The ECA study would not have been possible without the development of the Diagnostic Interview Schedule (DIS). The DIS is a fully structured interview instrument, administered by lay interviewers, that provides psychiatric diagnoses based on DSM-III criteria (Robins, Helzer, Croughan & Ratcliff, 1981). Computer algorithms generate DSM-III diagnoses based on the presence, severity, and duration of symptoms. Its structured nature allows for reliable data gathering without clinical judgment. A subset of 30 major psychiatric disorders was investigated in the ECA study. Prior to the DIS, the prohibitive costs of using clinical expertise in general population surveys made large-scale psychiatric epidemiology studies unfeasible.

Unless otherwise noted, all ECA data reported come from the recently published compendium of ECA findings (Robins & Regier, 1991). This edited volume uses a somewhat questionable strategy of weighting the 5-site data to the national demographic distribution, thus producing overall prevalence rates for the United States. Overall, the ECA study found little variation in rates of disorder by race. The findings for schizophrenia and depression are interesting in the light of previously conflicting findings in the literature. Blacks had rates of schizophrenia that were slightly higher than those of Whites, but this difference disappears when the data are adjusted for age, marital status, sex, and socioeconomic status (SES). Similarly, Black and White rates of depression are generally similar after adjustment for age, sex, and SES, with a tendency for the White rates to be higher.

Blacks and Whites were similar in their lifetime prevalence of alcohol abuse/dependence. At the same time there is a race-specific, age-related pattern to the lifetime rates of alcoholism for both men and women. The White lifetime rates were approximately double the Black rate in the youngest age group (18–29) but the Black lifetime rate exceeded the White rate in all remaining age groups. The contrast is largest in the age 45–64 age group. This finding should be further explored in relation to the norms of drinking across cultures, co-morbid psychiatric conditions, and stress.

Anxiety Disorders

The previously reported pattern of racial differences in phobias from studies using symptom checklists was also evident in the ECA study. In fact, the anxiety disorders category stands out as the one area where striking racial differences were found. African Americans had higher lifetime rates of simple phobia, social phobia, and agoraphobia than Whites. The one-month prevalence of phobia was 1.5 times higher for Blacks than Whites even after adjustment for demographic and socioeconomic factors (Brown, Eaton & Sussman, 1990). When reviewing the ECA findings regarding phobia, it should be recognized that it was relatively easy to be diagnosed as phobic. A respondent needed only to have responded ''yes'' to both having a single fear and reporting it to a physician or other health care provider.

The findings were less consistent for the other anxiety disorders. There were no consistent racial differences for panic disorder, although Blacks and Hispanics tended to have lower lifetime rates than Whites. However, comparisons of current and lifetime prevalence rates suggest longer durations of panic disorder among Blacks than Whites. In contrast, it appears that there are briefer durations of phobic disorders in Blacks and Hispanics than in Whites. Generalized anxiety disorder was also higher in the ECA data in Blacks than in Whites and was strongly related to several social risk factors. These researchers suggest that this ''disorder'' might be more appropriately conceptualized as a residual of symptoms reflecting poor life conditions and generalized stress.

Neal and Turner (1991) provide a comprehensive and insightful review of the relatively small body of research on specific anxiety disorders in African Americans. Studies have found higher rates of post-traumatic stress disorder (PTSD) among Black Vietnam veterans. There is also some evidence for a high rate of co-morbidity of isolated sleep paralysis and panic attacks in Blacks. Investigation into the links between hypertension and these two disorders may produce valuable hypotheses concerning the role of stress in the development of panic (Neal & Turner, 1991). Future research on anxiety disorders in Blacks must include the development of culturally sensitive instruments and the identification and assessment of potentially distinctive stressors and coping mechanisms.

This research is urgently needed because anxiety is a common psychiatric disorder that can have serious social, occupational, and marital sequelae. In addition, there is evidence from predominantly White samples that anxiety plays a role in the development and maintenance of alcoholism (Merikangas, Risch & Weissman, in press). Alcohol may be used as a method of self-medication in the presence of anxiety symptoms. The applicability of these findings to the

African-American population must be explored, because Blacks have more severe alcohol-related sequelae (Lex, 1987).

UNRESOLVED ISSUES

Despite the strengths of the ECA study, its findings with regard to health status differences between Blacks and Whites must be interpreted with caution. The ECA study highlights several important problems that must be resolved before we can obtain an accurate picture of the distribution of mental illness in the Black population.

Sampling

It is likely that, despite the ECA study, we still lack a complete picture of the mental health status of the Black population (Williams, Takeuchi & Adair, 1992b). The noncoverage of Black males in most epidemiologic surveys is a serious problem. African-American males tend to have low response rates in survey research studies. In addition, they are overrepresented in marginal and institutional populations that are likely to be characterized by poor levels of health. The ECA's use of post-stratification weights to make the sample corre- spond to Census estimates of the population does not solve these problems. Weighting would adequately address these problems only if we assume that nonrespondents are similar to respondents and that the Census has an accurate count of Black males.

Lifetime Measures

It is instructive that many of the racial differences in disorder in the ECA data were evident only for the lifetime prevalence measures. The validity of lifetime measures of psychiatric illness is questionable. The available evidence indicates that respondents have substantial difficulty in accurately recalling and dating psychiatric episodes that occurred over their lifetime (Rogler, Malgady & Tryon, 1992). Recall problems may differentially affect racial groups, as education level is probably associated with accuracy of recall.

Validity

Psychiatric diagnosis involves the classification of social behaviors and the use of clinical judgment regarding the individual's description of his or her symptoms. The DIS appears to eliminate observer subjectivity, but biases may still exist, because its criteria are based on studies of predominantly White patients (Neighbors, Jackson, Campbell & Williams, 1989). Diagnostic instruments cre- ated from these observations cannot be blindly transferred to minority mental health assessment without validation for the specific minority population. Only one DIS validation study in African Americans appears in the literature (Hendricks et al., 1983). The study compared lay-interviewer DIS diagnoses to psychiatrist chart diagnoses, using the clinician as the standard. Concordance between the two sources varied by diagnosis, with perfect concordance (Kappa = 1.00) for depression, but poor concordance for schizophrenia (Kappa = .24).

Full-scale validation studies are required to improve confidence in findings of studies that use the DIS. However, validation is not straightforward, because psychiatry lacks diagnostic standards. In addition, researchers have noted that clinical subjectivity including prejudice, stereotypes, and cultural distance between a psychiatric professional and client may influence the diagnostic process (Adebimpe, 1981). For example, differential self-disclosure may exist because of cultural distance between interviewer and interviewee. Malgady, Rogler, and Tryon (1992) have provided an excellent critique of current attempts at validation and outlined a comprehensive framework to establish content, criterion, and construct validity, in that order. There is a critical need for serious, sustained research efforts to validate current mental health measures to minimize the misdiagnosis of African Americans.

Misdiagnosis

When mental health research focuses on racial comparisons, misdiagnosis must be addressed. If races belong to different cultures, they may have distinct belief systems, values, and standards for acceptable behavior. Therefore, the domain of symptoms for any specific psychiatric disorder would be unlikely to remain identical across cultural groups. For example, depression may have a strong somatic component for individuals raised in cultures that frown at the free expression of emotion.

Differential rates of misdiagnosis by ethnicity have been proposed as an explanation for the higher treatment rates of psychiatric disorder among minorities (Neighbors et al., 1989; Adebimpe, 1981). The overdiagnosis of schizophrenia and underdiagnosis of affective disorders are the most frequently specified types of misdiagnosis for African Americans (Adebimpe, 1981). This error may be due in part to the higher incidence of hallucinations in manic-depressive Blacks (Jones & Gray, 1986). In addition, presentation with somatic (bodily complaints) rather than classic "psychological" depressive symptoms (such as guilt and hopelessness) may make diagnosis of depression in Blacks less straightforward (Adebimpe, 1981).

Some studies have found that Black and White schizophrenic patients have symptoms that differ in type and quantity. Adebimpe, Klein, and Fried (1981) reported higher levels of auditory and other hallucinations in Black schizophrenics in a state hospital. Similarly, Velasquez and Callahan (1990) found that Black schizophrenics had significantly higher scores on five MMPI scales (including schizophrenia and hypomania), with 56 percent of Black schizophrenics meeting MMPI criteria for schizophrenia compared to 33 percent of Whites. At the same time, Simon, Gurland, Stiller, and Sharpe (1973) found no symptom differences in Blacks and Whites diagnosed with a schizophrenic disorder. Fabrega, Mezzich, and Urich (1988) found no significant differences in psychotic symptoms, including hallucinations, but noted that, compared to their White counterparts, Black schizophrenics had significantly lower mean symptom scores as well as higher scores on conversion symptoms.

Symptom profile differences between Blacks and Whites have also been found for depression. Eaton and Kessler (1981) found that although there was no racial difference in mean CES-D scores after adjustment for socioeconomic factors, a larger percentage of Blacks had scores at the extremes of the distribution. Other studies find that depressed Blacks more often present with somatic symptoms than "psychological" symptoms (Adebimpe, 1981). Black ECA respondents who reported a sad mood in the two weeks prior to the interview experienced more physical symptoms (changes in appetite and retardation or agitation) while Whites more often reported dysphoria, fatigue, guilt, and thoughts of death (Robins & Regier, 1991). In addition, Fabrega et al. (1988) found symptom patterns for anxious patients to differ by race. Anxious Blacks endorsed more violent items than anxious Whites, but no differences were seen in symptoms specifically related to the diagnosis of anxiety.

The differential interpretation of similar symptoms that may arise from sociocultural distance and/or stereotyping may also contribute to misdiagnosis (Neighbors et al., 1989; Adebimpe, 1981). Formalized diagnostic criteria have not eliminated this problem. Loring and Powell (1988) demonstrated that diagnosis was related to the race and sex of client and to the race and sex of psychiatrist "even when clear-cut diagnostic criteria are presented." In this study, two case studies of undifferentiated schizophrenia were presented to psychiatrists, while varying the race and sex of the patients. Psychiatrists most often chose the model response for the case study of the same race and sex as themselves. Misdiagnosed case studies of Black males were given more severe diagnoses for both paranoid schizophrenia and paranoid personality disorder.

Cultural Sensitivity

The preceding discussion emphasizes that both research and service delivery efforts must be culturally relevant to the targeted group. Broadly defined, cultural sensitivity is the application of knowledge of culturally specific beliefs, values, experiences, and behavior to the development and adaptation of instruments, data collection methods, analysis, interpretation, or therapy for specific ethnic/racial groups (Rogler, 1989). A professional's development of self-awareness of his or her own prejudices, stereotypes and cultural background is also a key component in the acquisition of cultural sensitivity (Bradshaw, 1978). Cultural training should be stressed in psychiatric residency, continuing medical education, clinical psychology internships, and public health curricula. Standard diagnostic systems should provide details of cultural group findings, predispositions, and symptom presentations to alert clinicians to the important role of culture (Lopez & Nunez, 1987).

In addition to the training of mental health professionals, the recruitment of ethnic minority staff members may help to create more "user-friendly" and culturally appropriate services. Interestingly, one recent study found that the matching of clients and therapists on ethnicity was associated with a lower rate of dropout for Asian-American and Mexican-American clients, but not for African Americans (Sue, Fijino, Hu & Takeuchi, 1991). However, matching did increase the number of sessions attended by all ethnic groups. Subsequent research must identify the combination of components that would result in more productive utilization of mental health services by Blacks.

BEYOND RACE COMPARISON RESEARCH: EMERGING TRENDS

Heterogeneity of the Population

The overreliance of epidemiologic studies on a race comparison paradigm masks the heterogeneity of the Black population. The Black population is not monolithic, and the identification of its variation will help identify both preventive and risk factors. This level of detail would improve the targeting of effective intervention and prevention efforts.

Several studies have documented that there is considerable variation within the Black population in terms of health. Dressler and Badger (1985) compared risk factors for depressive symptoms within three Black communities located in different regions of the United States. They found that the effect of particular sociodemographic risk factors varied for different communities. Similarly, using the large nationally representative sample of the National Survey of Black Americans, Neighbors (1986) found that the association between SES and distress varied by problem type. Low-SES Blacks experienced more distress than their higher-SES peers in the wake of an economic crisis or physical illness. In contrast, in the presence of emotional adjustment problems, high-SES Blacks experienced more distress than their low-SES counterparts. However, research efforts that focus only on the Black population fail to document the extent to which observed patterns are unique.

Williams and colleagues (1992b) examined the relationship between SES and current and lifetime rates of psychiatric disorder among Blacks and Whites in the ECA study. They found that SES is inversely related to psychiatric disorder for both racial groups, but the association is weaker for Black males than for their White peers. There was some variation among specific disorders, but the strongest relationship with SES occurred for alcohol abuse. The strength of the association also depended on the particular SES indicator under consideration. Interestingly, income was unrelated to either current or lifetime rates of psychiatric disorder among African-American males. Depression was unrelated to SES among Blacks, but inversely related for Whites.

Williams et al. (1992a) also studied the association between marital status and psychiatric disorders for Blacks in the ECA study and explored the extent to which the patterns differ from those of Whites. Their analyses documented that there are distinctive patterns to the distribution of psychiatric disorders across race. All forms of marital dissolution (separation/divorce and widowhood) are associated with an increased rate of psychiatric illness for Blacks of both sexes and for White males, but the association is stronger for White men than for their Black peers. For White females, separation/divorce is the marital status category most strongly linked to elevated risk of disorder, and the association for Whites is stronger than that for Blacks. The pattern of gender vulnerability to psychiatric illness also contains race differences. Between-group ratios revealed that, among the widowed, Black women are worse off than Black men, while an opposite pattern is evident for Whites. The authors emphasize that the finding that unmarried Black women do not have higher rates of psychiatric illness than their married peers is especially noteworthy.

Adaptive Resources

The overall evidence on Black mental health is somewhat surprising. African Americans are disproportionately exposed to social conditions considered to be important risk factors for mental illness, but Blacks tend not to have higher rates of mental illness than Whites. This emphasizes the need for renewed attention to identify and understand the cultural strengths and health-enhancing resources within that population that provide protection from pathogenic risk factors. Much research focuses only on pathology and deficits. An exclusive focus on Black inadequacy provides a distorted view of the struggles and strengths of an oppressed community that continues to survive.

Strong family ties and extended kin networks have been frequently nominated as a support system that buffers the effect of adverse living conditions on African-American mental health. This is consistent with a large body of scientific evidence that indicates that the quantity and quality of social ties are among the most powerful determinants of health (House, Landis & Umberson, 1988). Consistent with this perspective, Dressler (1985) found an inverse association between the amount of kin support and depressive symptoms in a Southern Black community. Similarly, Neighbors (1985) reported a large reduction in the amount of unmet needs in the Black population when use of informal networks was included as help-seeking behavior. Sussman, Robins, and Earls (1987) also report that Blacks with major depressive episodes were more likely than Whites to consult only their informal social network of family and friends. At the same time, some studies suggest that levels of social support are higher among Whites than Blacks (Strogatz & James, 1986). Moreover, some researchers have romanticized the social networks of Blacks as if they were a panacea for a broad range of health issues. Although these networks facilitate survival (Stack, 1975), they provide both stress and support (Belle, 1982). The negative aspects of social ties have not received much research attention, but some limited evidence suggests that the conflictive aspects of social relationships are more strongly linked to health than the supportive ones (Rook, 1984). It is also likely that recent cutbacks in government-provided social services have increased the burdens and demands on the Black extended family. At the present time, we are largely unaware of how the Black family is coping with these new challenges in the face of declining economic resources.

The Black church is also a critical source of social relationships and can function as a type of extended family (Taylor & Chatters, 1988). In addition, some evidence suggests that religious involvement itself may also reduce some of the negative consequences of stress and promote psychological well-being. Studies of Wednesday-night prayer and testimony meetings indicate that participation by Black congregants in these religious services provide therapeutic benefits equivalent to those that individuals receive in formal therapy (Griffith, Young & Smith, 1984). More systematic efforts are needed to document the conditions under which particular kinds of religious involvement may either adversely or positively affects mental health.

Differential Vulnerability

Researchers have been giving increased attention to exploring interactions between race and SES. Kessler and Neighbors (1986) reanalyzed data from 8 epidemiologic surveys and demonstrated that the failure to test for an interaction between race and SES in statistical model-building results in an underestimation of the race effect and an overestimation of the SES effect. They found that low-SES Blacks had higher rates of distress than low-SES Whites.

Ulbrich, Warheit, and Zimmerman (1989) also found higher levels of psychological distress in Blacks with low income and occupational levels than in similarly situated Whites. On the other hand, Cockerham (1990) found no significant difference in psychological distress between Blacks and Whites at low income levels. Instead, lower levels of distress were found in high-income Blacks compared to high-income Whites. Surprisingly, recent analyses of the five-site ECA data document that low-SES White males have higher rates of psychiatric disorder than their Black counterparts (Williams et al., 1992b). Among women, low-SES Black females had higher levels of substance abuse disorders than their White peers. These findings suggest the importance of distinguishing distress from disorder, as well as the need to understand the interactions among race, gender, and class.

CONCLUSION: THE NEED TO UNDERSTAND THE SOCIAL
CONTEXT

Probably the most important need in future research on Black mental health is for researchers to give careful, considered attention to what race means and why race is related to health status. Much of the research on racial differences in health is based on assumptions that are without scientific merit. These are (1) that race reflects underlying genetic homogeneity, (2) that the genes that determine race also determine health status, and (3) that the health of a population is largely dependent on the genetic constitution of that population (Krieger & Bassett, 1986). Biologists and anthropologists indicate that the concept of races as human populations that differ genetically from others is without scientific basis (Lewontin, 1972; Polednak, 1989). There is more genetic variation within races than between them, and racial categories tend not to represent biological distinctiveness. Racial classification schemes are arbitrary, and race is more of a social category than a biological one (Cooper & David, 1986). Race is a gross indicator of distinctive histories and specific conditions of life that determine levels of health and the utilization of medical care. Research that will advance our understanding of race in health must seek to identify the ways in which social, economic, political, and cultural forces and racial discrimination shape the daily realities and experiences of individuals in ways that promote illness.

Research on alcoholism appears to be a particularly appropriate place to begin. First, the overall rates are high for alcohol abuse. The lifetime rate of alcohol abuse was 23 per 100 for Black and White males in the ECA study (Robins & Regier, 1991). Because of selective mortality, the underrepresentation of persons in transient and institutional populations, and problems of impaired recall, it is likely that the true prevalence of alcohol abuse is even higher. Second, of the specific disorders in the ECA, alcohol abuse displayed the most unambiguous association with SES (Williams et al., 1992b). For Blacks and Whites, males and females, for both 6-month and lifetime rates, there is a consistent inverse association between SES and alcohol abuse.

There is a tendency for research on alcohol use in particular, and health behaviors more generally, to focus only on the social-psychological factors that give rise to the initiation and maintenance of particular unhealthy practices. Scant attention is given to the macrosocial structures and processes that affect the rates of alcohol abuse in the Black population (Williams, 1991). Low-SES persons are more vulnerable to stress, face more stress, and have fewer resources to cope with it than their higher-SES peers (Williams & House, 1991). The consumption of alcoholic beverages increases during economic recessions and periods of increasing unemployment (Singer, 1986), suggesting that alcohol is frequently employed to provide relief from social and economic deprivation. Alcohol abuse is also positively associated with the availability of alcoholic beverages (Singer, 1986). In the United States, the availability of alcohol is controlled by government policies (Cowan & Mosher, 1985), which have facilitated a greater number of retail outlets for the sale of alcoholic beverages in poor and minority communities than in more affluent areas (Rabow & Watt, 1982). Moreover, the Black community has been specifically targeted by the alcohol industry to increase consumption of alcoholic beverages (Hacker, Collins & Jacobson, 1987).

It is also the case that feelings of powerlessness and helplessness are critical determinants of alcohol abuse (Seeman, Seeman & Budros, 1988). These individual predispositions are inversely linked to SES (Mirowsky & Ross, 1989), but inadequate attention has been given to the identification of the macrosocial structures and processes that shape these individual characteristics. What is needed at this time are rigorous prospective investigations that would seek to understand how macrosocial structures and processes, socializing mechanisms, and individual constitutional and dispositional factors are related to each other and how they combine within different sociocultural (e.g., racial) contexts, both additively and interactively, to give rise to particular patterns of disease distribution.

NOTE

Preparation of this chapter was supported by grant AG 07904 from the National Institute of Aging and training grant MH14235 from the National Institute for Mental Health. We wish to thank Molly Olsen for assistance in preparing the manuscript.

REFERENCES

Adebimpe, V. (1981). Overview: White norms and psychiatric diagnosis of black patients. *American Journal of Psychiatry, 138,* 279–285.

Adebimpe, V. R., Klein, H. E., & Fried, J. (1981). Hallucinations and delusions in black psychiatric patients. *Journal of the National Medical Association, 73,* 517–520.

Belle, D. E. (1982). The impact of poverty on social networks and supports. *Marriage and Family Review, 5,* 89–103.

Bradshaw, W. H., Jr. (1978). Training psychiatrists for working with blacks in basic residency. *American Journal of Psychiatry, 135,* 1520–1524.

Brown, D. R., Eaton, W. W., & Sussman, L. (1990). Racial differences in prevalence of phobic disorders. *Journal of Nervous and Mental Disease, 178,* 434–441.

Cockerham, W. C. (1990). A test of the relationship between race, socioeconomic status and psychological distress. *Social Science in Medicine, 31,* 1321–1326.

Cooper, R., & David, R. (1986). The biological concept of race and its application to public health and epidemiology. *Journal of Health Politics, Policy and Law, 11,* 97–116.

Cowan, R., & Mosher, J. F. (1985). Public health implications of beverage marketing: Alcohol as an ordinary consumer product. *Contemporary Drug Problems, 12,* 621–657.

Dressler, W. W. (1985). Extended family relationships, social support and mental health in a southern black community. *Journal of Health and Social Behavior, 26,* 39–48.

Dressler, W. W., & Badger, L. W. (1985). Epidemiology of depressive symptoms in black communities: A comparative analysis. *Journal of Nervous and Mental Disease, 173,* 212–220.

Eaton, W., & Kessler, L. (1981). Rates of symptoms of depression in a national sample. *American Journal of Epidemiology, 114,* 528–538.

Fabrega, H., Jr., Mezzich, J., & Urich, R. F. (1988). Black-white differences in psychopathology in an urban psychiatric population. *Comprehensive Psychiatry, 29,* 285–297.

Fischer, J. (1969). Negroes and whites and rates of mental illness: Reconsideration of a myth. *Psychiatry, 32,* 428–446.

Griffith, E., Young, J., & Smith, D. (1984). An analysis of the therapeutic elements in a black church service. *Hospital and Community Psychiatry, 35,* 464–469.

Hacker, A. G., Collins, R., & Jacobson, M. (1987). *Marketing Booze to Blacks.* Washington, DC: Center for Science in the Public Interest.

Hendricks, L. E., Bayton, J. A., Collins, J. L., Mathura, C., McMillan, S., & Montgomery, T. (1983). The NIMH Diagnostic Interview Schedule: A test of its validity in a population of black adults. *Journal of the National Medical Association, 75,* 667–671.

House, J. S., Landis, K. R., & Umberson, D. (1988). Social relationships and health. *Science, 241,* 540–545.

Jaco, E. G. (1960). *The Social Epidemiology of Mental Disorders.* New York: Russell Sage Foundation.

Jones, B. E., & Gray, B. A. (1986). Problems in diagnosing schizophrenia and affective disorders among blacks. *Hospital and Community Psychiatry, 37,* 61–65.

Kessler, R. C., & Neighbors, H. W. (1986). A new perspective on the relationships among race, social class and psychological distress. *Journal of Health and Social Behavior, 27,* 107–115.

Kessler, R. C. (1979). Stress, social status and psychological distress. *Journal of Health and Social Behavior, 20,* 259–272.

Krieger, N. (1987). Shades of difference: Theoretical underpinnings of the medical controversy on black/white differences in the United States, 1830–1870. *International Journal of Health Services, 17,* 259–278.

Krieger, N., & Bassett, M. (1986). The health of black folk: Disease, class, and ideology in science. *Monthly Review, 38,* 74–85.

Lewontin, R. C. (1972). The apportionment of human diversity. *Evolutionary Biology, 6,* 381–398.

Lex, B. W. (1987). Review of alcohol problems in ethnic minorities. *Journal of Consulting and Clinical Psychology, 55,* 293–300.

Lopez, S., & Nunez, J. A. (1987). Cultural factors considered in selected diagnostic criteria and interview schedules. *Journal of Abnormal Psychology, 96,* 270–272.

Loring, M., & Powell, B. (1988). Gender, race and DSM-III: A study of the objectivity of psychiatric diagnostic behavior. *Journal of Health and Social Behavior, 29,* 1–22.

Malgady, R. G., Rogler, L. H. & Tryon, W. W. (1992). Issues of validity in the diagnostic interview schedule. *Journal of Psychiatric Research, 26,* 59–67.

Merikangas, K. R., Risch, N. J., & Weissman, M. N. (in press). Comorbidity and cotransmission of alcoholism, anxiety and depression. *Psychological Medicine.*

Mirowsky, J., & Ross, C.E. (1989). *Social causes of psychological distress*. New York: Aldine de Gruyter.

Mollica, R. F., Blum, J. D. & Redlich, F. (1980). Equity and the psychiatric care of the black patient. *Journal of Nervous and Mental Disease, 168*, 279–285.

Neal, A. M., & Turner, S. M. (1991). Anxiety disorders research with African-Americans: Current status. *Psychological Bulletin, 109*, 400–410.

Neighbors, H. W. (1986). Socioeconomic status and psychologic distress in adult blacks. *American Journal of Epidemiology, 124*, 779–793.

Neighbors, H. W. (1985). Seeking professional help for personal problems: Black Americans' use of health and mental health services. *Community Mental Health Journal, 21*, 156–166.

Neighbors, H. W. (1984). The distribution of psychiatric morbidity in black Americans: A review and suggestions for research. *Community Mental Health Journal, 20*, 169–181.

Neighbors, H. W., Jackson, J. S., Campbell, L., & Williams, D. (1989). The influence of racial factors on psychiatric diagnosis: A review and suggestions for research. *Community Mental Health Journal, 25*, 301–311.

Pasamanick, B. (1963). Some misconceptions concerning differences in the racial prevalence of mental disease. *American Journal of Orthopsychiatry, 33*, 72–86.

Polednak, A. P. (1989). *Racial and ethnic differences in disease*. New York: Oxford University Press.

Rabow, J., & Watt, R. (1982). Alcohol availability, alcohol beverage sales and alcohol-related problems. *Journal of Studies on Alcohol, 43*, 767–801.

Robins, L. N., & Regier, D. A. (Eds.). (1991). *Psychiatric disorders in America: The Epidemiologic Catchment Area Study*. New York: Free Press.

Robins, L. N., Helzer, J. E., Croughan, J., & Ratcliff, K. (1981). National Institute of Mental Health Diagnostic Interview Schedule: Its history, characteristics and validity. *Archives of General Psychiatry, 38*, 381–389.

Rogler, L. H. (1989). The meaning of culturally sensitive research in mental health. *American Journal of Psychiatry, 146*, 296–303.

Rogler, L. H., Malgady, R. G., and Tryon, W. W. (1992). Evaluation of mental health: Issues of memory in the Diagnostic Interview Schedule. *Journal of Nervous and Mental Disease, 180*, 215–222.

Rook, K. S. (1984). The negative side of social interaction: Impact on psychological well-being. *Journal of Personality and Social Psychology, 46*, 1097–1108.

Seeman, M., Seeman, L., & Budros, A. (1988). Powerlessness, work and community: A longitudinal study of alienation and alcohol use. *Journal of Health and Social Behavior, 29*, 185–198.

Simon, R. J., Gurland, B., Stiller, P., & Sharpe, L. (1973). Depression and schizophrenia in hospitalized black and white mental patients. *Archives of General Psychiatry, 28*, 509–512.

Singer, M. (1986). Toward a political economy of alcoholism. *Social Science and Medicine, 23*, 113–130.

Snowden, L. R., & Cheung, F. K. (1990). Use of inpatient mental health services by members of ethnic minority groups. *American Psychologist, 45*, 347–355.

Stack, C. B. (1975). *All our kin: Strategies for survival in a black community*. New York: Harper and Row.

Strogatz, D. S., & James, S. A. (1986). Social support and hypertension among blacks

and whites in a rural, southern community. *American Journal of Epidemiology,*
    124, 949–956.
Sue, S., Fijino, D. C., Hu, L., & Takeuchi, D. T. (1991). Community mental health
    services for ethnic minority groups: A test of the cultural responsiveness hypoth-
    esis. *Journal of Consulting and Clinical Psychology, 59,* 533–540.
Sussman, L. K., Robins, L. N., & Earls, F. (1987). Treatment seeking for depression
    by black and white Americans. *Social Science and Medicine, 24,* 187–196.
Taylor, R. J., & Chatters, L. M. (1988). Church members as a source of informal social
    support. *Review of Religious Research, 30,* 193–203.
Ulbrich, P., Warheit, G., & Zimmerman, R. (1989). Race, socioeconomic status and
    psychological distress. *Journal of Health and Social Behavior, 30,* 131–146.
U.S. Bureau of the Census. *U.S. Census of Population: 1960. Inmates of Institutions
    Final Report PC 2-8A.* Washington, DC: Government Printing Office.
Velasquez, R. J., & Callahan, W. J. (1990). MMPIs of Hispanic, black and white DSM-
    III schizophrenics. *Psychological Reports, 66,* 819–822.
Vernon, S. W., & Roberts, R. E. (1982). Prevalence of treated and untreated psychiatric
    disorders in three ethnic groups. *Social Science in Medicine, 16,* 1575–1582.
Weissman, M. M., & Myers, J. (1978). Affective disorders in a U.S. urban community.
    Archives of General Psychiatry, 35, 1304–1311.
Weissman, M. M., Myers, J. K., & Ross, C. E. (Eds.). (1986). *Community surveys of
    mental disorders.* Series in Psychosocial Epidemiology, Vol. 4, New Brunswick,
    NJ: Rutgers University Press.
Weissman, M. M., et al. (1991). Affective disorders. In L. N. Robins, & D. A. Regier
    (Eds.), *Psychiatric disorders in America: The Epidemiological Catchment Area
    Study* (pp. 53–80). New York: Free Press.
Williams, D. H. (1986). The epidemiology of mental illness in Afro-Americans. *Hospital
    and Community Psychiatry, 37,* 42–49.
Williams, D. R. (1991). Social structure and the health behaviors of blacks. In K. Schaie,
    J. House, & D. Blazer (Eds.), *Aging, health behaviors and health status* (pp. 59–
    64). Hillsdale, NJ: Erlbaum.
Williams, D. R., & House, J. S. (1991). Stress, social support, control and coping: A
    social epidemiological view. In B. Badura and I. Kickbush (Eds.), *Health pro-
    motion research: Towards a new social epidemiology* (pp. 157–172). Copenhagen:
    World Health Organization.
Williams, D. R., Takeuchi, D., & Adair, R. (1992a). Marital status and psychiatric
    disorders among blacks and whites. *Journal of Health and Social Behavior, 33,*
    140–157.
Williams, D. R., Takeuchi, D., & Adair, R. (1992b). Socioeconomic status and psy-
    chiatric disorder among blacks and whites. *Social Forces, 71,* 179–194.

18

Nutrition Concerns of Black Americans

Deborah E. Blocker

INTRODUCTION

Good nutrition is crucial to the maintenance of health, and dietary factors contribute substantially to preventable chronic illness and premature death. The Surgeon General's Report on Nutrition and Health (1988) identifies the 10 leading causes of death in the United States. Of the 10, 5 are associated directly with nutrition (coronary heart disease, some types of cancer, stroke, diabetes mellitus, and atherosclerosis). Chronic diseases such as these disproportionately affect Black Americans and thus will be the focus of this chapter. These complex disorders are of multifactorial etiology involving interactions of environmental, behavioral, social, and genetic factors. The diet consumed by Black Americans is one of the environmental factors associated with the etiology and pathogenesis of these disorders that may predispose Blacks to an excess chronic disease burden.

It is difficult to characterize the nutritional status of Black Americans because they are a highly diverse group in terms of socioeconomic status, geography, and ethnicity; however, it is possible to make some generalizations. In general, Black Americans living in or near poverty consume diets that are marginal in vitamins A, D, E, B-complex, vitamin C, calcium, magnesium, iron, and zinc. Black Americans also tend to consume a greater percentage of calories from animal protein (meat) than do Whites. The diets of many Black Americans are low in foods that are good sources of complex carbohydrates and dietary fiber, namely, whole-grain products and fresh fruits and vegetables. Additionally, from 60 to 95 percent of adult Black Americans are lactose intolerant, and many of these individuals habitually avoid milk and milk products. Dairy products are the best source of calcium in the U.S. diet (Kumanyika & Helitzer, 1985; Kittler & Sucher, 1989). While acknowledging the nonmonolithic nature of the Black

American community, this chapter will do the following: describe the major diet-related chronic diseases affecting Black Americans, suggest recommendations for dietary and life-style modifications to prevent and/or ameliorate these disorders, and make suggestions for public health policy/interventions.

DIET-RELATED CHRONIC DISEASES DISPROPORTIONATELY AFFECTING BLACK AMERICANS

Coronary Heart Disease

Coronary heart disease (CHD) accounts for the largest number of deaths in the United States, and race is strongly associated with CHD morbidity and mortality (Surgeon General's Report on Nutrition and Health, 1988). An examination of the age-adjusted death rates (per 100,000) for coronary heart disease by race and sex in 1986 reveals the following rates: Black males (294.3) compared to White males (234.8) and Black females (185.1) compared to White females (119.0). A similar pattern is seen when age-adjusted death rates (per 100,000) for cerebrovascular disease by race and sex in 1986 are compared. The data show rates for Black males of 58.9 compared to White males of 31.1 and rates for Black females of 47.6 compared to White females of 27.1 (National Center for Health Statistics, 1989). Black Americans also suffer from cardiovascular morbidity at a higher rate than Whites (Report of the Secretary's Task Force on Black and Minority Health, 1985).

The major diet-related risk factors for coronary heart disease are hypertension, obesity, and elevated serum cholesterol level. Elevations in total serum cholesterol, low density lipoprotein (LDL) cholesterol, and/or a reduced high density lipoprotein (HDL) cholesterol are considered to increase CHD risk. For the risk factor of hypertension, adult Black Americans are clearly at higher risk because they have much higher rates of hypertension than do Whites (Lewis, Raczynski, Oberman & Cutter, 1991). Obesity is also more prevalent in the Black community and affects Black women most severely. A preponderance of abdominal fat may be an even more important determinant of CHD risk than total body weight or body fat. Folsom et al. (1991) analyzed data collected on African American subjects in the Coronary Artery Risk Development in Young Adults (CARDIA) study and the Atherosclerosis Risk in Communities (ARIC) Study and found that the waist-to-hip ratio, which measures abdominal adiposity, was lower in Black men than White men at all ages. On the other hand, Black women were found to be considerably more obese than White women at all ages, and Black women also had higher waist-to-hip ratios than White women.

The research findings appear to be more favorable with respect to serum cholesterol levels in Black Americans. Wilson et al. (1983) examined a sample of 100 highly educated Black adults and found significantly lower total cholesterol levels than in a comparable White sample. However, when the National Health and Nutrition Examination Survey II 1976–1980 (NHANES II) data were analyzed by Sempos et al. (1989), no racial differences in total cholesterol were noted. Freedman, Strogatz, Eaker, Joesoef, and DeStefano (1990) report that although total serum cholesterol levels are similar among Black and White males, Black males appear to have a higher level of high density lipoprotein (HDL) cholesterol than White males; however, the racial differential in HDL cholesterol does not hold true at higher educational levels. Srinivasan, Frerichs, Webber, and Berenson (1976) reported that adolescent and young adult Black males participating in the Bogolusa heart study had higher levels of HDL cholesterol than their White counterparts. Kumanyika and Savage (1986) found that Blacks of both sexes apparently have higher levels of high density lipoprotein cholesterol (HDL-C) and lower levels of low density lipoprotein cholesterol (LDL-C) and triglycerides than Whites. Black males appear to have a more favorable lipid profile than Black females.

The major pathology in CHD results from inadequate circulation of blood to the heart muscle. This is almost always due to atherosclerosis, which in turn is strongly associated with elevated serum cholesterol levels and elevated LDL-C. The principal nutrition-related factors identified with high blood cholesterol and the development of CHD are obesity and dietary fat intake. Obesity will be discussed in detail later in this chapter. For dietary fat there is strong and consistent clinical, epidemiologic, and experimental animal evidence that high intakes of saturated fat increase serum total and LDL-C, which increases the risk of coronary heart disease. Dietary cholesterol intake has a less significant effect on serum cholesterol levels than does saturated fat intake (National Research Council, 1989). Factors shown to reduce serum cholesterol levels include monounsaturated fatty acids and polyunsaturated fatty acids (PUFAs), soluble fiber, and vegetarian diets (Kris-Etherton, Krummel, Dreon, Mackey & Wood, 1988; National Research Council, 1989).

Block, Rosenberger, and Patterson (1988), in a review of NHANES II data, report that Black Americans consume 35 to 38 percent of their calories as fat, with 11 to 13 percent as saturated fat. These percentages are similar to those reported for Whites. However, dietary cholesterol intake is higher for Blacks than for Whites. In reviewing research on Black eating patterns and their relation to CHD risk, Kumanyika and Adams-Campbell (1991) report that Black American food patterns are similar to those of White Americans; however, some areas where these patterns diverge include lower consumption of dairy products by Blacks resulting in a decreased calcium intake, decreased consumption of total fruits and vegetables resulting in a decreased consumption of dietary fiber and potassium, and a higher consumption of vitamin A from both animal and plant sources. Additional research is needed to clarify the dietary determinants of serum lipid levels and the long-term effects of dietary modifications on CHD risk and human health.

Hypertension

Current reports estimate that at least 58 million Americans are hypertensive, that is, have blood pressure readings higher than 140/90. Hypertension

(HTN) disproportionately affects Black Americans. In fact, the Intersalt Co-operative Research Group (1988) reports that the highest rates of hypertension worldwide occur in Black Americans. HTN is an important risk factor for CHD and stroke. The major dietary correlates of HTN are obesity and salt (sodium) intake. Population studies reveal that in societies where diets contain in excess of 6 grams of salt per day it is associated with a higher prevalence of HTN (National Research Council, 1989). This susceptibility to salt-induced HTN is probably genetically determined. The concept of salt or sodium sensitivity means that these individuals will have increased blood pressure in response to high sodium intake. One-third of the U.S. population is thought to be salt sensitive; however, this subgroup cannot yet be reliably identified. Freis, Reda, and Materson (1988) report there is a greater frequency of salt-sensitive hypertension in Black Americans, which according to Blaustein and Grim (1991) suggests that decreasing dietary sodium intake can be beneficial in lowering blood pressure in this salt-sensitive subgroup. The dietary recommendation is to limit total salt intake to less than 6 grams per day (National Research Council, 1989). In the general population, decreasing salt intake should not cause any detrimental effects because there is no known benefit from consuming large amounts of salt.

Because of traditional Black American eating patterns it could be assumed that there is a higher sodium intake among Blacks, which would increase the likelihood of expressing the genetic predisposition to hypertension existing in the Black community. Data from the Intersalt (1988) study show no consistent evidence of higher sodium intake among Blacks; however, the data do suggest that there is a lower potassium intake among Blacks of both genders and among both urban and rural Blacks versus Whites. This results in a lower sodium:potassium ratio, which has been shown to be associated with an increased risk of hypertension. The diets of many Black Americans are low in fresh fruits and vegetables, which contribute potassium (Kumanyika & Helitzer, 1985; Kittler & Sucher, 1989).

Epidemiologic and clinical evidence also suggests an inverse, albeit inconsistent, association between dietary calcium intake and blood pressure. This further suggests that a deficiency of dietary calcium may have implications for increased hypertension risk. Blacks may be at particular risk because most adult Black Americans are lactose intolerant and therefore tend to avoid milk and milk products rich in calcium (Kumanyika & Helitzer, 1985; Kittler & Sucher, 1989).

There may also be positive effects of increased intakes of magnesium, omega 6 and omega 3 PUFA, and dietary fiber on blood pressure. Psychosocial stressors are also likely greater among Blacks than Whites. In reviewing research on psychosocial factors predisposing Blacks to higher CHD risk, Kumanyika and Adams-Campbell (1991) report that several psychosocial factors have been associated, but not in a consistent fashion, with blood pressure and hypertension in Blacks.

Diabetes Mellitus

Diabetes mellitus is an endocrine disorder characterized by an insufficient and/
or ineffective secretion of insulin, accompanied by an elevation in plasma glucose
levels as well as abnormalities in lipoprotein and amino acid metabolism (Anderson, 1988). The prevalence of diabetes in the United States is estimated at
11 million (Hollenbeck & Coulston, 1988). There are two major types of diabetes,
Type I, or insulin-dependent diabetes mellitus (IDDM), and Type II, or non-
insulin-dependent diabetes mellitus (NIDDM).

IDDM accounts for approximately 10 percent and NIDDM for approximately
88 percent of all cases of diabetes. IDDM is the predominant form of the disease
in children, adolescents, and young adults. The onset of diabetic symptoms tends
to be rapid. As these symptoms are the result of insufficient insulin secretion,
patients require exogenous insulin injections to control the disease. NIDDM, on
the other hand, appears most commonly after the age of 40 and is often associated
with obesity. The onset of diabetic symptoms is gradual, often evolving over a
span of several years. The primary cause of hyperglycemia in NIDDM is apparently reduced insulin sensitivity of peripheral tissues (insulin resistance) as
opposed to decreased insulin secretion. NIDDM is most often controlled by diet,
weight reduction, and the use of oral hypoglycemic agents (Harris, Hadden,
Knowler & Bennett, 1987).

In diabetes, the absence or ineffectiveness of insulin and the resultant hyperglycemia engender numerous metabolic aberrations affecting many body systems. The prevalence of IDDM is 1.5 times higher among Whites than Blacks
(National Research Council, 1989). However, the reverse is true of NIDDM.
According to Harris, Hadden, Knowler, and Bennett (1987), NIDDM is 33
percent more common among Blacks than Whites. The highest rates are among
overweight Black women, and the complications of diabetes are all more prevalent among Blacks than Whites with diabetes. Pi-Sunyer (1990) reviewed data
on obesity and diabetes in Blacks and reports that the prevalence of NIDDM
among Blacks is increasing. Mortality rates from diabetic complications are also
higher among Blacks; and they experience a greater (i.e., versus Whites) severity
of diabetic complications, including diabetic atherosclerosis, diabetic retinopathy, diabetic neuropathy, and diabetic nephropathy. Black women are more
seriously affected by these complications than are Black men. Pi-Sunyer points
out that both genetic predisposition and environment are likely involved in the
pathogenesis of obesity and diabetes and that more research is needed to clarify
this interrelationship in Blacks. Hyperinsulinemia and insulin resistance may be
a common pathogenic mechanism relating NIDDM, obesity, and hypertension—
all of which have a higher prevalence rate in Blacks (Douglas, 1990).

Diet is a major environmental factor in the pathogenesis of diabetes because
it is a major determinant of obesity. Obesity is the only factor that has been
consistently related to the prevalence of NIDDM. Diets with high total caloric
intake, high percentage of calories from fat, and low percentage of calories from

carbohydrates are positively associated with diabetes prevalence (National Research Council, 1989).

Obesity

The data from the 1976–1980 NHANES II revealed that 34 million Americans aged 20–75 years were overweight. In general, people of color were more obese than Whites, women were more obese than men, and the poor were more obese than the affluent.

For U.S. males aged 20–74 years, NHANES II data show that in the middle-aged group (35–54 years) Black males have a higher prevalence of overweight and severe overweight than their White counterparts. For males aged 20–34 and 55–64 years, Black men are less obese; for men aged 65–74 years, obesity rates are roughly the same for Black and White men (Foster & Burton, 1985).

These same data show that 44 percent of Black women aged 20–74 years can be classified as overweight (Van Itallie, 1985). Gillum (1987b) reviewed published data from the National Center for Health Statistics and reported that the age-adjusted prevalence of overweight for Black women is much higher than for White women or for males of either race. For U.S. females aged 25–74 years, Black women have approximately twice the prevalence of obesity as White women in every age group compared. In 1976–1980, the prevalence of overweight in Black women aged 25–74 years was 48.1 percent. This means that over a decade ago, nearly half of all adult Black females were overweight, and the data indicate that the prevalence of overweight in this group is increasing. Overweight was found to be inversely related to education and income; however, the excess of overweight in Black women is reported in all income levels. Southern and rural Black women were more likely to be overweight than northern, western, or urban Black women.

Obesity is a major risk factor for mortality as well as being a risk factor for hypertension, non-insulin-dependent diabetes mellitus, cardiovascular disease, hypertriglyceridemia, decreased high density lipoprotein cholesterol, elevated total and low density lipoprotein cholesterol, gallbladder disease, osteoarthritis, gout, and compromised pulmonary function as well as cancers of the breast, endometrium, gallbladder, ovaries, and cervix in women and colorectal cancer in men (Pi-Sunyer, 1991).

Kumanyika and Adams-Campbell (1991) note that obesity is a complex disorder involving genetic predisposition, diet, and nondietary environmental exposures. Obesity can be defined as 20 percent above desirable body weight. However, this definition is problematic. To date, a definition of obesity that takes into account the degree of excess body fat does not exist. Body mass index (body weight in kilograms divided by the square of height in meters), which considers both weight and height measurements, is a widely used surrogate measurement for obesity. What may be as important as the amount of adiposity is the distribution of body fat. Abdominal fat is associated with an increased risk of chronic diseases. Accordingly, an increased waist-to-hip circumference ratio is associated with an increased chronic disease risk (Healthy People 2000, 1990). The waist-to-hip circumference ratios are higher in Black than in White women, especially in middle age (Gillum, 1987b). Waist-to-hip circumference ratios are similar in Black and White males before age 65. After 65, Black males have, on average, lower waist-to-hip circumference ratios than do White males (Gillum, 1987a).

The traditional Black American diet, which stresses the consumption of meat (particularly pork), fried foods, and eggs (Sanjur, 1982; Kittler & Sucher, 1989), would imply that there is a higher intake of cholesterol and saturated fat among Blacks. However, Block et al. (1988) report that total fat consumption is similar among Blacks and Whites. An examination of dietary energy intake among Black females reveals an unexpected finding, that the energy intake of Black females is in fact lower than that of their White counterparts. This paradoxical finding is surprising: considering the higher prevalence of obesity among Blacks, especially women, a higher energy would have been anticipated (Kumanyika, 1987). This paradox can be clarified by examining the energy expenditure of Black females. Evidence suggests that the higher prevalence of obesity in Black females can be linked to lower levels of energy expenditure. Wing et al. (1989), reporting on the Pittsburgh Healthy Women Study, showed that Black women were more likely to be sedentary than White women. Schoenborn (1988) reporting findings from the National Health Interview Survey (NHIS) found that Black females were less likely to participate in regular physical activity than White females. However, it is important to note that the decreased physical activity reported by Black females may be the result and not the cause of obesity. Among males, findings showed that young (ages 18–30) Black males were more likely than White males in that age group to engage in regular physical activity, but that among older Black males activity rates were similar or slightly lower than their White counterparts (Schoenborn, 1988).

Additional research is needed on the effects of body fat distribution, metabolic derangements in obesity, and the relationship between energy intake and energy expenditure, as well as the identification of genetic, environmental, and lifestyle antecedents of obesity in Black women.

Certain Cancers

Cancer is the second leading cause of death in the United States, causing nearly 500,000 deaths a year. Cancer is not one but many diseases, with multifactorial etiologies and associated with a variety of risk factors (Surgeon General's Report on Nutrition and Health, 1988).

Boring, Squires, and Heath (1992) summarized cancer statistics for Black Americans and report that cancer is also the second leading cause of death among Blacks, exceeded only by cardiovascular disease. Age-adjusted cancer mortality rates are higher for Blacks than for all races (217 per 100,000 versus 170 per

100,000). The authors cite several reasons for this disparity, noting that it probably reflects not a genetic predisposition to cancer among Blacks but a host of environmental factors including poverty, inadequate education, and limited access to health care. These factors result in diagnosis at a later stage of cancer and, as a consequence, reduced cancer survival rates.

Cancer incidence rates are also higher in Blacks compared with Whites. Of new cancer cases diagnosed in 1991, the major sites affected, in decreasing order, were lung, female breast, prostate, colorectal, pancreas, oral cavity, and stomach. Boring et al. (1992) point out that despite the fact that cancer mortality rates were comparable for all races 30 years ago, since then cancer mortality has increased for Black men and women by 66 and 10 percent, respectively. Much of this cancer burden can be attributed to cigarette smoking. There is a higher prevalence of cigarette smoking among Blacks; however, smoking among Blacks now appears to be on the decline, especially in the adolescent age group. There is also encouraging evidence that Blacks are participating more fully in early cancer detection initiatives. In fact, Black American women receive more frequent Pap tests than women of other racial/ethnic groups (Harlan, Bernstein & Kessler, 1991). Despite these positive trends, Black men currently experience an increased risk of cancer versus non-Black males with a 25 percent higher risk of all cancers and a 45 percent higher incidence of lung cancer. Only 39 percent of Blacks with cancer survive 5 years after diagnosis, compared to 50 percent of Whites (Healthy People 2000, 1991).

Although it is impossible to quantify the percentage of human cancer attributable to diet, at least one-third of all cancer mortality is thought to be related to nutrition. The role of dietary factors in the pathogenesis of various types of cancer were summarized in *Diet and Health: Implications for Reducing Chronic Disease Risk* (National Research Council, 1989). Dietary fat intake (via epidemiologic and experimental animal evidence) is associated with increasing risk of certain cancers (e.g., breast, colon, rectum, endometrium, prostate). Increased intake of fruits and vegetables is associated with a lower risk of several cancers, most notably mouth, bladder, colon, lung, and stomach. Dietary fiber may have a beneficial effect, especially on colon cancer.

Vitamin A has been reported to protect against epithelial cancers, apparently by promoting normal cellular differentiation. B-carotene also exerts a protective effect, presumably through its role as an antioxidant. Nutrient antioxidants (like B-carotene, Vitamins E and C, and selenium) can quench free radicals and their oxidative products and may minimize carcinogenesis. B-carotene has also been reported to enhance several aspects of immune function. There is also encouraging recent evidence that several water-soluble vitamins, including riboflavin, folic acid, and vitamin B12, may block the initiation or promotion of cancer.

The major dietary associations for cancers that have the highest prevalence in the Black community can also be identified. For lung cancer, the predominant cause is exposure to tobacco smoke. Breast cancer is still more common among White women than Black, but rates are increasing among Black women. There is evidence that breast cancer mortality is positively correlated with total caloric intake and dietary fat, especially animal fats, and negatively correlated with intake of complex carbohydrates and dietary fiber. Obesity, which is twice as prevalent for Black women than for White women, is also positively associated with breast cancer risk. Prostate cancer rates are especially high in Black males. Several studies show a positive correlation between this type of cancer and total dietary fat intake. Data on diet and colorectal cancer are inconsistent; however, many studies report that high meat intake, low vegetable intake, high saturated fat intake, and low dietary fiber intake are all positively correlated with colorectal cancer risk. Research must provide increased evidence of different diet and cancer interactions. Also, we must increase nutrition education in diet modification (e.g., increased green and yellow vegetable intake).

RECOMMENDATIONS FOR DIETARY AND LIFE-STYLE MODIFICATIONS

Cardiovascular Disease

Blacks suffer from higher rates of cardiovascular disease morbidity and mortality than do Whites. *Recommendations:* The prevalence of obesity should be decreased by weight reduction. Saturated fat and cholesterol intake should be decreased and dietary fiber intake increased by consuming less meat and greater amounts of whole grains and fresh fruits and vegetables.

Hypertension

Black Americans have the highest rates of hypertension in the world. *Recommendations:* Although there is no consistent evidence of high sodium intake among Blacks, it is prudent to recommend decreasing salt consumption. Increasing consumption of fresh fruits and vegetables will increase potassium intake. Additional research is needed on decreasing the sodium content of processed foods and to clarify the apparent positive effects of increased intakes of potassium, calcium, magnesium, omega 6 and omega 3 PUFA, and fiber on blood pressure.

Diabetes Mellitus

The prevalence of non-insulin-dependent diabetes is increasing among Black Americans. Black women are more severely affected by diabetes, a disease that is positively correlated with obesity. *Recommendations:* Weight reduction should be facilitated by consumption of a diet that is low in fat, moderate in protein, and high in complex carbohydrates; physical activity should be increased.

Obesity

Obesity is the major chronic disease problem affecting Black American women. Nearly half of all Black women can be classified as obese. *Recommendations:* Weight reduction should involve a holistic approach combining diet, increasing physical activity, and behavior modification. Implementation of nutrition education initiatives should be designed within the cultural context of the Black community and specifically target Black women.

Certain Cancers

Cancer incidence and mortality are increasing for Blacks, especially for Black men. *Recommendations:* Smoking prevention/cessation activities in the Black American community should be undertaken to decrease the risk of lung cancer. The prevalence of obesity should be lessened by modifying food intake and increasing physical activity, increasing the consumption of fresh fruits and vegetables and whole grains, while decreasing dietary fat, especially saturated fat intake.

RECOMMENDATIONS FOR PUBLIC HEALTH POLICY/ INTERVENTIONS

Efforts to improve the nutritional and health status of Black Americans must include increased nutritional surveillance and longitudinal prospective studies with large sample sizes, reflecting the socioeconomic, geographic, and cultural diversity in the Black American community. These surveillance activities will provide data to document Black American dietary patterns, correlate those findings with the prevalence of chronic diet-related diseases in this community, and facilitate evaluation of the efficacy of nutrition intervention programs.

Further research is needed on nutrition intervention programs targeting the Black community. For many reasons, programs designed for White Americans may not be appropriate for Black Americans. Nutrition education aimed at Black Americans must take into account Black dietary patterns, specifically targeting weight control, reducing the percentage of calories from fat, lowering salt intake, increasing fruit and vegetable intake, and increasing the intake of complex carbohydrates and dietary fiber. These efforts must be designed and implemented within the context of Black culture and with the full participation of members of the Black American community at every stage of the process. Nutrition intervention programs should be coordinated with activities and programs existing in schools, community centers, and churches. Maximal impact on the Black community will be achieved by programs that target young children and their parents as the recipients of nutrition education, with the goal of empowering Black families to adjust their eating patterns in a more health-promoting direction. The most effective education programs will advocate and support gradual modifications in diet and life-style that enable Black Americans to enjoy and celebrate many of the foods in their traditional diet prepared in more healthful ways. Increased funds must be made available to finance existing and new nutrition research and education initiatives aimed at Black Americans. An important correlate is the need to increase the numbers of Black nutrition professionals. This country must also aggressively address the societal correlates of poor health status among Blacks, namely persistent institutional racism, poverty, and inadequate access to quality health care. This will require a major and unwavering commitment of resources and a reorganization of our national priorities.

REFERENCES

Anderson, J. W. (1988). Nutrition management of diabetes mellitus. In M. E. Shils & V. R. Young (Eds.), *Modern nutrition in health and disease* (7th Ed.). Philadelphia: Lea & Febiger.

Blaustein, M. P., & Grim, C. E. (1991). The pathogenesis of hypertension: Black-white differences. *Cardiovascular Clinics, 21,* 97–114.

Block, G., Rosenberger, W. F., & Patterson, B. H. (1988). Calories, fat and cholesterol: Intake patterns in the U.S. population by race, sex, and age. *American Journal of Public Health, 78,* 1150–1155.

Boring, C. C., Squires, T. S., & Heath, C. W. (1992). Cancer statistics for African Americans. *CA—A Cancer Journal for Clinicians, 42,* 7–17.

Douglas, J. G. (1990). Hypertension and diabetes in blacks. *Diabetes Care, 13* (11, Supp. 4), 1191–1195.

Folsom, A. R., Burke, G. L., Byers, C. L., Hutchinson, R. G., Heiss, G., Flack, J. M., Jacobs, D. R., & Caan, B. (1991). Implications of obesity for cardiovascular disease in blacks: The CARDIA and ARIC studies. *American Journal of Clinical Nutrition, 53,* 1604S–1611S.

Foster, E. R., & Burton, B. J. (Eds.) (1985). Health implications of obesity. National Institute of Health Consensus Development Conference. *Annals of Internal Medicine, 103,* 981–1077.

Freedman, D. S., Strogatz, D. S., Eaker, E., Joesoef, M. R., & DeStefano, F. (1990). Differences between black and white men in correlates of high-density lipoprotein cholesterol. *American Journal of Epidemiology, 132,* 656–669.

Freis, E. D., Reda, D. J., & Materson, B. J. (1988). Volume (weight) loss and blood pressure following thiazide diuretics. *Hypertension, 12,* 244–250.

Gillum, R. F. (1987a). The association of body fat distribution with hypertension, hypertensive heart disease, coronary heart disease, diabetes and cardiovascular risk factor in men and women aged 18–79 years. *Journal of Chronic Diseases, 40,* 421–428.

Gillum, R. F. (1987b). Overweight and obesity in black women: A review of published data from the National Center for Health Statistics. *Journal of the National Medical Association, 79,* 865–871.

Harlan, L. C., Bernstein, A. B., & Kessler, L. G. (1991). Cervical cancer screening: Who is not screened and why? *American Journal of Public Health, 81,* 885–890.

Harris, M. I., Hadden, W. C., Knowler, W. C., & Bennett, P. H. (1987). Prevalence of diabetes and impaired glucose tolerance and plasma glucose levels in U.S. population aged 20–74 years. *Diabetes, 36,* 523–534.

Healthy People 2000. (1991). National health promotion and disease prevention objectives. DHHS Publication No. (PHS) 91-50212. Washington, DC: Government Printing Office.

Hollenbeck, C. B., & Coulston, A. M. (1990). Diabetes mellitus. In Brown, M. (Ed.), *Present knowledge in nutrition* (6th Ed.). International Life Sciences Institute, Nutrition Foundation, Washington, DC.

Intersalt Cooperative Research Group. (1988). Intersalt: An international study of electrolyte excretion and blood pressure. Results for 24 hour urinary sodium and potassium excretion. *British Medical Journal, 297,* 319–328.

Kittler, P. G., & Sucher, K. (1989). *Food and Culture in America.* New York: Van Nostrand Reinhold.

Kris-Etherton, P. M., Krummel, D., Dreon, D., Mackey, S., & Wood, P. D. (1988). The effect of diet on plasma lipids, lipoproteins, and coronary heart disease. *Journal of the American Dietetic Association, 88,* 1373–1400.

Kumanyika, S. (1987). Obesity in black women. *Epidemiologic Reviews, 9,* 31–50.

Kumanyika, S., & Adams-Campbell, L. L. (1991). Obesity, diet, and psychosocial factors contributing to cardiovascular disease in blacks. *Cardiovascular Clinics, 21,* 47–73.

Kumanyika, S., & Helitzer, D. L. (1985). Nutritional status and dietary pattern of racial minorities in the United States. In *Report of the Secretary's Task Force on Black and Minority Health.* (Volume II), USDHHS, Washington, DC: Government Printing Office.

Kumanyika, S. K., & Savage, D. D. (1986). Ischemic heart disease risk factors in black Americans. In *Report of the Secretary's Task Force on Black and Minority Health* (Volume IV): Cardiovascular and Cerebrovascular Disease. USDHHS, Washington, DC: Government Printing Office.

Lewis, C. E., Raczynski, J. M., Oberman, A., & Cutter, G. R. (1991). Risk factors and the natural history of coronary heart disease in blacks. *Cardiovascular Clinics, 21,* 29–45.

National Center for Health Statistics. (1989). *Health, United States, 1988.* USDHHS, Publication No. (PHS) 89-1232. Washington, DC: Government Printing Office.

National Research Council. (1989). *Diet and health: Implications for reducing chronic disease risk.* Committee on Diet and Health. Food and Nutrition Board. Commission on Life Sciences. Washington: National Academy Press.

Pi-Sunyer, F. X. (1990). Obesity and diabetes in blacks. *Diabetes Care, 13* (11, Supp. 4), 1144–1149.

Pi-Sunyer, F. X. (1991). Health implications of obesity. *American Journal of Clinical Nutrition, 53,* 1595S-1603S.

Report of the Secretary's Task Force on Black and Minority Health. (1985). USDHHS. Washington, DC: Government Printing Office.

Sanjur, D. (1982). *Social and Cultural perspectives in Nutrition.* Englewood Cliffs, NJ: Prentice-Hall.

Schoenborn, C. A. (1988). National Center for Health Statistics, *Health Promotion and Disease Prevention United States, 1985.* Vital and Health Statistics, Series 10, No. 163, DHHS, Publication No. (PHS) 88-1591, Washington, DC: Government Printing Office.

Sempos, C., Fulwood, R., Haines, C. V., Carroll, M., Anda, R., Williamson, D. F., Remington, P., & Cleeman, J. (1989). The prevalence of high blood cholesterol levels among adults in the United States. *Journal of the American Medical Association, 262*, 45–52.

Srinivasan, S. R., Frerichs, R. R., Webber, L. S., & Berenson, G. S. (1976). Serum lipoprotein profile in children from a biracial community: The Bogalusa Heart Study. *Circulation, 54*, 309–318.

Surgeon General's Report on Nutrition and Health. U.S. Department of Health and Human Services. (1988). Public Health Service, DHHS (PHS) Publication No. 88-50210, Washington, DC: Government Printing Office.

Van Itallie, T. B. (1985). Health implications of overweight and obesity in the United States. *Annals of Internal Medicine, 103*, 983–988.

Wilson, P. W. F., Savage, D. D., Castelli, W. P., Garrison, R. J., Donahue, R. P., & Feinleib, M. (1983). HDL-cholesterol in a sample of black adults: The Framingham Minority Study. *Metabolism, 32*, 328–332.

Wing, R. R., Kuller, L. H., Bunker, C., Matthews, K., Caggiula, A., Meihlan, E., & Kelsey, S. (1989). Obesity-related behaviors and coronary heart disease risk factors in black and white premenopausal women. *International Journal of Obesity, 13*, 511–519.

IV

Sociopolitical Conditions and Related Issues

19

The Epidemiology of Homelessness in Black America

Gregg Barak

INTRODUCTION

Nobody knows how many people are homeless and nobody knows the rate of homelessness growth in this country, although most observers and service providers agree that homelessness has been growing for the past two decades. Trying to measure the number of homeless or the rates and trends in the growth of homelessness in the United States is a dubious exercise at best. Ultimately, the variation in the estimates of the magnitude of the problem are influenced by the definitions of homelessness that one employs. Definitions, for example, range from the more narrow and restrictive, that is, from the number of people, counted during one or two nights a year, found sleeping at a shelter for the homeless to the more broad and inclusive definitions of homelessness that include the number of people found in shelters, on the street, in welfare hotels, and doubling and tripling up with friends and family. Accordingly, throughout the 1980s most estimates of the number of homeless in the United States ranged from a low of some 250,000 to a high of 3 million (Barak, 1991).

Similarly, when it comes to projecting the number of homeless in America at the turn of the century, the variations in estimates reveal an even larger divergence. Here the numbers, with lows of some one million and highs of 20 million homeless by the year 2000, are affected by whether or not one's projections are based on data regarding trends in unemployment and underemployment, health care in all its manifestations, education, crime and incarceration, the cost of housing, levels of counseling, shelter, and public and/or private ventures in low-income housing. Some experts have suggested an approximate 5 percent growth in the homeless population a year (Mathews, 1992).

Even a 5 percent growth figure dwarfs the projected 1 percent growth in the general population, from 255 million in 1990 to 275 million in 2000. On the other hand, estimates as late as 1990 and 1991, by those who were fixing the number of homeless in the United States at around 3 million, were projecting as many as 20 million homeless by the turn of the century or more than a 50 percent growth rate per year. For example, a 1988 congressionally funded study by the Neighborhood Reinvestment Corporation informed us that unless immediate action was taken to preserve and expand the supply of affordable housing in the United States, then by the end of the century there could be as many as 19 million homeless residents.

In 1992 the Urban Institute was placing the number of homeless in the United States at 600,000. The federal government's current estimate of some 700,000 or even the Urban Institute's more conservative figure, along with the latter's 5 percent annual growth estimate, still predicts some one million homeless persons in the year 2000. There are, of course, those persons who would like to debate whether or not such figures constitute a homeless crisis in America, let alone one of epidemic proportions.

Anna Kondratas, the assistant secretary at the Department of Housing and Urban Development in charge of homelessness, has said that ''600,000 homeless people represent 'a national shame,' but that it is 'a manageable problem' '' (Mathews, 1992, p. 29). From the perspective of homeless people in general and from that of Black homeless people in particular, however, the problem of homelessness and its associated conditions of abject poverty, lack of health care, drug addiction, alcoholism, AIDS, violence, and mental and physical debilitation is anything but manageable. For example, between 1970 and 1980 the disproportionate percentage of poor Blacks who lived in extreme poverty tracts in the 10 largest American cities rose from 22 percent to 38 percent; similarly, unemployment rates for Blacks were at record-setting levels of between 16 percent and 30 percent (Wacquant & Wilson, 1989). These same indicators of social marginality today are also reflected in the disproportionate number of Blacks in the homeless population, constituting 32 percent in Los Angeles, 26 percent in San Francisco, 33 percent in Chicago, and 64 percent in New York City, when Blacks represent only 12 percent of the U.S. population as a whole (Ropers, 1988).

ON THE NATURE OF THE CONDITION

The overrepresentation of Black homelessness in the United States is not confined just to urban America but also includes rural and especially Southern America. As James H. Carter, professor of psychiatry at Duke University Medical Center, has suggested, there is ''a critical need for health care policymakers, shelter operators, and educators to make a thorough assessment of the impact of homelessness, racism, and poverty on the health of rural Southern African Americans'' (Carter, 1991, p. 981). Part of the omission has to do with the fact that most of our information on the homeless has been gathered from sheltered populations, and the South simply does not shelter the homeless populations as do the Northern, Eastern, and Western regions of the country. Part of the omission has to do with the fact that the plight of the rural homeless has been overshadowed by the more conspicuous urban homelessness chronicled by academicians, government reports, and the mass media.

In discussing the convergence of homelessness, AIDS, drug abuse, and other social problems engulfing low-income Blacks in urban America, James S. Jackson, director of the University of Michigan's Program for Research on Black Americans, predicts that many of the inner-city neighborhoods that have been decimated by the gradual withdrawal of middle-class Blacks to the suburbs will someday be bulldozed so that they can start over again. "But in the meantime," as he says, "urban black families are beset by so many different pathologies that 'it's very difficult to figure out what's causing what' " (Morganthau, 1992, p. 22).

Unraveling the nature of the condition as well as the causes of homelessness among Black people in America today is complicated, to say the least. Homeless people, regardless of color, are essentially poor people; variations do exist, stemming from differences with respect to one's age, gender, psychiatric well-being, and racial composition and from structural transformations in the global political economy as reflected by changes in the job market. For example, mental illness/disorder is more prevalent among Whites than among either Blacks or Hispanics, and it is also more common among women in each racial group. At the same time, with the exception of the elderly, all women, whether they are classified as psychiatric or nonpsychiatric, are more likely than men to receive money from the state in one form or the other (i.e., food stamps, Medicaid, AFDC). Accordingly, in their study of New York City's homeless shelter population in the mid-1980s, Crystal et al. (1986) found two very different portraits of homeless people: One group of homeless clients consisted of young (mid-30s) Black males who had lived in apartments of their own or with family during the 6 months before entering the shelter. These Black men had been victimized by the structural changes in the job market that had produced service-type employment whose wages had not kept up with the cost of living in general and with the cost of low-income housing in particular. A second group of homeless clients consisted of White women (also in their mid-30s), who had been living independently, receiving financial entitlements, and residing for more than a year in a shelter. These White women had become victimized by the feminization of psychiatric disorders, especially as related to formerly nonmarginal women.

Virtually all studies conducted on homelessness in the United States during the 1980s noted the overrepresentation of minorities in general and of Blacks in particular in an emerging homeless population that had dramatically changed from the 1960s. Three decades ago or in 1965, 90 percent of the homeless (sheltered) population was White and male. By 1985 the composition of homelessness in America had become younger, darker, and much more heterogenous, including a rapidly growing percentage of homeless families, especially single mothers with children. These trends have continued into the 1990s, and there is nothing to suggest that they will not continue into the next century.

As Wright (1989 pp. 66–67) has argued, "representation of racial and ethnic composition of a city's homeless population usually reflects that of the city's larger poverty population." Moreover, in cities with high proportions of Blacks, the homeless are overwhelmingly Black. For example, Blacks represent 54 percent and 75 percent of the homeless sheltered population in Chicago and in New York City respectively. "In many demographic respects, the GA [General Assistance] clients strongly resemble the homeless; like the homeless studied in the 1985–86 Chicago survey, the GA recipients are predominantly male (68 percent), Black (76 percent), and unmarried (92 percent). Economically, GA clients and the homeless were very similar: both groups had nonexistent or very small incomes, and both groups also were characterized by high unemployment and erratic employment histories" (Rossi, 1989).

While there is regional variation according to racial and ethnic composition, roughly half of the homeless populations in most areas are members of minority groups, primarily Black and Hispanic. For example, in a 1986 study of 16 cities by the National Health Care for Homeless Program, it was found that Whites represented 45 percent, Blacks represented 40 percent, and Hispanics represented 11 percent of the homeless sheltered populations. In those cities studied the percentage of Blacks and Hispanics was 11.7 and 6.4 respectively, meaning that overrepresentation in the homeless population was 3.33 for Blacks and 1.7 for Hispanics (Wright, 1989). Clearly, Blacks are the most overrepresented or victimized group of homeless people in America. This being the case, the following question can be asked: What are some of the more obvious and negative health consequences of this overrepresentation for homeless Blacks in America?

Selected Health Problems and Black Homelessness

Morbidity and Related Problems

We know, for example, that like the general needs of children raised in poverty for primary health care and access to appropriate referral services, the needs of children, Black or White, raised in homeless poverty are at least as severe. That is to say, both groups of children are at increased risk for adverse health and developmental outcomes when compared to children raised in nonpoor families (Lewis and Meyers, 1989). While the evidence is mixed as to whether homeless poor children are appreciatively worse off than other poor children; studies in New York City have shown that poor children who are homeless have a higher prevalence of health problems than those poor children who are not homeless, including iron deficiency, plumbism (lead poisoning), child abuse and neglect, immunization delay, and hospital admissions (Alperstein, Rappaport & Flanigan, 1988). However, studies of homeless children (or adults) have not measured the psychological and emotional stress that affects the so-called normal residents of the shelters. Of course, nobody is examining the health and welfare of those homeless persons who have not found their way to shelter facilities or county hospitals, but who are still surviving somewhere on the "streets" beyond the official counts. In all likelihood there is a tendency to underestimate the long-term and permanent damage, developmental and otherwise, done to children raised in homeless poverty. The severity of the homelessness problem, like so many other social problems in America, impacts most negatively on young Blacks and other disjointed and discounted minorities who are disproportionately overerrepresented among the homeless.

Another prominent group of homeless Black persons includes those who are both veterans and suffering from chronic mental illness. Available data from 11 surveys of homeless adults indicate that a substantial number of the homeless, from 18 to 51 percent, are veterans. While it remains unclear whether veterans, who constitute 31 percent of the adult male population, are overrepresented among the homeless, it is clear that Blacks are overrepresented (33.6%) among the homeless chronic mentally ill (Rosenheck et al., 1989). As to the need for specialty examinations, Rosenheck et al. (1989) found in their study of 10,529 homeless veterans that 67.8 percent were judged to need further specialized psychiatric evaluation or treatment and that 71.6 percent were felt to need medical evaluation or treatment.

Among the more significant findings in the study by Rosenheck and his colleagues were the data collected at the time of initial assessment pertaining to the various living arrangements, substance usage, and psychiatric symptomatology of the homeless chronic mentally ill veterans: 47.3 percent were living in shelters, 35.2 percent had no residence at all, 9.1 percent were living intermittently with family or friends, and 7.6 percent had a room or apartment. Slightly more than 46 percent of all veterans reported a significant substance abuse problem—broken down as 33.4 percent alcohol, 4.7 percent drugs, and 8.1 percent both alcohol and drugs. Nearly 33 percent had reported that they had been hospitalized at some time for a psychiatric problem, and 64.8 percent had been hospitalized for either a psychiatric or a substance abuse problem. Moreover, 48.9 percent of those assessed by outreach clinicians manifested or reported one or more of 10 (psychiatric) symptoms, and 34.7 percent were positive for two or more of them (Rosenheck et al., 1989).

Other corroborating evidence on the health care needs of the homeless suggest an even higher overrepresentation of Black persons. For example, a document published in 1989 by the National Association of Community Health Centers, Inc. (NACHC), reported on the study of 109 projects offering health care services for the homeless in 41 states, the District of Columbia, and the Commonwealth of Puerto Rico. It revealed that just under 60 percent of the homeless served by the Health Care for the Homeless Program (HCHP) were "members of minority racial/ethnic groups. Blacks constitute[d] about 42 percent of those served, Whites about 40 percent, Hispanics just over 10 percent, and other minority groups (Asians, Native Americans, etc.) about 8 percent" (NACHC, 1989). The absolute numbers of homeless Blacks served by the HCHP in 1988 and 1989 (the first two years of the program's availability) were 64,000 and 128,000, respectively. Among the more common health conditions exhibited by the homeless adults who received services were skin disorders, mental illness, hypertension, pulmonary disease, and substance abuse. Among the needy homeless children, common suffering resulted from anemia, undernutrition, incomplete immunizations, skin disorders, pulmonary disease, and developmental delay.

Mortality

Finally, when it comes to health problems in general and to mortality in particular, homeless people suffer a great deal. For example, regarding virtually every category of chronic health problems, with the exception of obesity, stroke, and cancer, homeless people are far more likely to have higher rates than the general housed population. Moreover, by comparison with housed persons, homeless persons, adults and children alike, suffer from at least one chronic health problem almost twice as often as the housed (Wright & Weber, 1987). While a perusal of the literature does not show any breakdowns of mortality and homelessness by race or ethnicity, it is reasonable to assume from all the other available data that Blacks are, once again, overrepresented in this category.

With respect to the general problem of mortality and homelessness, the National Coalition for the Homeless has summarized the contemporary state of affairs: "These deaths provide a stark reminder of the havoc caused by the current crisis of affordable housing and perhaps the most compelling evidence that the nation's health care system and so-called 'safety net' are in shambles (Williams, 1991, p. iii).

Although complete national counts are not available on the number of people who die homeless in the United States each year, estimates run into the thousands. A national study involving 19 cities nationally, excluding the city of New York, where the most homeless people die annually, documented that at least 750 homeless persons died during 1991. Of these deaths, about 50 percent happened outside, and most of the deaths were premature; the average age of a person dying homeless was 41 years. Common causes of homeless deaths included exposure, AIDS, complications resulting from alcoholism, accidents, homicide, and other violence. "Homeless people also died of cancer, pneumonia, tuberculosis, heart disease, and suicide. Of 191 [homeless] deaths in Atlanta, 44 were homicides, 26 were accidental, 40 were from AIDS, 10 were suicides, and 15 were from exposure" (Williams, 1991, p. iii).

In the only national study on mortality rates among the homeless population, Wright and Weber analyzed the records of Health Care for the Homeless patients. They reported that the death rate among the homeless was 3.1 times higher than the standard mortality rate for the same age group in the general population (average age = 34); the average age of death was 51 years, approximately 20 years lower than the general life expectancy for this age group; and the homeless people were 20 times more likely than the general population to be murdered (Wright & Weber, 1987).

THE POLITICAL ECONOMY OF HOMELESSNESS

The root causes of homelessness in America can be located in the changing relations of competing social policy formations, individual versus collective rights of justice for all, and class, race, and gender interests. More fundamentally, homelessness in the United States during the 1980s and 1990s reflects the developing income inequality in relation to a changing global political economy as represented by de- and reindustrialization, peripheralization of labor, and internationalization of capital. As the United States moves from an industrial economy to a service economy and as the number of jobs in the manufacturing sector continues to decline, along with the polyethnic internationalization of labor and the development of immigrant-based urban capitalism (e.g., family-owned businesses from Asian and Middle Eastern countries), Blacks have, in effect, lost two historical economic bases, namely, an indigenous economy based on Black-owned businesses and a relatively well-paid wage-labor force grounded in manufacturing and industry. The results have been increased participation by young Blacks in crime, welfare, and homelessness.

Analyzing and addressing the relations of homelessness necessitates the study of changing cultural values, social structures, political systems, technological developments, and distributions of income and wealth. More specifically, as I have argued elsewhere, homelessness in America is caused by the unequal control of investment and economic allocations of social (public) revenues. I have also argued that the solution to homelessness in the United States lies in democratizing the entire process of social investment for purposes of satisfying the basic needs of life. In other words, the elimination of homelessness requires that our domestic policies confront the necessity of creating noncapitalist spheres of economic and social activity; at the same time, they must decommodify certain goods and services such as housing and education for the working and nonworking poor (Barak, 1991).

Homelessness and the homeless are typically attributed to four factors: (1) individual characteristics such as alcoholism, mental illness, and the lack of marketable skills; (2) family disruption involving runaway children or elderly persons who lose family support; (3) institutional policies affecting dependent populations, such as deinstitutionalization of the chronically mentally ill; and (4) market forces related to housing affordability, such as tightening of the low-income housing market, rising mortgage interest rates, declining wages, or job shortfalls. In short, the nature of homelessness in America over the past 20 years has changed significantly as a function of a global political economy in transition. An example is the changing faces of the "old" and "new" homeless that correspond with the movement away from an industrial-oriented economy and toward a service-oriented economy. The "new" homeless are the products of underconsumption and a surplus of technically unskilled workers. The "old" homeless were the products of a depressed, industrial economy struggling with underproduction and experiencing a temporary labor surplus (Barak, 1991).

Although each of the contributing factors to homelessness must be addressed by social policy, especially in the context of a changing political economy, market forces related to housing affordability is particularly important because it reveals the fallacy of the mean-spirited argument that large numbers of families remain homeless because of personal traits rather than structural constraints. For example, in one national study of families with children, real income declined by 34 percent between 1973 and 1984 for those families in the lowest income quintile (Danzinger & Gottschalk, 1985). Also, in the state of New York, Hirschl (1987) found that "of the 535,800 households below the 75 percent poverty level, 421,500 are renters. Of these renters, 77.3 percent pay more than 50 percent of their income in rent. . . . [I]f income drops for one of these households by more than 50 percent for any given month, housing costs alone could swamp the household budget." Using 1983 New York State households who fell below the 75 percent poverty level and the number of poor households that spend more than half their incomes on housing costs, Hirschl calculated the number of people who are not currently homeless but who are economically vulnerable to homelessness (884,400) and then compared it to the number of homeless people living in shelter facilities (20,210). A vulnerability ratio of 44 to 1 was reported.

Hirschl's vulnerability thesis is not reductionist. It does not argue that housing affordability is the only cause of homelessness, nor does it predict that those who are economically vulnerable to homelessness will, in fact, become part of the homeless population. His thesis is that reduced housing affordability is the single most important condition for the persistence of a large homeless population. Hirschl's thesis is certainly warranted when it comes to the realities of the past Reagan and Bush administrations' policy on public housing. As part of an attempt to help manage the fiscal crisis of the 1980s, cutbacks in the welfare state generally and in low-income housing in particular increased throughout the period. When Carter left office in 1980, $32 billion a year was being authorized for low-income housing. Eight years later, when Reagan's administration came to an end, the number of dollars spent on low-income housing had been reduced to about $8 billion. As the first term of Bush's administration came to a close, the number of dollars spent in 1992 was approximately $9.6 billion.

More generally, the changing worldwide political economy of the 1970s and 1980s has historically recorded both the end of the postwar boom in the development of U.S. transnational capital and the decline of U.S. hegemony in international relations, each coming to pass during the so-called Vietnam era (Sherman, 1976; Mandel, 1980; Berberoglu, 1987). These changing global realities have had the effect of contributing to what now appears to be a permanent U.S. fiscal crisis brought about by overproduction and the downward turns in the business cycle (Batra, 1987). In addition, this crisis has been fueled by the rise to world prominence of the European and Asian economies, coupled with the effects of the transnational corporate expansion abroad on the domestic economy. For example, these structural transformations in the U.S. and global economies produced the most severe recession since the 1930s in 1974. Moreover, the U.S. economy sunk into recessions in 1979, in 1982, and in 1991.

Hence, for the past 20 years or so, the general trend in domestic business activity has been in a downward direction while the rates in unemployment and underemployment have been in upward directions. Throughout the current period of "adjustment," real wages of workers have continued to decline, especially for those at the bottom end of the income scale. The effect has been that a greater number of both employed and unemployed persons are unable to afford the rising costs of U.S. housing. During this period of economic decline, these negative trends in the standards of living for the average American have impacted marginal groups most severely. Constituting a disproportionate minority of marginal America, Blacks have been particularly vulnerable to the crisis in affordable housing. In addition, Blacks continue to suffer from the legacies of racism and discrimination that serve to further exacerbate their plight to find decent paying jobs and low-income housing.

As John Calmore in his 1986 study of housing policies and Black Americans, writes, "The 'disadvantageous distinction' of being Black in America probably presents its most diverse, complex, and intractable problems in our attempts to secure viable property rights and housing opportunities" (1986, p. 115). Alphonso Pinkney has also discussed the housing discrimination practices that have faced minorities in general and Blacks in particular. After citing studies conducted by the Department of Housing and Urban Development, Pinkney (1984) concluded his analysis by stating, "Discrimination in housing is a function of many factors, including broker practices and years of ingrained cultural attitudes. But one of the major causes is the lack of enforcement of the law by the Department of Housing and Urban Development" (p. 71).

THE SOCIAL AND POLITICAL UNDOING OF HOMELESSNESS

In my book *Gimme Shelter,* I argued that the social and political undoing of homelessness in America would come about only when the strengths of capitalism and socialism were brought together in a hybrid system or when the development of a "free-market socialism" had occurred, in which individuals were limited by government "to accumulating wealth only to the extent that accumulation [did] not deprive another coproducer or coconsumer of a minimal and humane share of the created wealth, based on what [was] commonly regarded as 'fair' were their positions reversed" (Barak, 1991, p. 181). In "Homelessness and the Case for Community-Based Initiatives" I argued that there were models of social-service deployment that not only were of revolutionary potential, providing a critique of bourgeois values and society, but also exerted serious effort "to develop progressive alternatives to the existing human-service delivery systems'' (Barak, 1991a, p. 64).

These are not the only arguments that I have made about social change, public policy, and homelessness. But these are representative arguments that contrast with the two other policy approaches to addressing the homelessness crisis in America. I refer to the reactionary approach that maintains that the homeless are volunteers and are responsible for their own fates and that, therefore, the role of the state and private sector becomes one of non-intervention and laissez-faire. I also refer to the liberal approach that suggests that there are societal conditions associated with homelessness and calls for temporary shelters as part of the ''healing'' process involved in getting homeless people back on their feet and into permanent residences.

The problems with the reactionary and liberal approaches to homelessness are many, but fundamentally they may be critiqued on their shortsightedness and on their tendency to ignore the changing structural conditions of society. By contrast, the radical approach, as called for in this chapter, not only recognizes the need for long-term commitment to the low-cost housing crisis in America but also expresses a fundamental appreciation for the dilemmas and contradictions surrounding the resolution of homelessness in the United States. Specifically, I refer not only to the continuities and discontinuities between long-term and short-term public policy but also to the differences between ''structuralist'' reform and ''reformist'' reform. Hence, the social and political undoing of homelessness in America is dependent upon the development of a ''grass-roots'' or ''popular'' movement whose vision is for long-term, radical social change and whose practice involves the immediate struggle for the empowerment of ordinary people, including the homeless.

The resolution of homelessness and the low-income housing crisis in the United States requires that the nation as a whole make a long-term commitment to eliminating the lack of adequate and affordable housing. Such a goal, not yet the object of U.S. public policy, would take about a generation or 20 years to realize. This goal necessitates the collective transformation of the cultural ethic of American individualism. It also necessitates a sustained drive to address the underlying or root causes of homelessness in America. Without this kind of national policy or political commitment, however, it is still possible to struggle for the eradication of homelessness. As Zarembka (1990, p. 46) has argued: ''even if the nation as a whole will not make a long-term commitment, it may be possible to design long-term goals and policies to achieve some of the goals on a state-by-state or city-by-city basis.''

The undoing of homelessness demands fundamentally new policies on housing (as well as on health care and education). At the heart of a new domestic policy on housing and homelessness is the basic need to establish a Social Housing Sector where the construction of housing for use, rather than profit, coexists with the private, for-profit housing market. The provision of a sector for social housing allows participants to escape the spiraling costs of housing brought about by the constant cycle of mortgaging and remortgaging of property at ever-higher prices.

The creation of social housing breaks the cycle of escalating housing costs; hence, once the initial costs of construction are paid off the only future expenses are for repairs, maintenance, management, and utilities. The ownership of property under such a plan becomes "mixed" with the majority in private hands, but with a portion set aside for local governments, public housing authorities, limited-equity cooperatives, mutual housing associations, community land trusts, and nonprofit organizations. Financing a Social Housing Sector requires the establishment of a nonprofit Housing Bank that provides low-interest, low-down-payment loans to homebuyers and low-interest loans to builders. Such a housing system also requires resale price controls, antispeculation laws, and rent control to help stabilize housing prices. Finally, social housing recognizes the need to subsidize low-income households (Zarembka, 1990).

In the meantime, while we wait for U.S. domestic policy to come of age, there are plenty of things that both individuals and organizers can do to alleviate the misery and suffering of the homeless. For starters, concerned citizens can get to know homeless people in their communities. In the process they can learn how these people became, in reality, homeless. In addition, there are many voluntary roles that individuals can occupy. In shelters, throughout the country people can work with the homeless: helping displaced families find affordable housing; assisting the unemployed in their quest for employment; reading to pre-schoolers, doing homework with school-age children, and tutoring young mothers studying for their high school equivalency exams; and providing emotional support to those people in need. Finally, for individuals disinclined to interact with the homeless, there is always the need for political advocacy and consciousness raising at both the local and national levels. In short, people are always needed to act as emissaries to spread the message, throughout their communities and to their elected officials, that the problems associated with homelessness are getting worse and that the housing crisis in America needs immediate attention (Whitaker, 1989).

In a more politically engaging way, interested persons can join with other like-minded persons who have developed programs and/or coalitions to assist the homeless. At the national level and in virtually every state in the union organized groups are currently involved in a number of projects and activities that address the immediate needs of homeless people. In the area of homelessness and health care, for example, there is the ongoing movement of activism in what has been termed the "new urban health crisis." This movement aims to empower poor and oppressed people who are in need of fundamental human and social services. It is located largely in low-income minority communities and strives to build support systems and self-help groups, emphasizing the common needs of "personal transformation, provision of help in nonhierarchical and noncontrolling ways by virtual peers, and identification with communities in struggle" (Bale, 1991, p. 3).

In resisting the current epidemic in drug abuse, violence, AIDS, homelessness, seriously ill newborns, overcrowded hospitals, and compromised care, the movement recognizes that "the crisis builds upon growing economic, racial and spacial polarization, intensified poverty, and badly organized and overloaded service systems" (Bale, 1991: 4). Consequently, activism to counter the health crisis aims to reverse the tendencies of an expanding system of services and social control that seeks to manage people variously labelled as at-risk, sick, and dangerous. Health care activists, in other words, "develop and advocate models of care and service that draw upon and expand the abilities of people in difficult circumstances to control their lives. They struggle against the alternative models of collective policing and crisis management of objectified persons addressed principally as threats to public health and social order" (Bale, 1991, p. 4).

In a similar fashion, Ellen Baxter, homeless activist and director of Supportive Housing for the Community Service Society in New York City, also appreciates the fact that the prevailing governmental policies on homelessness have been "committed to keeping people in a transitional state until their personal problems are solved, rather than seeking to develop supportive housing alternatives that provide additional social services as well" (Merzel, 1991, p. 6). During the 1980s, Baxter and her colleagues were able to successfully establish and have maintained five buildings in Washington Heights and Upper Harlem, accommodating 220 men and women, all of whom have leases. These nonprofit owned and managed entities have been renovated with bank loans and/or state grants from New York. They have been legally protected as low-income housing for a minimum of 30 years, and they have mortgages attached to federal Section 8 rent subsidies.

What is particularly noteworthy about these not-for-profit low-income housing ventures are two things: (1) those who own and manage these properties are not like private landlords (profit or nonprofit organizations), who often are antagonistic or adversarial in their relations with tenants; and (2) the residents, former homeless people, are part of an integrated and multicultural housing structure that includes men, women, and children. While there are some paid people (i.e., superintendents, maintenance people, bookkeepers, project directors) and on-site social services provided for tenants, for the most part the tenants themselves do as much as possible to run these apartments. However, active participation in any part of the running of these buildings is not required.

IMPLICATIONS FOR THE FUTURE

While the U.S. low-cost housing crisis and problems of the homeless in America vary from city to city, from rural to urban, and from the Midwest and the South to the West and East coasts, a common feature is the structural nature of the problem as it is surrounded by an established discourse, ideology, public policy, and economic pattern of development. Unless these relationships are addressed and changed, then the further victimization of the growing number of homeless people in general and of Black homeless in particular will continue unabated throughout the 1990s and into the next century. The solutions to homelessness for "Black" or "White" America are not, in other words, to be found in the development and reproduction of ideal models of shelterization.

These kinds of necessary emergency/temporary shelters may provide humane short-term alternatives to living in a subway or alley or to selling oneself into sexual servitude, but they do not provide for the development of long-term permanent housing for all U.S. residents. Although we need to support and further expand those grass-roots efforts, such as Project Habitat or the congressionally chartered Neighborhood Reinvestment Corporation, that provide small-scale refurbishing of abandoned homes and buildings and facilitate the independent living of small groups of formerly homeless persons, these models of public-private initiatives at the local level without a fundamental change in our national housing policy will prove themselves inadequate for the task of eradicating homelessness in America.

What is called for is the creation of a sector for social housing. Of course, bringing this into fruition involves politically challenging the vested interests of property, business, and defense. For example, in 1988 expenditures to subsidize low-income housing accounted for one cent of every revenue dollar collected. Expenditures to subsidize middle-income and affluent housing through mortgage interest write-offs also accounted for one cent of every dollar of revenue collected. By contrast, the expenditures for defense/military spending accounted for 82 cents of every tax dollar. The current homelessness problem in the United States could virtually be eliminated if the amount of the subsidy for low-income housing was tripled from one cent to three cents per tax dollar collected (Low Income Housing Information Service, 1988).

When it comes to resisting Black homelessness in America, Black homeless activists need to engage the Black community in the struggle to empower marginal Black people. These activists must also form coalitions of solidarity with the Black church and with the Congressional Black Caucus. At the same time, Black homeless volunteers and advocates need to be careful not to ghettoize the problem of Black homelessness in America.

In the final analysis, William Julius Wilson (1980) was correct in his analysis of *The Declining Significance of Race* and its relationship to the development of a domestic policy in America that would truly benefit all marginal people in the United States. For in the end, Black homelessness (like street crime) is not essentially a Black problem. More fundamentally, it is a problem of expanding class conflict and marginality in the context of a developing global economy. Hence, the resolution of homelessness in America demands new domestic policies that challenge both the assumptions and the practices of a hegemonic multinational monopoly capitalism. Until the time comes when there is a development of an alternative economic and domestic agenda grounded in a national commitment not only to end homelessness in the United States but also to provide the basic necessities of life (e.g., food, shelter, education, health care, human dignity, and self-determination), an ever-growing number of Americans will continue to suffer from the state of being without a place to call home.

REFERENCES

Alperstein, G., Rappaport, C., & Flanigan, J. M. (1988). Health problems of homeless children in New York City. *American Journal of Public Health, 78,* 1232–1233.

Bale, T. (1991). Activism in the new urban health crisis. *Health/PAC Bulletin, 21,* 3–4.

Barak, G. (1991). *Gimme shelter: A social history of homelessness in contemporary America.* New York: Praeger.

Barak, G. (1991a). Homelessness and the case for community-based initiatives: The emergence of a model shelter as a short term response to the deepening crisis in housing. In H. E. Pepinsky and R. Quinney (Eds.), *Criminology as peacemaking.* Bloomington: Indiana University Press.

Batra, R. (1987). *The great depression of 1990.* New York: Simon and Schuster.

Berberoglu, B. (1987). Labor, capital, and the state: Economic crisis and class struggle in the United States in the 1970s and 1980s. Paper presented at the annual meeting of the American Sociological Association, Chicago.

Calmore, J. (1986). National housing policies and black America: Trends, issues, and implications. In *The State of Black America in 1986.* New York: National Urban League.

Carter, J. H. (1991). Mental health needs of rural homeless African Americans. *Hospital and Community Psychiatry, 42* (October), 981.

Crystal, S., Ladner, S., & Towber, R. (1986). Multiple impairment patterns in the mentally ill homeless. *International Journal of Mental Health, 14,* 56–72.

Danzinger, S., & Gottschalk, P. (1985). How families with children have been faring. Paper prepared for the Joint Committee, United States Congress.

Hirschl, T. A. (1987). Homeless in New York State: A demographic and socioeconomic analysis. Paper presented at the annual meeting of the American Sociological Association, Chicago.

Lewis, M. R., & Meyers, A. F. (1989). The growth and development status of homeless children entering shelters in Boston. *Public Health Reports, 104,* 247–250.

Low Income Housing Information Service. (1988). *The 1989 Low Income Housing Budget.* Washington, D.C.: LIHIS.

Mandel, E. (1980). *The Second Slump.* London: Verse.

Mathews, J. (1992). Rethinking homeless myths. *Newsweek,* April 6.

Merzel, C. (1991). Rethinking empowerment. *Health/PAC Bulletin, 21,* 5–6.

Morganthau, T. (1992). Losing ground: New fears and suspicions as black America's outlook grows bleaker. *Newsweek,* April 6.

National Association of Community Health Centers (NACHC). (1989). *The health needs of the homeless: A report on persons served by the McKinney act's health care for the homeless program.* Washington, DC: NACHC, Inc.

Pinkney, A. (1984). *The myth of black progress.* Cambridge: Cambridge University Press.

Ropers, R. H. (1988). *The invisible homeless: A new urban ecology.* New York: Human Sciences Press.

Rosenheck, R., Leda, C., Callup, P., Astrachan, B., Milstein, R., Leaf, P., Thompson,

D., & Errara, P. (1989). Initial assessment data from a 43-site program for homeless chronic mentally ill veterans. *Hospital and Community Psychiatry, 40,* 937–942.

Rossi, P. (1989). *Without shelter: Homelessness in the 1980s.* New York: Priority Press Publications.

Sherman, H. (1976). *Stagflation.* New York: Harper and Row.

Wacquant, L. J. D., & Wilson, W. J. (1989). The cost of racial and class exclusion in the inner city. *The Annals of the American Academy of Political and Social Science, 501,* 8–25.

Whitaker, C. (1989). What we can do about the homeless. *Ebony,* June.

Wilson, W. J. (1980). *The declining significance of race.* Chicago: University of Chicago Press.

Williams, L. (1991). *Mourning in America: Health problems, mortality, and homelessness.* Washington, DC: National Coalition for the Homeless.

Wright, J. (1989). *Address unknown: The homeless in America.* New York: Aldine de Gruyter.

Wright, J., & Weber, E. 1987. *Homelessness and health.* New York: McGraw Hill.

Zarembka, A. (1990). *The urban housing crisis: Social, economic, and legal issues and proposals.* Westport, CT: Greenwood Press.

20

The Physical, Psychological, and Social Health of Black Older Americans

Ron C. Manuel

During 1990, about 45 percent of the 2.5 million Black Americans aged 65 and over lived on incomes falling below or near (within 125% of) the poverty threshold.[1] Nearly two-thirds (64.2%) of these elderly persons were economically vulnerable, that is, within 200 percent of the threshold. About 16 percent of the White older population lived on incomes below or near the poverty threshold in 1990 (U.S. Bureau of the Census, 1991).

Highlighting racial differences in old-age poverty rates fuels questions about similar differences in the quality of life and chances in life that result for Black older Americans who have had to live their life course as a sociological minority.[2] The purpose of this chapter is to examine the effect of being old and Black (and thus having experienced the cumulative life-course effects of being systematically denied opportunities normally available in society) on each of the following life-quality indicators: physical, psychological, and social health. The pursuit of this general question permits testing a number of hypotheses, several of which have not been heretofore systematically considered. Racial differences in health ultimately have practical implications for the approach taken to health education, health promotion, advocacy, and policy.

The report begins with a brief summary of key issues in the existing literature on race, health, and old age. Limitations in this literature serve to focus attention next on the extent to which a true health disadvantage exists for older Black Americans, unconfounded by class. The consistency of the hypothesized Black disadvantage effect is then examined across data sets, as is also a hypothesis about trends in this effect. The hypothesized Black disadvantage effect, in the context of federal retrenchment policies of the early 1980s, is particularly noted. Next, several hypotheses about heterogeneity within the older Black population are examined. The data to test these hypotheses come from a diverse array of nationally representative, methodologically well-respected surveys. Finally, a theoretical model is presented from which new hypotheses may be generated to direct future research and policy considerations.

THE BACKGROUND

A Growing Population

An understanding of the growth and expected growth of the Black older population highlights the significance of systematically studying this population. For several decades, the growth of the older Black population has been distinctive. Between 1960 and 1980, for example, the number of Black persons aged 65 and over increased 83 percent, while their older White counterparts increased 57 percent. Between 1980 and 1990, the respective older Black and White percentage increases were 20.9 percent and 15.4 percent (U.S. Bureau of the Census, 1991). In 2020, about the time the baby-boom generation (roughly, persons born between 1946 and 1956) has retired, the 5.6 million older Black persons living during that year will represent a 121.2 percent increase beyond the 1990 population. Between 1990 and 2020, their White counterparts, will also experience a phenomenal increase, at 64.7 percent.[3] Clearly, the study of the current and projected growth in the older Black population remains as relevant today as for Smith (1957), when he called attention to the Black elderly as an exceptionally fast-growing, but impoverished, segment of the population.

Some Major Conclusions in the Literature

Understanding the health of older Black Americans has most frequently depended on the study of survival and mortality data. Comparative study of mortality rates have provided and continue to provide unambiguous, reliable, and easily ascertained indicators of the relative general condition of health within the older Black population. The paucity of data on morbidity and functioning (including physical, psychological, and social functioning), as well as the limited number of Black respondents, in many early national samples contributed to this trend. A relatively rich literature on (race) differential mortality thus has undergirded many of the issues and concepts concerning health and minority aging. As will later become clear, health as indicated by mortality patterns does not tell the entire story about health. That is, health as indicated by patterns in mortality is not necessarily equivalent to health as indicated by patterns in morbidity and functioning.

At risk of oversimplification, the early literature generally concludes that, while the mortality rate for both Blacks and Whites has lessened over time, the rate remains consistently higher among Blacks than Whites for all of the major causes of death. Keith and Smith (1988) found 60 percent of the racial differential in mortality attributable to the black disadvantage in experiencing cardiovascular disease, homicide, malignant neoplasms, and infant mortality. Black life expectancy (at birth), accordingly, generally lags behind White life expectancy by about six to seven years. For example, in 1989, White life expectancy, at birth, was 76 years while Black life expectancy was 69. Indeed, Black males, at birth, have never been expected to live beyond 65 years, the most frequent indicator for defining the beginning of old age.

The concept of double jeopardy is frequently invoked in the early literature to describe the relatively disadvantaged health status of older Blacks. According to the double jeopardy thesis, injustices associated with being old act to compound the effects of racially based economic and social indignities experienced throughout the earlier life course (National Urban League, 1964). The thesis has received both confirmation (Dowd & Bengtson, 1978) and disconfirmation (Ferraro, 1987), but has remained largely undeveloped as a possible theoretical orientation (in essence a theory about the interaction of age and race). Also, the term has served more frequently as a euphemistic concept for drawing attention, politically, to the special plight of the Black aged.

In addition to the concepts of differential mortality and double jeopardy, a third focal point has been the study of the crossover effect. While, generally, the Black American death rate exceeds the White rate, after about age 75 (the crossover point) the White rate surpasses the Black rate for several causes of death (Manton, 1982). An hypothesis not yet systematically tested is that the oldest of older Blacks represent an elite group. These are persons who have survived because they presumably possess special coping skills or resources, or perhaps have a unique biological composition. Skills used for coping with racial injustices, hypothetically, may have consequences for coping with the stressors of old age.

An alternate hypothesis, that the crossover effect is a methodological artifact resulting from inflated age reports by older Blacks, has been noted (Manton, 1982). Recent evidence, however, shows little support for the artifact thesis (Wing, Manton, Stallard, Hames & Tyroler, 1985).

The crossover effect is a dynamic phenomenon, however. In 1960, the crossover had occurred by age 65 to 85 on each of the leading causes of death. In 1989, the effect, where present, appeared only for the cohort aged 85 and over. A clear need exists for research to examine age cohort psychosocial differences that might explain the dynamic nature of the crossover effect. An elite survival hypothesis, for example, might suggest that decreases in patterns of racism and discrimination (say, more equitable medical treatment during youth and midlife for recent Black age cohorts of Blacks) led to changes in coping with the consequences of racism. Having perhaps had to develop fewer skills for coping with racism early in the life cycle, Black Americans may be increasingly similar to their White counterparts in coping with the special stressors associated with old age.

Racial differences in mortality, as noted, have been the primary hub around which conclusions about the health of the Black aged have been based. Recently, however, Jackson and Perry (1989) and others, including Gibson and Jackson (1987) and Gibson (1991), have done much for beginning the development of a stream of research that focuses on the health conditions and functioning of Black Americans who survive to experience old age. From this literature, a fourth conclusion about the health of older Blacks appears to be taking shape, namely, that as a consequence of the dynamic nature of the mortality crossover, the health status of Black survivors will vary by age cohort. Gibson's (1991) review of the literature on this topic highlights a narrowed Black (to White) health disadvantage among persons aged 85 and over, but greater Black disadvantage among persons aged 65 to 74. The focus in this chapter is on expanding the scope of the data, the hypotheses, and the issues pertaining to this question of heterogeneity, as well as other conclusions in the literature about the health of the Black aged.

EXPANDING THE FOCUS ON HEALTH OF THE BLACK AGED

Health is a state of complete physical, mental, and social well-being and not just the absence of disease or infirmity (World Health Organization, 1959). Ideally, then, a concise reliable index of older Black health would measure not only physical capacity and functional independence but also economic, psychological, and social independence, including social integration or role functioning, psychological self-esteem, and life satisfaction. Space limitations in this chapter prevent studying a systematic array of indicators under each of these health domains. The study here of selected physical, psychological, and social indicators of health, however, will extend existing analyses, contributing to the evolving systematic understanding of the relation of health and race in old age.

Physical Health

Data for the physical health indicators come from the National Center for Health Statistics' (NCHS, 1986a) 1984 National Health Interview Survey (NHIS), Supplement on Aging (SOA). Racial contrasts (Black versus White) are studied where race has both statistical (from a two by two—that is, a dichotomous health status by race—chi square analysis) and substantive (a percentage-point difference of at least seven points) significance.[4]

Conditions and Impairments

The analysis begins with a study of seven chronic health conditions, selected from the SOA to match data appearing in the 1987 and the 1974–75 National Health and Nutrition Examination Surveys (NHANES). (The 1987 and 1971–74 NHANES data will be used in subsequent analyses, respectively, to examine the reliability of, and trends over time in, the conclusions from the 1984 SOA.) The data do not show a distinctive Black disadvantage for any of the chronic conditions associated with the major causes of death (i.e., heart disease, cancer, and stroke). The Black disadvantage is shown on three of the four remaining health conditions: arthritis, diabetes, and hypertension.

Hypertension and arthritis were the most prevalent conditions affecting the health of both Blacks and Whites aged 65 and over, in 1984 (NCHS, 1986b). Diabetes ranked as the fourth most prevalent condition among Blacks. When studied relative to 52 of the most common chronic health conditions in 1984, arthritis, hypertension, and diabetes together accounted for about 44 percent of the excess disadvantage experienced by black older persons.[5]

While no important contrasts appear in the impairment data, an interesting trend occurs for vision impairment. More older Black Americans than White Americans have problems seeing television, as well as seeing newsprint. Older Black Americans, however, are less likely to use any type of eyeware. Branch and Jette (1982) note that unattended vision impairment, besides contributing to a lesser quality of life, increases the likelihood of eventual dependence.

Physical Functioning and Self-rated Health

As in the selection of the health conditions chosen for this study, the selection of functional (physical) ability measures depended on whether they appeared in the other surveys examined for this report. It is seen that the data for the five functional health indicators do not vary by race. While a consistent trend (across the indicators) exists for Black persons to be less functionally able than their White counterparts, in each of these cases the rate difference is less than 7 percentage points.

Finally, the physical health data includes a measure of overall subjective health. Two-thirds more Blacks than Whites in the SOA evaluated their health as poor or fair, a finding that is consistent with the current literature. Krause (1987), for example, documented the effect of race on self-rated health under a number of control conditions, including education. The study of this general subjective indicator of health, with controls for other variables, will be discussed in later sections. It is nevertheless perplexing (and thus a fertile ground for hypothesis formulation) to note the rather clear-cut Black disadvantage on subjectively evaluated health. Yet, few disparities appeared between Blacks and Whites on the actual conditions, disabilities, and impairments studied.

Health as Social and Psychological Well-being

Little consensus exists on the meaning of social well-being. One sociological circumstance often studied, although not necessarily as a dimension of health, is the older person's integration in his or her family and community. It is this dimension of social well-being that the SOA data permit examining. Clearly, both the quantity and quality of informal supportive environments have implications for the demand on formal health care provisions.

For behavior occurring two weeks prior to being interviewed, older Black

Americans visited less and talked (by telephone) less with relatives than did their White counterparts. Black older persons get together less often with friends and are less likely to have done volunteer work or to have gone to the movies or other social outings. They, however, attend church more often than their White counterparts. In general, contrary to the literature (e.g., Taylor & Chatters, 1991), these data do not support the thesis that older Black persons are relatively more integrated in their family and friendship networks. The assumption that the Black aged depend on an informal care community needs much additional research. A model suggestive of the lines of research potentially important here is discussed in a subsequent section.

Though less pronounced than the case for social well-being, psychological well-being also is not often a target for profiling the health of the population. Carter (1982) counsels that many of the psychological defensive maneuvers of older Blacks, including suspiciousness and distrust (often diagnosed as paranoia), may not be necessarily unhealthy. Rather, the psychological solutions used to cope by older Black persons may make the experience of racism bearable.

The limited number of indicators in the SOA permit only brief discussion at this point. Two of the five contrasts on psychological health support the Black disadvantage hypothesis. Older Black Americans report distinctively greater confusion compared to a year earlier. They also more often acknowledge experiencing increased memory difficulties (during the year prior to being interviewed). However, the data from the 1989 NHIS Supplement on Mental health (NCHS, 1991a) show that older Black persons neither report significantly more mental health disorders nor, among persons with a disorder, are they distinctively unable to cope with life stressors.

In sum to this point, 4 of the 20 physical health indicators, 6 of the 9 sociological indicators, and 2 of the 8 psychological health indicators support the Black disadvantage hypothesis. It is noteworthy that 11 of 18 (excluding use of seeing and hearing aids) physical health indicators, 8 of the 9 social health indicators, and 7 of the 8 psychological indicators reflect a rather consistent trend supportive of the Black disadvantage hypothesis. The trends do not all meet the significance criteria. Nonetheless, the analyses illustrate, again, that racial contrasts do not follow a random pattern of relative Black and White risks.

THE QUESTION OF RACE VERSUS CLASS

A question often considered (Jackson, 1971; Markides, 1989), but seldom systematically studied (for an exception, see Wallace, 1990), asks whether the race effect on health is spurious. The data show that older Black Americans, both persons having less than 12 years and those having 12 or more years of schooling, disproportionately acknowledge having an arthritic or hypertensive condition.[6] They also more often evaluate their health unfavorably. The race effect earlier noted for diabetes now appears only for the Black subsample having less than 12 years of schooling. Wallace (1990) counsels that to find race effects, in spite of class controls, means that economic focused policies or programs alone (e.g., Medicare) will not be sufficient to create a more random distribution of health problems across race categories.

With education controlled, race differences remain in 4 of the 5 initially highlighted sociological indicators (i.e., failure within the two weeks prior to the interview to get together with friends/relatives, to talk on the telephone with relatives, to go to the movies, and partake in other recreational events) and both of the psychological indicators (i.e., having more trouble this year than last remembering and getting confused). Contingent, rather than independent, race effects predominate among the sociological indicators, however. Interestingly, the racial contrasts occur as frequently among the better educated as among the less educated. Contrary to Jackson and Perry (1989), these data suggest that the race effect is not simply a lower socioeconomic class phenomenon. In short, race effects, whether independent or interactive, remain in these data even with social class, that is education, controlled.

THE CONSISTENCY OF RECENT EVIDENCE

Credible and reliable conclusions should be repeatable in other samples under closely matched circumstances. To examine the reliability of the preceding conclusions, data were additionally assembled from the 1987 National Health and Nutrition Examination Survey (NHANES) longitudinal follow-up to 1971–75 NHANES (NCHS, 1991b). Both the 1987 NHANES and the SOA, in 1984, occurred closely enough in time so that one might speak of circumstances in the mid-1980s. However, beyond potential caveats about the comparable representativeness of the SOA and the maturing, attrition-influenced 1987 NHANES data, a question remains about the comparability of some indicator wording. For example, the 1987 NHANES, unlike the SOA, explicitly asks respondents about physician-diagnosed, not respondent-evaluated, conditions. The data, nevertheless, are considered valuable for the hypothesis being tested: The Black disadvantaged effects, noted in the SOA, will also appear in the 1987 NHANES.

Findings from the 1987 NHANES confirm that the same 4 effects on physical health (class controlled) noted in the SOA also occurred in the NHANES. Hypertension, arthritis, and diabetes are distinctively more characteristic of the older Black community; and older Blacks more often unfavorably evaluate their health.

The remaining, comparable (across surveys) physical health indicators were consistent in that no class-controlled racial effects could be demonstrated. Two exceptions are notable. The 1987 NHANES, unlike the SOA, shows a significant Black disadvantage (among persons having less than 12 years of schooling) in the use of aids to enable sight and also hearing. This occurred despite, for example, the higher percentage of older Black persons unable to see newsprint.

The unavailability of sufficiently relevant or timed data prevented testing the consistency of the SOA findings on psychological and social well-being.

THE QUESTION OF TRENDS

The next hypothesis posits that the health of the older Black population, relative to their White counterparts, has declined in recent years or, at a minimum, has not improved over the last 10 to 15 years. With the 1981 Omnibus Budget Reconciliation Act and other legislation driven by the early 1980s New Federalism, federal retrenchment from the Great Society programs of the 1960s is unmistakable. Program changes, such as the change of Medicare and Medicaid from cost-based retrospective to fixed-priced prospective payment systems—for the reimbursement of physician and hospital costs—have led many to express concern about lower-quality care and restricted access to health care (Haber, 1989). Thus, a research hypothesis is that the direction of domestic policy, starting in the early 1980s, negatively influenced the health of the older Black population more than their economically better-situated White counterpart. Of course, any hypothesis here must be interpreted in the context of the dynamic nature of the older population resulting from age cohort flow. If, hypothetically, Black survivor cohorts are increasingly less special as elitist copers, time-related changes in Black versus White health may have as much to do with changing, nonpolitical, relative cohort experiences as with changing policies.

Nationally representative data from the 1972–74 NHANES (NCHS, 1985), in conjunction with the preceding 1984 SOA data, permitted studying relative changes in physical health conditions. No 1970s data to match the 1984 health-impairment data could be located, however; and only one indicator of psychological well-being (health worry) could be studied. Data on functional well-being to match the 1984 data come from the 1974 National Council on Aging Survey (NCOA, 1979). Matching indicators for social integration appeared in the 1968 National Senior Citizens Survey (Schooler, 1979).

The pattern of the data provides general confirmation for the hypothesis. First, the Black (class controlled) disadvantage effects shown in the mid-1980s, are not present in the early to mid-1970s, with the exception of hypertension. Indeed, the only health condition in the 1972–74 NHANES showing a Black disadvantage is hypertension. Race also does not influence overall self-rated health in the 1970s. The contrasts on the functional well-being indicators remain stable, with no widening or closing (except for the "ability to prepare a meal") of the racial gap.

Two social well-being indicators for which 1987 data were present also supported the thesis of a widening or stable Black disadvantage. Whereas the Black disadvantage in 1968 did not occur for either "getting together with relatives" or "friends," in 1984, the disadvantage is clear. Worrying about health, on the other hand, varies much by race in the 1980s than in the 1970s. Generally, to the extent that pre-1980 data could be found that matched the 1984 SOA (or 1987 NHANES) data, there is evidence that the hypothesized Black disadvantage has recently become more evident and clearly has not improved.

THE QUESTION OF HETEROGENEITY

Older Black Americans are not a homogeneous collective. Failure to consider subgroup variations within the older Black population transfers into failure to respond to the longstanding special circumstances of many of these subgroups within the population.

Age Cohort Differences

Persons aged 75 and over (the old-old) must be distinguished from the young-old, persons aged 65 to 75 (Neugarten, 1974). The assumption underlying this distinction is that good health becomes more problematic with increasing age. With larger and larger numbers of people living to join the ranks of the oldest old, the health of this population becomes even more special. Gibson (1991), however, identifies a younger (age 65 to 69) and relatively more sick Black (than White) cohort and an older (age 85 and older) relatively more healthy group. Cross-sectional and longitudinal sampling sequences are obviously needed to untangle the confounded age-differences and age-changes implied by these findings. The data make clear, however, the importance of examining age and cohort-related heterogeneity within the Black older population.

The cross-sectional SOA data suggest that Black Americans aged 75 and over suffer neither more nor fewer chronic conditions than their Black counterparts aged 60 to 74. Moreover, neither social nor psychological well-being varies by age cohort. Persons aged 75 and over consistently experience more functional disability, however—as is also true for three of the impairment indicators (cataracts, seeing newsprint, and hearing).

This analysis of the SOA data thus does not support Gibson's (1991) emphasis that there may be both younger and more sickly and older and more healthy Black age cohorts. Fruitful additional study would begin by untangling the age, cohort, and time-related differences confounded in much of the existing data.

Marital Status Differences

About 37 percent of the Black aged were married in 1990, compared to 56 percent of their White counterparts. Spousal support and thus the advantage to good health offered by being married is less available to older Blacks than Whites. But does marital status, as a supposed risk factor for health, vary with the health of older Black Americans?

The SOA data show that neither sociological nor psychological dimensions of health vary by marital status, as is also true for all but 4 of the physical health indicators. Only the nonmarried prevalence rates for arthritis, cataracts, problems walking, and problems preparing meals exceed the corresponding rates among married persons. These findings are perhaps most useful for hypothesizing about the circumstances that influence the relationship of marital status and health. Spousal fear may contribute to the denial that a heart attack is a possibility, thus leading to a delay in seeking health care for heart-related symptoms (Harvard Medical School, 1992). Alternatively, for symptoms of less-threatening conditions, constant spousal prodding may contribute to seeking health care early.

Gender Contrasts

Women outlive men in industrial societies by about 8 years. Women, however, experience more illnesses than men. Verbrugge (1989) observes that men's lives are shortened by their higher rates of fatal illnesses, while women are left with added years of life in which to experience the aches and pains associated with numerous less-often fatal illnesses. With longer years of life also come the added risks of loneliness and social isolation.

The hypothesized female health disadvantage occurs for 5 of the 18 physical health indicators (arthritis, hypertension and diabetes, cataracts, and problems walking). Male physical health is uniquely disadvantaged only in that a significantly higher percentage of males report hearing problems. These findings for the older Black subsample agree with patterns in the larger (White) population (Verbrugge, 1989). Two of the four female disadvantaged health conditions in the Black subsample, however, are for fatal conditions. Also, a clear picture emerges as to whom reference is made when speaking of the Black disadvantage in arthritis, hypertension, and diabetes: older Black women.

No gender differences occur among the psychological health indicators, and a male disadvantage appears in four of the nine social integration indicators (failure in the past two weeks to talk on the telephone with friends/relatives and to go to church or a senior center). Females, on the other hand, are more likely to be dissatisfied with their level of social contact.

CONCLUSIONS

Summary

Do older Black Americans shoulder a disproportionately higher burden of health problems than their White counterparts? The answer is yes and no. No, in the sense that, among the indicators studied, relatively few significant differences distinguish Black and White older persons in the prevalence of chronic physical and psychological conditions and limitations in daily functioning. Published data from the 1984 NHIS (NCHS, 1986b) show an excess older White (not Black) prevalence rate on 26 of 52 analyzable chronic health conditions and impairments, including the number-one cause of death, heart disease. However, with the exception of cancer, the White prevalence rate excesses are largely insignificant, however.

From a different perspective, besides experiencing relatively less social integration, the health conditions unfavorable for Black older Americans are major causes of, or precursors to, death (hypertension and diabetes) or are among the most disabling conditions (arthritis). These three conditions accounted for close to half of the excess burden experienced by older Black Americans on the chronic health conditions reported by NCHS (1986b). Two of these conditions, arthritis and diabetes, grew (since the mid-1970s) as sources of distinction between older Black and older White health.

The findings confirm, refine, and in some measure challenge conclusions in the existing literature. Certainly, as shall be argued in the next section, far too few analyses have been completed to suggest that health problems in old age are randomly distributed with regard to race.

Directions for Further Study

The health of the Black aged is most often presented as a descriptive profile based on studying a bivariate relation between race and health outcomes. While the analyses in this chapter adjusted for a few of the often-overlooked third variables, the study of race and health in old age remains incomplete.

Figure 20.1 presents an overall model for specifying specific hypotheses about missing, yet unformulated, psychological and biomedical mechanisms that link race and health. It is beyond the scope of this presentation to use the model to specify even a small sampling of hypotheses implied by the model. Rather, the immediate expectation is that the model may serve the purpose of orienting investigators to the variety of possible hypotheses that heretofore have not been considered.

Consider that arthritis, for example, consistently correlated with race in the preceding analyses. Why? What is it about the conditions of life of young and middle-aged Black females that sets in motion the special problems of arthritis seen in old age? Following a life-course perspective, it can be hypothesized that the current cohort of Black older females spent a lifetime engaging in at-risk experiences, for example, as domestic workers, repeatedly crawling and bending, thereby affecting the cartilage of their joints. Therefore, denial of opportunity for other occupational choices by virtue of race is an obvious mediating link between race and arthritis. Hypothetically, this process is facilitated by the unavailability, or the conditioned expected unavailability, of medical care.

A developing literature emphasizes the importance of numerous personal health practices and resources (e.g., the extent of social support) acting to facilitate or impede disease and illness onset (German & Fried, 1989). Thus the model in Figure 20.1 implies, in addition to the now frequently studied single direct effect of race on health, the importance of specifying and testing a plethora of interactive, mediational, and reciprocal-effect hypotheses.

Figure 20.1
A Multicausal Model for Deriving Hypothetical Effects of Race on Health

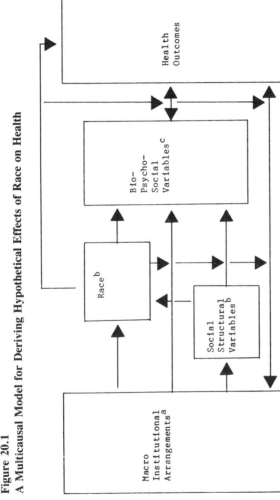

[a]Economic and political structures in society.

[b]Race, as a social structural variable among other socially stratifying variables, is indicative of: 1) a life course of minority group (sociologically defined) experience; and 2) the social psychological significance of existing experiences.

[c]These variables reflect a multidisciplinary set of conditions ranging from social support to personal health practices to personality characteristics.

The causative agents underlying health outcomes, however, include more than simply matters of personal responsibility or personal reactivity. Additional linkages shown in Figure 20.1 suggest that life course-related, macro-level institutional arrangements shape the distribution of health problems in old age (Olson, 1982). The links among cultural, political, and economic arrangements also influence the impact of being Black on health outcomes. Governmental failure, for example, to support a reasonable minimum wage in the interest of industry profits suggests the importance of the interaction of race-based discrimination with political and economic conditions.

In short, the need for a strong knowledge base about the interacting and meditating links of race and health with numerous sociological and social psychological and, indeed, biological, mechanisms must be preliminary to concluding that older Black and White health is more similar than dissimilar. The challenge is to maximize the chance that as many persons as possible may expect to live for as many years as possible, with the best possible quality of health, functioning, and well-being.

NOTES

The data used in this chapter come from the National Center for Health Statistics (NCHS) and the Inter-University Consortium for Political and Social Research (ICPSR). The conclusions from this data are those of the author and do not necessarily reflect the views of NCHS or ICPSR.

1. The older population typically includes persons aged 65 and over, as is the meaning here. The samples used for testing hypotheses in this report, however, include persons aged 60 and over.

2. Race is a proxy indicator of the sociological significance of living life as a Black or White person in America. Being Black or White subsumes a complex range of cultural experiences, including minority (or nonminority) status (see Manuel, 1982).

3. The conclusions about percentage increases are based on tabulations from the U.S. Bureau of the Census (1991) and Manuel (1988).

4. The alpha criterion for statistical significance is set at .01 to adjust the chances (1) that purely chance-significant chi squares were being observed, given the large number of tests being made; (2) that significant effects are an artifact of the large sample size in several of the analyses; and (3) that inflated standard errors (resulting from the complex multistaged sampling) may be influential.

A percentage difference of at least seven units defined substantive significance. A recent NCHS (1992) report describes a 7 percent contrast as evidence that Blacks are "far more likely" than Whites to report their health as poor or fair. Moreover, an informal survey among sociologists suggested that percentage differences between 5 and 10 percent typically are interpreted as credible effects.

Statistical summary measures (percentages and chi squares) are not tabularly presented in order to conserve space.

5. Calculations of Black and White excess prevalence on the chronic conditions followed procedures noted in the 1985 U.S. Department of Health and Human Services Report (Report of the Secretary's Task Force on Black and Minority Health, 1985).

6. Social class is measured by a single indicator: years of schooling, operationalized to reflect persons having less than twelve years of schooling versus those having twelve or more years of schooling. Education was the one variable common to the several data sets used throughout the analyses. In 1990, close to 72 percent of Black persons, aged 65 and over, had fewer than twelve years of schooling. Thirty-nine percent of their White counterparts were similarly situated (U.S. Bureau of the Census, 1991).

REFERENCES

Branch, L. G., & Jette, A. M. (1982). A prospective study of long-term care institutionalization among the aged. *American Journal of Public Health, 72,* 1373–1379.

Carter, J. H. (1982). The significance of racism in the mental illnesses of elderly minorities. In R.C. Manuel (Ed.), *Minority aging: Sociological and social psychological issues* (pp. 89–93). Westport, CT: Greenwood Press.

Dowd, J. J., & Bengtson, V. L. (1978). Aging in minority populations: An examination of the double jeopardy hypothesis. *Journal of Gerontology, 33,* 427–436.

Ferraro, K. F. (1987). Double jeopardy to health for black older adults. *Journal of Gerontology, 42,* 528–533.

German, P. S., & Fried, L. P. (1989). Prevention and the elderly: Public health issues and strategies. *Annual Review of Public Health, 10,* 319–332.

Gibson, R. C. (1991). Age-by-race differences in the health and functioning of elderly persons. *Journal of Aging and Health, 3,* 335–351.

Gibson, R. C., & Jackson, J. S. (1987). The health, physical functioning, and informal supports of the black elderly. *The Milbank Quarterly, 65,* 421–454.

Haber, D. (1989). *Health care for an aging society: Cost-conscious community care and self-care approaches.* New York: Hemisphere Publishing Corporation.

Harvard Medical School. (1992). *Harvard Health Letter* (August, 1992). Boston: Harvard Medical School Health Publications Group.

Jackson, J. J. (1971). Negro aged: Toward needed research in social gerontology. *Gerontologist, 11,* 52–57.

Jackson, J. J., & Perry, C. (1989). Physical health conditions of middle-aged and aged blacks. In K. S. Markides (Ed.), *Aging and health: Perspectives on gender, race, ethnicity, and class* (pp. 111–176). Newbury Park, CA: Sage Publications.

Keith, V. M., & Smith, D. P. (1988). The cultural differential in black and white life expectancy. *Demography, 25,* 625–632.

Krause, N. (1987). Stress in racial differences in self-reported health among the elderly. *Gerontologist, 27,* 72–76.

Manton, K. G. (1982). Differential life expectancy: Possible explanations during the later ages. In R. C. Manuel (Ed.), *Minority aging: Sociological and social psychological issues* (pp. 63–68). Westport, CT: Greenwood Press.

Manuel, R. C. (1982). The minority aged: Providing a conceptual perspective. In R. C. Manuel (Ed.), *Minority aging: Sociological and social psychological issues* (pp. 13–25). Westport, CT: Greenwood Press.

Manuel, R. C. (1988). The demography of older blacks in the United States. In J. S. Jackson (Ed.), *The black American elderly: Research on physical and psychosocial health* (pp. 25–49). New York: Springer Publishing Company.

Markides, K. S. (Ed.). (1989). *Aging and health: Perspective on gender, race, ethnicity, and class.* Newbury Park, CA: Sage Publications.

National Center for Health Statistics (NCHS). (1985). Public Use Tape Documentation, Medical History Questionnaire, Ages 12–74, National Health and Nutrition Examination Survey, 1972–74 (machine readable data file and documentation). Hyattsville, MD.

National Center for Health Statistics. (1986a). Public Use Tape Documentation, National Health Interview Supplement on Aging (SOA Person file), 1984 (machine readable data file and documentation). Hyattsville, MD.

National Center for Health Statistics. (1986b). P. W. Ries: Current Estimates from the National Health Interview Survey, United States, 1984 (*Vital and Health Statistics, Series 10, N. 156*). Washington DC: Government Printing Office.

National Center for Health Statistics. (1991a). Public Use Tape Documentation, National Health Interview Survey of Mental Health, 1989 (machine readable data file and documentation). Hyattsville, MD.

National Center for Health Statistics. (1991b). Public Use Tape Documentation, National Health and Nutrition Examination Survey, Epidemiologic Follow-up Study, 1987 (machine readable data file and documentation). Hyattsville, MD.

National Center for Health Statistics. (1992). *Health, United States, 1991*. Hyattsville, MD: Public Health Service.

National Council on Aging. (PI). (1979). *Myth and Reality of Aging*, 1974 (machine readable data file and documentation). Ann Arbor, MI: Inter-University Consortium for Political and Social Research.

National Urban League. (1964). *Double jeopardy: The older Negro in America today*. New York: National Urban League.

Neugarten, B. L. (1974). Age groups in American society and the rise of the young-old. *The Annals of the American Academy of Political and Social Science, 415*, 187–198.

Olson, L. K. (1982). *The political economy of aging: The state, private power, and social welfare*. New York: Columbia University Press.

Report of the Secretary's Task Force on Black and Minority Health. (1985). (Volumes I–VII). USDHHS. Washington, DC: Government Printing Office.

Schooler, K. K. (PI). (1979). *National Senior Citizens Survey*, 1968 (machine readable data file and documentation). Ann Arbor, MI: Inter-University Consortium for Political and Social Research.

Smith, T. L. (1957). The changing number and distribution of the aged Negro population of the United States. *Phylon, 18*, 339–354.

Taylor, R. J., & Chatters, L. M. (1991). Extended family networks of older black adults. *Journal of Gerontology: Social Sciences, 46*, s210–s217.

U.S. Bureau of the Census. (1991). *Poverty in the United States: 1990*. Current Population Reports, Series P-60, No. 175. Washington, DC: Government Printing Office.

Verbrugge, L. M. (1989). Gender, aging and health. In K. S. Markides (Ed.), *Aging and health: Perspectives on gender, race, ethnicity, and class* (pp. 23–78). Newbury Park, CA: Sage Publications.

Wallace, S. P. (1990). Race versus class in the health care of African-American elderly. *Social Problems, 37*, 517–534.

Wing, S., Manton, K. G., Stallard, E. C., Hames, C. G., & Tyroler, H. A. (1985). The black/white mortality crossover: Investigation in a community-based study. *Journal of Gerontology, 40*, 78–84.

World Health Organization. (1959). The public health aspects of the aging of the population. Copenhagen: World Health Organization (Regional Office for Europe).

21

Urban Infrastructure: Social, Environmental, and Health Risks to African Americans

Robert D. Bullard

The nation's urban infrastructure is crumbling at the seams. Nowhere is this more apparent than in America's large urban centers, where the majority of African Americans are concentrated. More than 57 percent of African Americans live in central cities, the highest concentration of any racial and ethnic group. Even affluent African American families—those with household incomes of $50,000 or more—are more likely to live in central cities than their White counterparts. For example, 56 percent of affluent African Americans live in central cities and 40 percent live in the suburbs. The patterns for affluent Whites reveal that 25 percent live in central cities and 61 percent live in the suburbs.

In general, the physical infrastructure of central cities is old and in need of repair. The physical infrastructure includes roads and bridges, housing stock, schools, job centers, public buildings, parks and recreational facilities, public transit, water supply, wastewater treatment, and waste disposal systems. Taken as a whole, this infrastructure condition determines the well-being of our society. At present, too many of our cities and their inhabitants are at risk from infrastructure decay, environmental degradation, health threats, and economic impoverishment.

This chapter examines the factors that contributes to the nation's decaying urban infrastructure and the accompanying social, environmental, and health risks to African Americans.

IMPACT OF INSTITUTIONAL DISINVESTMENT

Urban America continues to be segregated along racial lines. The legacy of institutional racism lowered the nation's gross national product by almost 2

Reprinted and reformatted by permission of the National Urban League from *The State of Black America 1992*, pp. 183–196.

percent a year, or roughly $104 billion in 1989 (Updegrade, 1989). A large share of this loss is a result of housing discrimination. The "roots of discrimination are deep" and have been difficult to eliminate (James, McCummings & Tynan, 1984). Housing discrimination contributes to the physical decay of inner-city neighborhoods and denies a substantial segment of the African-American community a basic form of wealth accumulation and investment through homeownership. The number of African-American homeowners would probably be higher in the absence of discrimination by lending institutions (see Darden, 1989; Bullard, 1986). Approximately 59 percent of middle-class African Americans own their own homes, compared with 74 percent of Whites.

Studies over the past 25 years have clearly documented the relationship among redlining and divestment decisions and neighborhood decline (e.g., Bradbury, Case & Dunham, 1989; Feagin, 1990). From Boston to San Diego to urban centers all across the nation, the pattern is clear: African Americans still do not have full access to lending by banks and saving institutions as do their White counterparts.

A 1991 report by the Federal Financial Institutions Examination Council (FFIEC) found that African Americans were rejected for home loans more than twice as often as Anglos (FFIEC, 1991). After studying lending practices at 9,300 U.S. financial institutions and more than 6.4 million loan applications, the federal study discovered that the rejection rates for conventional home mortgages were 33.9 percent for African Americans, 21.4 percent for Latinos, 22.4 percent for American Indians, 14.4 percent for Anglos, and 12.9 percent for Asians.

Loan denial rates for African Americans varied widely among large urban centers (see Table 21.1). For example, one in three African-American loan applicants was rejected in the Boston, Houston, St. Louis, Pittsburgh, and Phoenix metropolitan areas. The lowest loan-rejection rate for African Americans occurred in the District of Columbia, Baltimore, Oakland, and San Diego metropolitan areas.

Federal regulators continue to ignore discrimination in lending. These alarming loan-rejection statistics still leave some government and industry officials in doubt as to whether the culprit is a function of discrimination. Discriminatory lending practices subsidize the physical destruction of African-American communities. Today, these same communities must share in paying hundreds of billions of dollars to bail out failed savings-and-loan institutions, many of which engaged in redlining African-American communities (Bullard & Feagin, 1991).

THE ROOT OF INFRASTRUCTURE DECLINE

Racism and residential segregation are facts of life in urban America. Eight out of every ten African Americans live in neighborhoods where they are in the majority. Residential segregation decreases for most racial and ethnic groups (but not for African Americans) with additional education, in-

Table 21.1
Mortgage Rejection Rates in 19 Large Metropolitan Areas

Metro Area	Asian	Black	Latino	Anglo
Atlanta	11.1	26.5	13.6	10.5
Baltimore	7.3	15.6	10.1	7.5
Boston	15.4	34.9	21.2	11.0
Chicago	10.4	23.6	12.1	7.3
Dallas	9.3	25.6	19.8	10.7
Detroit	9.1	23.7	14.2	9.7
Houston	13.3	33.0	25.7	12.6
Los Angeles	13.2	19.8	16.3	12.8
Miami	16.9	22.9	17.8	16.0
Minneapolis	6.4	19.9	8.0	6.1
New York	17.3	29.4	25.3	15.0
Oakland	11.6	16.5	13.3	9.6
Philadelphia	12.1	25.0	21.0	8.3
Phoenix	12.8	30.0	25.2	14.4
Pittsburgh	12.2	31.0	13.9	12.0
St. Louis	9.0	31.8	13.5	12.1
San Diego	11.2	17.8	15.1	9.8
Seattle	11.6	18.3	16.8	10.7
Washington, DC	8.7	14.4	8.9	6.3

Source: Federal Reserve Bank Board, 1991.

come, and occupational status (Denton & Massey, 1988). An African American with an earned income of $50,000 is as segregated as a Latino American who earns $5,000.

African Americans, no matter what their educational or occupational achievement or income level, are exposed to higher crime rates, less effective educational systems, higher mortality risks, more dilapidated surroundings, and greater environmental threats because of their race (Bullard, 1990).

Institutional barriers make it difficult for many African Americans to buy their way out of health-threatening physical environments. For example, in the heavily populated South Coast air basin of Los Angeles, it is estimated that over 71 percent of African Americans and over 50 percent of Latinos reside in areas with the most polluted air, while only 34 percent of Whites live in highly polluted areas (Mann, 1991).

The development of spatially differentiated metropolitan areas where African Americans are segregated from other Americans has resulted from governmental policies and marketing practices of the housing industry and lending institutions. Millions of African Americans are geographically isolated in economically depressed and polluted urban neighborhoods away from the expanding suburban job centers (Bullard & Wright, 1990).

The infrastructure conditions result from a host of factors, including the distribution of wealth, patterns of racial and economic discrimination, redlining, housing and real estate practices, location decisions of industry, and differential enforcement of land use and environmental regulations. All communities are not treated equally. Apartheid-type housing-development policies limit mobility, reduce neighborhood options, diminish job opportunities, and decrease environmental choices for African Americans (Bullard, 1989).

It is difficult for millions of African Americans in segregated neighborhoods to say "not in my backyard" (NIMBY) if they do not have a backyard (Bullard & Wright, 1987; Bullard, 1989). Nationally, only 44 percent of African Americans own their homes, compared to over two-thirds of the nation as a whole. Homeowners are the strongest advocates of the NIMBY positions taken against locally unwanted land uses, or LULUs, such as garbage dumps, landfills, incinerators, sewage-treatment plants, recycling centers, prisons, drug-treatment units, and public housing projects. Generally, White communities have greater access to and influence over land use and environmental decision making than do their African-American counterparts.

The ability of an individual to escape a health-threatening physical environment is usually related to affluence. However, racial barriers complicate this process for millions of African Americans (Denton & Massey, 1988). The imbalance between residential amenities and land uses assigned to central cities and suburbs cannot be explained by class factors alone. Blacks and Whites do not have the same opportunities to "vote with their feet" and escape undesirable physical environments (Bullard, 1990). Those who are less fortunate must suffer the double jeopardy of poverty and pollution.

Institutional racism continues to influence housing and mobility options available to African Americans of all income levels and is a major factor that influences the quality of neighbors available to them. The "web of discrimination" in the housing market is a result of action and inaction of local and federal government officials, financial institutions, insurance companies, real-estate marketing firms, and zoning boards. More stringent enforcement mechanisms and penalties are needed to combat all forms of discrimination.

UNEVEN DEVELOPMENT AND UNEQUAL OPPORTUNITIES

Uneven development between central cities and suburbs combined with the systematic avoidance of inner-city areas by many businesses has heightened social and economic inequalities. For the past two decades, manufacturing plants have been fleeing central cities and taking their jobs with them. Many have moved offshore to Third World countries, where labor is cheap and environmental regulations are lax or nonexistent.

Industry flight from central cities has left behind a deteriorating urban infrastructure, poverty, and pollution. What kinds of replacement industry can economically depressed African-American communities attract? Some planners have suggested enterprise zones as a development strategy. Many of these communities do not have a lot of choices available to them. Some community leaders and workers have become so desperate that they see even low-paying hazardous industries as better than no industry at all.

These communities and their workers are forced to choose between unemployment and jobs that may result in risks to their health, their families health, and the health of their community. This practice amounts to "economic blackmail" (Kazis & Grossman, 1983). Economic conditions in many African-American communities make them especially vulnerable to this practice.

Some polluting industries have been eager to exploit this vulnerability. Some have even used the assistance of elected officials in obtaining special tax breaks and government operating permits. For example, public officials in Robbins, Illinois—a small Black village located 6 miles south of Chicago—are using their enterprise zones to attract industry. Robbins has been selected as the site for an incinerator that will burn garbage from 600,000 south-suburban residents (Ritter, 1990). The Illinois Environmental Protection Agency has given its preliminary approval of the $200 million project.

Reading Energy Company of Philadelphia is scheduled to begin burning garbage in 1993 at the Robbins site. The incinerator is being designed to burn 1,600 tons of garbage a day, enough to fill 160 garbage trucks. The incinerator will create 500 construction jobs and 80 permanent jobs. Because of the low skill level of workers in Robbins, it is unclear how many of the construction and permanent jobs will go to local residents. The incinerator, however, will pay the community at least $750,000 a year in taxes, rentals, and fees (Ritter, 1990). Local citizens who oppose having other people's garbage barged into Robbins and burned feel they are having to give up too much in terms of health risks for a new job-producing industry.[1]

Clearly, economic development and environmental policies flow from forces of production and are often dominated and subsidized by state actors. Numerous examples abound where state actors have targeted cities and regions for infrastructure improvements and amenities, such as water irrigation systems, sewer treatment plants, ship channels, road and bridge projects, and mass transit systems. On the other hand, state actors have done a miserable job in protecting central-city residents from the ravages of industrial pollution and nonresidential activities valued as having a negative impact on the quality of life.[2]

REGULATING URBAN LAND USE

Racial and ethnic inequality is perpetuated and reinforced by local governments in conjunction with urban-based corporations. In general, "at a certain point in community development . . . trajectories of economic growth and quality of life converge" (Gottdiener, 1988). Race continues to be a potent variable in explaining urban land use, street and highway configuration, commercial and industrial development, and industrial facility siting. Moreover, the question of "who gets what, where, and why" often pits one community against another.

Competition intensifies for the residential amenities and infrastructure improvements that are not always distributed equitably along racial and class lines. Some residential areas and their inhabitants are at a greater risk than is the larger society from unregulated growth, ineffective regulation of industrial toxins, and public-policy decisions authorizing industrial facilities that favor those with political and economic clout.

Zoning is probably the most widely applied mechanism to regulate urban land use in the United States (Kelly, 1988). Zoning laws broadly define land for residential, commercial, or industrial use and may impose narrow land-use restrictions (e.g., minimum and maximum lot size, number of dwellings per acre, and square feet and height of buildings).

Zoning ordinances, deed restrictions, and other land-use mechanisms have been widely used as a NIMBY (not in my backyard) tool, operating through exclusionary practices. Thus, exclusionary zoning has been used to "simply zone against something rather than for something" (Marshall, 1989). Exclusionary zoning is "one of the most subtle forms of using government authority and power to foster and perpetuate discriminatory practices" (Marshall, 1989). With or without zoning, deed restrictions, or devices, various groups are "unequally able to protect their environmental interests" (Logan & Molotch, 1987). More often than not, African-American communities get shortchanged in the neighborhood protection game.

DUMPING GROUNDS IN A BOOMTOWN

One of the best examples of environmental discrimination against an African-American community has been documented in Houston, where well-established waste facility practices allowed Black neighborhoods to become the dumping ground for the city's garbage (Bullard, 1983). Houston, the nation's fourth-largest city with a population of 1.6 million inhabitants, had the distinction of being the only major American city without zoning.

From the mid-1920s to the late-1970s, all the city-owned landfills were located

in African-American neighborhoods; six of the eight city-owned garbage incinerators were located in African American neighborhoods during this same period.
The city closed its waste disposal facilities in the early 1970s and contracted out
this service with private firms. During Houston's booming years, from the early
to late 1970s, four privately owned sanitary landfills were used to dispose of
Houston's solid waste. Three of these facilities were located in mostly African-
American neighborhoods, although African Americans made up just one-fourth
of the city's population. The private waste disposal industry followed the discriminatory facility-siting pattern established by Houston's government.

Concentrating landfills, incinerators, and garbage dumps in Houston's African-
American neighborhoods during the boom era of the 1970s lowered residents'
property values, accelerated physical deterioration, and increased disinvestment
practices. Moreover, the discriminatory siting of landfills and incinerators stig-
matized the neighborhoods as "dumping grounds" for a host of other unwanted
facilities, including salvage yards, recycling operations, cement plants, paint
shops, and used-automobile storage facilities (Bullard, 1987).

PAYING THE PRICE FOR RISKY TECHNOLOGIES

The problems identified in Houston are not unique. Risky technologies such
as lead smelters, hazardous waste landfills, and incinerators pose health and
environmental threats to African-American communities from West Dallas to
South Central Los Angeles.

The case of hazardous incinerators is one that has drawn much attention in
recent years. For example communities with hazardous waste incinerators generally have large minorities populations, low incomes, and low property values.
A 1990 Greenpeace report found that (1) the minority proportion of the population
in communities with existing incinerators is 89 percent higher than the national
average, (2) communities where incinerators are proposed have a minority population 60 percent greater than the national average, (3) average income in
communities with existing incinerators is 15 percent less than the national average, (4) property values in communities with incinerators are 38 percent lower
than the national average, and (5) average property values are 35 percent lower
in communities where incinerators are proposed (Costner & Thornton, 1990).

African-American residents have begun to treat their struggle for a clean
environment as an extension of their struggle for basic human rights. Just as
social justice activists fought for equal access to education, employment, and
housing, they are now defining the opportunity to live in an unpolluted physical
environment as a basic right.

Moreover, many community leaders are now convinced that targeting their
communities with risky technologies, such as waste disposal facilities, contributes to urban infrastructure decline comparable to housing discrimination, redlining practices, and disinvestment decisions of lending institutions.
Environmental discrimination mirrors other forms of discrimination.

Industries employing risky technologies often make location decisions in African-American communities with little or no input from local or community leaders. When questions are raised by concerned citizens, the argument of jobs for local residents is used to quell dissent. Promises of jobs and a broadened tax base in economically depressed communities are presented as acceptable trade-offs for potential health and environmental risks. This "dangling carrot" scenario has proven to be the rule for African-American people in this country and for peoples in the Third World.

Many industrial firms, especially waste disposal companies and industries that have a long history of pollution violations, have come to view the African-American community as a pushover, lacking community organization and environmental consciousness. The strong (and sometimes blind) pro-jobs stance—a kind of "don't bite the hand that feeds you" sentiment—has aided institutionalizing "unacceptable risks" and environmental inequities (Bullard & Wright, 1987).

TOXIC TIME BOMBS

The hazardous waste problem continues to be one of the most "serious problems facing the industrial world" (Epstein, Brown & Pope, 1983). The nation's Love Canals persist. Millions of tons of hazardous waste still end up at municipal landfills designed for household garbage, are released from tank trucks onto back roads, or are dumped directly into sewer systems. Sewage treatment plants are not designed for industrial chemicals. Toxic pollutants from these plants are discharged into the environment via wastewater discharge, air emissions, and sludge.

Over one-fourth of the Super Fund sites on the National Priority List had been used as municipal landfills. These toxic time bombs are not randomly scattered across the urban landscape. Nor is it a great mystery as to who is most likely to live next to a municipal landfill, incinerator, or toxic-waste dump. These facilities are often located in communities that have high percentages of poor, elderly, young, and minority residents (Greenberg & Anderson, 1984).

Do waste facilities just happen to end up in poor and minority communities? The nonrandom pattern of waste facility siting is not due to chance or the luck of the draw. Location decisions often involve cooperation between government and industry officials. In the case of siting waste-to-energy facilities (incinerators), Cerrell Associates, a Los Angeles-based consulting firm, advised the California Waste Management Board to push incinerators off on "neighborhoods least likely to express opposition—older and lower socioeconomic neighborhoods" (Cerrell Associates, 1984). Recommendations of this type offer a green light to government and industry to target African-American and other communities of color for incinerators.

The Commission for Racial Justice's landmark "Toxic Wastes and Race" study found race to be the single most important factor (i.e., more important than income, homeownership rate, and property values) in the location of abandoned toxic waste sites (Commission for Racial Justice, 1987). The study also found that (1) three out of five African Americans live in communities with one or more abandoned toxic waste sites; (2) 15 million African Americans (60 percent) live in communities with one or more abandoned toxic waste sites; (3) three of the largest commercial hazardous waste landfills are located in predominantly African-American or Latino communities and account for 40 percent of the nation's total estimated landfill capacity; and (4) African Americans are heavily overrepresented in the populations of cities with the largest number of abandoned toxic-waste sites, which include Memphis, St. Louis, Houston, Cleveland, and Atlanta (Commission for Racial Justice, 1987).

There are hundreds of examples of urban environmental problems confronting African Americans in cities. However, only a few examples will be highlighted in this paper.

Atlanta

Often referred to as the "capital of the New South," Atlanta has a total of 94 abandoned toxic waste sites. Nearly 83 percent of the city's African-American population live in zip codes where these sites are found, while 60 percent of White Atlantans live in waste-site areas. Atlanta is also one of the most segregated cities in the South. More than 86 percent of the city's African-American population live in mostly Black areas. Atlanta's residential patterns and waste-site location are closely related.

Chicago

Chicago is the nation's third-largest city, with a population of more than 3 million inhabitants. The city's 1.1 million African Americans make up 39 percent of its total population. Chicago has the reputation of being the most segregated big city in America. Some 92 percent of the city's African Americans live in segregated neighborhoods in 1980 (i.e., a figure down from 93 percent in 1970) (Taeuber, 1983).

Institutionalized discrimination by the housing industry and lending institutions has trapped many of the city's African-American residents in deteriorating older neighborhoods. For example, the city's southside neighborhoods not only are threatened by economic stagnation and infrastructure decline but also must contend with heavy use by polluting industries. Industrial encroachment into residential areas has turned Chicago's southside area into an urban "sacrifice zone."

The Altgeld Gardens housing project, located on Chicago's southeast side, lies within this sacrifice zone. Residents have described the project as a "toxic donut" because it is encircled by municipal and hazardous-waste landfills, incinerators, grain elevators, sewage-treatment facilities, and a host of other polluting industries.[3] The southeast-side Chicago neighborhood is home to 150,000 residents (of whom 70 percent are African American and 11 percent are Latino), 50 active or closed commercial waste landfills, 100 factories (including seven chemical plants and five steel mills), and 103 abandoned toxic waste dumps (Greenpeace, 1991). The southeast area is also scheduled to host the 1,600-ton-per-day Robbins municipal incinerator, which will be allowed to release two tons of mercury and a half-ton of lead into the air each year.

Los Angeles

Los Angeles is the nation's second-largest city, with a population of 3.5 million persons. It is one of the most culturally and racially diverse big cities in the country. Persons of color (Latinos, Asian and Pacific Islanders, African Americans, and Native Americans) now constitute a majority (63 percent) of the city's population.

Residential segregation continues to be the dominant housing pattern in Los Angeles. For example, eight out of every ten African Americans live in segregated areas. The South Central Los Angeles area is one of these segregated neighborhoods, at over 52 percent African American and 44 percent Latino. The neighborhood suffers from years of systematic neglect, infrastructure decay, high unemployment, poverty, and heavy industrial use.

A recent article in the San Francisco *Examiner* described the zip code in which South Central Los Angeles lies as the "dirtiest" in the state (Kay, 1991). The population in the zip code is 59 percent African American and 38 percent Latino. The one-square-mile area is saturated with abandoned toxic-waste sites, freeways, smokestacks, and wastewater pipes from polluting industries. South Central Los Angeles is a haven for locally unwanted land uses. Some 18 industrial firms in 1989 discharged more than 33 million pounds of waste chemicals in the environment.

Los Angeles' growing population has meant a mounting municipal solid-waste and hazardous waste problem. In an effort to deal with its bulging garbage problem, the city (under a grant from the federal EPA) developed a plan in 1979 to build three waste-to-energy incinerators.[4] A number of advisory councils and committees were appointed by the mayor and City Council between 1981 and 1984 to coordinate the Los Angeles City Energy Recovery (LANCER) project. Ogden-Martin was selected to build the incinerators that would handle a capacity of 1,600 tons of waste per day. The first of the three incinerators, or LANCER 1, was to be built in South Central Los Angeles.

Although the LANCER project had been in the works for more than 6 years, neighborhood residents were informed about the city-sponsored project in August of 1985. Local residents organized themselves into a group called Concerned Citizens and, along with their allies, clearly demonstrated that it is possible for grass-roots groups to defeat discriminatory facility-siting proposals.

Richmond (California)

Located in Contra Costa County along the eastern shore of the San Francisco Bay, Richmond has a population of about 80,000 residents. More than half are African American, and about 11 percent are Latino. The median income of Richmond residents is one-third of that of all Contra Costa County residents. One in four Richmond residents lives below the poverty line, a figure that is three times the county average.

Richmond is a highly industrialized area with over 350 industrial facilities that handle hazardous materials. These industrial firms generate over 800,000 pounds of toxic air contaminants, nearly 18,000 pounds of toxic pollutants in wastewater, and about 179,000 tons of hazardous waste each year (Citizens for a Better Environment, 1989). Most of Richmond's African-American population lives adjacent to the city's petrochemical corridor. For example, African Americans comprise "72 percent to 94 percent of the local population in 14 Richmond neighborhoods" that are closest to the city's heavy industrial zone (Citizens for a Better Environment, 1989). Local residents for years have suspected that pollution from the petrochemical plants is responsible for all kinds of community health problems, from skin rashes to cancer.

In 1987, Richmond residents organized themselves into a group called the West County Toxics Coalition. The group was initiated with support from the Boston-based National Toxics Campaign. Today, the West County Toxics Coalition is the leading environmental and social justice advocate in Richmond.

Dallas

Dallas is the seventh-largest city in the nation, with a population just under one million. The city's African-American population grew from 265,594 in 1980 to 296,262 (an 11.5% increase) in 1990. African Americans make up about 30 percent of the city's population.

Over the years, Dallas's African-American neighborhoods have had to cope with the problem of lead smelters operating in their midst. All of the lead smelters in the city were located in mostly African-American and Latino neighborhoods. For example, the 63-acre Murph Metals secondary lead smelter (later known as RSR Corporation) operated in the West Dallas neighborhood, beginning in the mid-1930s.

West Dallas has a population of 13,161 residents, of which more than 85 percent are African American. The lead smelter is located next door to an elementary school and across the street from the West Dallas Boys Club and a 3,500-unit public housing project. The housing project is located just 50 feet from the sprawling lead smelter's property line and is in the direct path of the prevailing southerly winds.

During the peak period of operation in the mid-1960s, the plant employed more than 400 persons (few of whom lived in the neighborhood). The smelter pumped more than 269 tons of lead particles each year into the West Dallas air. Lead particles were blown by prevailing winds through the doors and windows of nearby residents and onto the West Dallas streets, ballparks and children's playgrounds.

Dallas officials were informed as early as 1972 that lead was finding its way into the bloodstreams of children who lived in two mostly African-American and Latino neighborhoods: West Dallas (RSR lead smelter) and East Oak Cliff (Dixie Metals smelter). The city's health department found that living near the smelters was associated with a 36 percent increase in blood lead level. The city was urged to restrict the emissions of lead to the atmosphere and to undertake a large screening program to determine the extent of the public health problem. The city failed to take immediate action.

The community organized itself into the West Dallas Neighborhood Committee on Lead Contamination in 1981. The city took action only after a series of lead-related articles made the headlines in the local newspapers, triggering widespread concern, public outrage, several class-action lawsuits, and legal action by the Texas attorney general against the smelter. West Dallas plaintiffs won an out-of-court settlement worth over $45 million. The lawsuit was settled in June 1983, with the firm agreeing to a soil cleanup in West Dallas, a blood-testing program for children and pregnant women, and the installation of new anti-pollution equipment.

The anti-pollution equipment was never installed. In May 1984, the Dallas Board of Adjustments—a city agency responsible for monitoring land-use violations—requested the city attorney to order the smelter permanently closed for violating the zoning law. The West Dallas smelter was shut down (but not cleaned up) in 1984 under a zoning ordinance; the smelter operator had never obtained the necessary use permits to operate in the neighborhood.

The Dixie Metals smelter, on the other hand, was allowed to continue operating in the East Oak Cliff neighborhood under a phase-down agreement. The plant was shut down in 1990.

CONCLUSIONS

African-American communities are beginning to mobilize around quality-of-life issues. These issues range from fair housing to anti-redlining to environmental equity strategies. Institutional barriers and discriminatory public policies contribute to urban infrastructure decline, reduce wealth accumulation, and add risks for African Americans.

A national urban policy is needed to begin addressing the nation's decaying urban infrastructure. A new form of activism has emerged that is not limited to attacks on well-publicized toxic contamination issues; these activists have begun to seek remedial action on neighborhood disinvestment, housing discrimination and residential segregation, urban mass transportation, pollution, and other urban problems that threaten public safety.

It is in the national interest that we have healthy cities. An economic, environmental, and infrastructure crisis exists in Urban America. This crisis has been created, in part, by the systematic withholding of investments and infrastructure improvements, while allowing some urban neighborhoods to become municipal and hazardous waste dumping grounds. Many African-American communities are subsidizing, with their health, the siting of risky industries other communities refuse to accept.

The current emphasis on waste-management and pollution-control regulations encourages dependence on disposal technologies that are themselves sources of toxic pollution. Pushing incinerators off on people is not economic development. It is, however, a cruel hoax that exploits the economic vulnerability of desperate communities.

Pollution regulations have done little to rid African-American communities of toxic pollutants. African-American communities have received few tangible benefits from current waste-management strategies. Pollution prevention holds the greatest promise for protecting human health and the environment of all communities.

African Americans in urban areas are tired of their communities becoming toxic wastelands for polluting industries that promise jobs and an expanded tax base. Too often, the communities that host landfills and incinerators remain impoverished. All communities must deal with their waste. For example, federal, state, and local garbage prevention programs need to be funded that set goals for recycling, composting, using recycled materials, and eliminating throw-away products. Small and minority businesses should be encouraged to explore the pollution-prevention field as a possible expansion market.

Because of the inherent inequities associated with waste-facility siting, a national moratorium is needed on the construction of new commercial hazardous-waste treatment, storage, and disposal facilities and new municipal solid-waste incinerators and landfills in communities already saturated with environmental problems.

Clearly, institutional arrangements influence land-use policies and perpetuate the separate and unequal quality of residential areas for Whites and African Americans. Racial discrimination reduces the options available to African Americans in terms of where they live, work, and play. The problems associated with a nearby lead smelter and lead in drinking water must be addressed as quality of life issues.

The nation must redefine "environment" to include infrastructure problems that threaten the fabric of our cities and their inhabitants. An inadequate sewer treatment plant is an environmental and health threat. The repairing or replacing of decayed sewer lines and upgrading existing and building new sewer plants are investments in America.

The rebuilding of urban America must involve people who live in cities. Public officials must take leadership roles in calling for new investments in housing, mass transit, and pollution-prevention programs.

Social justice and equity must be incorporated into all infrastructure improvement and pollution-prevention plans. No segment of society should have to bear a disproportionate burden of the nation's pollution problem.

In addition to the standard "technical" requirements, equity proposals will need to require implementation of a "fair share" plan that takes into account sociodemographic, economic, and cultural factors of impacted communities.

Finally, the problems associated with environmental racism need to be elevated to the national agenda. The time is long past when institutional racism can be dismissed as a figment of someone's imagination. A number of action steps are recommended to address the problem of environmental injustice and disproportionate impact: (1) hold congressional hearings; (2) establish a blue-ribbon commission or think tank; (3) select the National Academy of Sciences to conduct a comprehensive study; and (4) create a permanent division within the federal EPA that examines environmental equity, disproportionate impact, and pollution strategies.

NOTES

1. Reverend Adolph Coleman. (1991). A resident of Robbins and associate pastor of the West Pullman Church of God. Personal interview, November 17.

2. See Bryant, B., and Mohai, P. (forthcoming). *Race and the incidence of environmental hazards.* Boulder, Colorado: Westview Press.
Logan, J. R., and Molotch, H. L. (1987). *Urban Fortunes: The political economy of place.* Berkeley: University of California Press, pp. 95–96
Bullard, R. (1990). *Dumping in Dixie: Race, class, and environmental quality.* Boulder, Colorado: Westview Press, pp. 33.

3. Johnson, H. (1991). Resident of Chicago's Altgeld Gardens and executive director of People for Community Recovery. Personal interview, November, 17.

4. For detailed discussions of the LANCER project, see Blumberg, L., and Gottlieb, R. (1989). *War on waste: Can America win its battle with garbage?* Washington, DC: Island Press, pp. 155–188.
Russell, D. (1989). Environmental racism. *Amicus Journal* (Spring), 22–29.

REFERENCES

Bradbury, K. L., Case, K. E., & Dunham, C. R. (1989). Geographic patterns of mortgage lending in Boston, 1982–1987. *New England Economic Review,* September/October, 3–30.

Bullard, R. D. (1983). Solid waste sites and the black Houston community. *Sociological Inquiry, 53,* 273–288.

Bullard, R. D. (1986). Blacks and the American dream of housing. In J. A. Momeni (Ed.), *Race, ethnicity, and housing in the United States* (pp. 53–68). Westport, CT: Greenwood Press.

Bullard, R. D. (1987). *Invisible Houston: The black experience in boom and bust.* College Station, TX: Texas A & M University Press.

Bullard, R. D. (1989). Environmentalism, economic blackmail, and civil rights. In J.

Gaventa & A. Willingham (Eds.), *Communities in economic crisis* (pp. 190–199). Philadelphia: Temple University Press.

Bullard, R. D. (1990). *Dumping in Dixie: Race, class, and environmental quality.* Boulder, CO: Westview Press.

Bullard, R. D., & Wright, B. H. (1987). Environmentalism and the politics of equity: Emergent trends in the black community. *Mid-America Review of Sociology, 12,* 21–38.

Bullard, R. D., & Wright, B. H. (1990). Toxic waste and the African American community. *Urban League Review, 13,* 67–75.

Bullard, R. D., & Feagin, J. R. (1991). Racism and the city. In M. Gottdiener & C. V. Pickvance (Eds.), *Urban life in transition.* Newbury Park, CA: Sage.

Cerrell Associates. (1984). Political difficulties facing waste-to-energy conversion plant siting. Report prepared for the California Waste Management Board, p. 65.

Citizens for a Better Environment. (1989). Richmond at risk: Community demographics and toxic hazards from industrial polluters. San Francisco: C > B > E > Report, pp. 1, 121.

Commission for Racial Justice. (1987). Toxic wastes and race in the United States. New York: United Church of Christ Commission for Racial Justice, pp. xiii–xiv, 18–19.

Costner, P., & Thornton, J. (1990). Playing with fire. Washington, DC: Greenpeace Report, pp. 48–49.

Darden, J. T. (1989). The status of urban blacks 25 years after the Civil Rights Act of 1964. *Sociology and Social Research, 73,* 160–173.

Denton, N. A., & Massey, D. S. (1988). Residential segregation of Blacks, Hispanics, and Asians by socioeconomic status and generation. *Social Science Quarterly, 69,* 797–818.

Epstein, S. S., Brown, L. O., & Pope, C. (1983). *Hazardous waste in America.* San Francisco: Sierra Club Books, pp. 33–39.

Feagin, J. R. (1990). *Building American cities: The urban real estate game.* Englewood Cliffs, NJ: Prentice-Hall.

Federal Financial Institutions Examination Council (FFIEC). (1991). Home Mortgage Disclosure Act: Expanded data on residential lending. *Federal Reserve Bulletin,* November, 859–881.

Gottdiener, M. (1988). *The social production of urban space.* Austin, TX: University of Texas Press, p. 172.

Greenberg, M. R., & Anderson, R. F. (1984). *Hazardous waste sites: The credibility gap.* New Brunswick, NJ: Rutgers University Center for Urban Policy Research, pp. 158–159.

Greenpeace. (1991). Home street, U.S.A. *Greenpeace Magazine,* October–December, 8–13.

James, F. J., McCummings, B. I., and Tynan, E. A. (1984). Minorities in the Sunbelt. New Brunswick, NJ: Rutgers University Center for Urban Policy Research, p. 138.

Kay, J. (1991). Fighting toxic racism: L.A.'s minority neighborhood is the "dirtiest" in the state. *San Francisco Examiner,* April 7, p. A1.

Kazis, R., & Grossman, R. (1983). *Fear at work: Job blackmail, labor, and the environment.* New York: The Pilgrim Press, chapters 1 & 2.

Kelly, E. D. (1988). Zoning. In F. S. So & J. Getzels (Eds.), *The practice of local government planning,* 2nd ed. (pp. 251–284). Washington, DC: International Management Association.

Logan, J. R., & Molotch, H. L. (1987). *Urban fortunes: The political economy of place.* Berkeley: University of California Press, p. 158.

Mann, E. (1991). L.A.'s lethal air: New strategies for policy, organizing, and action. Los Angeles: Labor/Community Strategy Center, p. 31.

Marshall, P. G. (1989). Not in my back yard. *Editorial Research Reports, 1,* 312–313.

Ritter, J. (1990). Robbins to get incinerator. *Chicago Sun Times,* January 31, 3.

Taeuber, K. (1983). Racial residential segregation, 28 cities, 1970–1980. Center for Demography and Ecology. Working Paper 83-12. University of Wisconsin, Madison, p. 3.

Updegrade, W. L. (1989). Race and money. *Money, 18,* 152–172.

22

Black Children: Growth, Development, and Health

Dionne J. Jones and Veronica A. Roberts

INTRODUCTION

In 1990, Black Americans represented 15.0 percent of the population under 19 years old (U.S. Department of Commerce, 1992a, p. 18). Recent research indicates that some general conditions endemic to Blacks in the areas of health and welfare continue to place large numbers of Black children and youth at risk for medically based school problems. For example, Black children are far more likely than their White counterparts to experience health-related difficulties that impinge on their physical, emotional, and educational development. A number of the health problems experienced by Black children are directly related to their socioeconomic status. In 1991, more than two-thirds of all African American children (68.2%) living in female-headed households were poor. The comparable rate for White children was 47.2 percent (U.S. Department of Commerce, 1992b).

The aims of this chapter are (1) to highlight some salient indicators of the general condition of Black children, (2) to assess the impact of malnutrition and other health risk factors on the growth and development of Black children, (3) to present some prescriptive strategies for reducing the vulnerabilities of Black children, and (4) to make recommendations useful to policy makers in instituting changes that can systematically improve the condition of Black children.

GENERAL CONDITION OF BLACK CHILDREN

Health, Education, and Welfare

From even a cursory look at the data, it can be surmised that a disproportionately large number of Black children are not faring well. On almost every major indicator of health, education, and welfare, Black children are worse off than their White counterparts.

Health

A recent study by the National Black Child Development Institute (NBCDI) (1990) found that only 45 percent of Black children 5 years and younger enjoy excellent health. This compares with 57 percent of White children in that age group. As the children get older, the disparity widens. In fact, there is a 17.4 percentage-point gap between Black and White parents who reported that the health status of their 6 to 17 year-old children was excellent (39.5% for Black parents vs. 56.9% for White parents).

Black school-age children are more likely than Whites to experience activity limiting health conditions. One reason is that Black children do not have access to preventive health care services at the younger ages. Access to health care is determined largely by health insurance. Many Black families do not have adequate health insurance, and some have none. While one in ten infants in the United States has no routine source of health care, the proportion of Black infants in that situation is one in five. A 1988 survey indicated that just over half (56%) of Black children 17 years of age and younger had health insurance coverage, and about one-third of them were covered by Medicaid. By way of comparison, 82.9 percent of White children 17 years and younger had health insurance coverage, and only 7.3 percent of them were covered by Medicaid (NBCDI, 1990, p. 45). The lack of insurance is usually a primary reason for the failure of many Blacks to seek preventive health care services.

Prenatal care and infant health are closely related. Indeed, early prenatal care significantly reduces the risk of infants with low birth weight as well as infant mortality. It was shown that Black women delivered 61 percent of live-birth babies when they received prenatal care during the first trimester compared with only 11 percent of live births when they received prenatal care during the third trimester only or where there was no prenatal care (NBCDI, 1990, p. 47). The infant mortality rate (per 1,000 live births) among Blacks was 18.6 in 1989, and the rate of low-birth-weight infants for Black mothers was 13.2 in 1989 (U.S. Department of Health and Human Services, 1992).

The death rate (per 100,000 children) for Black children ages 1 to 14 years was 48.4 in 1989, a 12.6 percent decrease from the 1980 rate (55.1%). The death rate due to violence among Black teenagers (15 to 19 years per 100,000 teens) increased sharply, by 62 percent, between 1984 (53.0%) and 1989 (86.1%) (Center for the Study of Social Policy, 1992, p. 21). A large proportion of teenage deaths were drug related.

Education

With a life-start ridden with health care setbacks of such magnitude, it is not surprising that Black children continue to be plagued by many health-related problems in their developing years. Health-related problems such as malnutrition and anemia, lead poisoning, child abuse and neglect, and frequent episodes of acute illnesses during early childhood often have a devastating impact on the cognitive development of Black children. In fact, some educators have concluded that even relatively infrequent serious illnesses have far-reaching social consequences because of their potential for interference with the crucial stages of the child's social and cognitive development (Miller, Fine, Adams-Taylor & Schorr, 1986).

To illustrate, school problems such as truancy as well as the more chronic absenteeism among some Black children have been traced to health-related problems such as malnutrition and early childhood diseases, both physical and psychopathological (Schorr & Schorr, 1988). Persistent absenteeism often functions as a precursor to disruptive behaviors associated with school failure. There is consensus among scholars that, given the proper health care and educational conditions, school performance among Black children is comparable with that of their White counterparts, particularly at the elementary level (Senior, 1991; Roberts, 1992).

Risk factors such as the absence of immunization and exposure to lead poisoning are prime factors in the low-achievement equation (Agency for Toxic Substances and Disease Registry, 1988). Learning disabilities (LD) are often shown to be medically based, resulting from inappropriate responses to minor illnesses in the early childhood years or poor health management of chronic illnesses (Schorr & Schorr, 1988).

National standardized tests illustrate continuing large gaps in educational attainment measures between Black and White school-age children, despite improvements by Blacks over the last decade. Disparities occur largely in national achievement test scores in critical subject areas such as reading, mathematics, and science (U.S. Department of Education, 1992, p. 122). Aligned to the failure in academic subjects by many Black students is the high dropout rate, which is due to a number of factors including teenage pregnancy, involvement in illicit activities, and incarceration. In addition, many Black students are "turned off" by school; with a curriculum that has little meaningful application to them and, more often than not, devalues them and their culture. These students receive confirmation of their devaluation daily as Black students continue to be disproportionately represented in special-education classes for the learning disabled, while White students continue to be overrepresented in gifted/talented classes and other enrichment programs.

A truncated educational experience diminishes prospects for students' success in employment and leads, ultimately, to an increased risk of continued poverty (Turner, Grindstaff & Phillips, 1990). Deficits in critical cognitive skills restrict opportunities for competitive jobs, improved salary and, ultimately, social and economic mobility. Without supporting relationships, poor Black children who have been denied this support are more frequently at risk for prolonged poverty than their more well-off Black or White counterparts (Schorr & Schorr, 1988).

Welfare

The greatest risk factor for Black children is poverty. As defined by the federal government, children are poor when they are living in families whose income is below a predetermined amount necessary for existence. The official poverty line for a family of four was $12,675 per year, and 43.2 percent of children lived in families below the poverty level (U.S. Department of Commerce, 1992b, p. 462). This condition was not eased despite the fact that many of the heads of these households worked either full-time or part-time at some point during the year. But with a stagnant minimum wage, wage inequities, high unemployment, and the high rate of female-headed families, the proportion of poor children and their families is increasing.

Poverty and the stresses (from role overload) of motherhood are shown to impact on the health of children (U.S. Department of Health and Human Services, 1991). Many poor families turn to public assistance to ease their financial burden, but they find the payments inadequate to fully meet their needs. Indeed, the maximum benefit paid through Aid to Families with Dependent Children (AFDC) was less than one-half of the federal poverty line for a family of three in July 1988 in 31 states (Children's Defense Fund, 1989, p. 20). An increasing number of AFDC families are becoming homeless. The AFDC benefits are so low and the cost of housing so high that many families simply cannot afford to live independently. For example, a mere 22 percent of all AFDC families received housing assistance in 1988 (Children's Defense Fund, 1989, p. 23).

MALNUTRITION, ANEMIA, AND OTHER HEALTH RISKS

Malnutrition

The conditions of poverty evidenced by hunger and overcrowding contribute to the incidence of illness among Black children, thus restricting the quality and quantity of life. The relationship between inadequate nutrition and health damage has been well established. A pregnant woman who is malnourished has a high likelihood of giving birth to a low birth weight infant, that is, a baby weighing less than 5.5 pounds. Low birth weight is a leading cause of infant death, and those babies who do survive have an increased risk to being impaired for life by conditions such as retardation, autism, learning disabilities, vision or hearing loss, cerebral palsy, and epilepsy (NBCDI, 1990).

The Physician Task Force on Hunger in America, which was coordinated through the Harvard University School of Public Health, traveled the nation in 1985 to examine the hunger problem. At that time, the Task Force found that many millions of Americans experience hunger at some point each month and that malnutrition affects almost 500,000 children (Children's Defense Fund, 1989). Updating its report in 1987, the Task Force found that hunger had failed to abate and, in addition, that an increasing number of working Americans living in depressed regions of the nation had been forced to turn to bread lines and soup kitchens to feed themselves and their children. This is especially true for Black children.

Anemia

Other developmental limitations associated with poverty are iron deficiency and growth retardation. Iron deficiency, for instance, is more than twice as common in one- and two-year-old low-income children, a large proportion of whom are Black, as it is among children at higher socioeconomic levels. Growth retardation, on the other hand, affects 16 percent of low-income children younger than 6 years old (U.S. Department of Health and Human Services, 1990).

The long-term effects of iron deficiency have been well documented. For example, it has been recently established that iron deficiency can cause abnormal behavior and reduced learning and mental functioning in children (Youdim, Ben-Shachar & Yehuda, 1989). It is also reported that iron deficiency interferes with mental processes, especially those involved with visual attention and learning of concepts (Soewondo, Husaini & Pollitt, 1989). The evidence, therefore, points to the need for increased funding for nutritional programs to families, including school lunch programs.

Lead Poisoning

Lead poisoning has been identified as one contributor to developmental problems in Black children (Schwartz & Otto, 1991). In 1984, more than 3 million children in the United States between the ages of 6 months and 5 years of age were found to have dangerously high blood lead levels. Lead poisoning became one of the nation's most prevalent childhood threats in 1984. One of the primary sources of this toxin is thought to be old flaking lead-based paint found in substandard housing areas (U.S. Department of Health and Human Services, 1991). Such housing conditions are found in low-income Black and minority communities. Profound mental retardation, coma, seizures, and death can and do result from severe lead poisoning. Indeed, even low levels of lead poisoning can result in impaired central nervous system functioning and cause delayed cognitive development, hearing problems, growth retardation, and metabolic disorders (Agency for Toxic Substances and Disease Registry, 1988).

A total of 796 cases of childhood lead poisoning were identified in 1988 by the New York City Bureau of Lead Poisoning Control, and 59 percent of these cases were Black children (Daniel, Sedlis, Polk, Dowuona-Hammond, McCants & Matte, 1990). One- and two-year-old children accounted for 61 percent of all the cases. Although lead is also toxic to adults and affects all organ systems, it adversely affects cognitive development and behavior in young children. Toddlers are especially liable to ingest lead in contaminated environments (i.e., peeling paint) because of normal mouthing behavior and increased hand contact with dirt and dust. It is for this reason that children in this age group are more susceptible than older children to lead-related neurobehavioral toxicity.

If New York can be used as an example of a severe problem, Daniel et al. (1990) report that the magnitude of the problem of excessive lead absorption among children in New York City is underestimated. In the first place, not all children in the high-risk age group of 9 months to 5 years of age are screened. Second, the screening coverage and results of children utilizing noncity-affiliated providers is unknown. Third, in most of the new cases identified by the Bureau of Lead Poisoning Control, the children's blood lead levels were too low to cause overt symptoms, although they were toxic.

Immunization

The incidence of measles increased dramatically among preschool-aged children in inner cities in 1989 and 1990. The largest outbreaks occurred primarily among unvaccinated Black and Hispanic children in large cities, such as Chicago, Dallas, Houston, Los Angeles, Milwaukee, and New York (Measles vaccination levels, 1991). Overall, in the inner-city public schools studied, the percentage of children vaccinated by the second birthday ranged from 51 percent in Jersey City to 79 percent in Pittsburgh. In two cities with predominantly White schools, first-graders in White schools had higher vaccine coverage levels than first-graders in other schools (Measles vaccination levels, 1991).

Similarly, the Connecticut Department of Health Services studied 666 urban first-grade students in Hartford and 810 in New Haven to determine which children had received early-childhood vaccinations in Fall 1990 and Spring 1991. The results indicated that 23 percent and 33 percent of students, respectively, in the two cities had not begun the series of vaccinations by the age of three months. Children who had not been vaccinated by that time were more likely to fail to complete the entire series of vaccinations (Measles vaccination levels, 1991).

Some parents avoid vaccinating their children either because they are worried about side effects or because they feel that childhood diseases are no longer dangerous. There may, however, be some validity to these fears in the wake of the ongoing debate surrounding the diphtheria-pertussis-tetanus vaccine (Ince, 1991; Stern, 1989).

Dental Care

Dental care appears to be even more infrequent than other forms of medical care among Black children. Based on interviews with parents in the National Health Interview Survey of Child Health, approximately 38 percent of Black children in 1988 had not seen a dentist within the previous year (NBCDI, 1990). Sinkford (1988) analyzed the data bases of three national surveys to assess the status of dental health in Black and White Americans. The surveys were the Health and Nutrition Examination Survey (HANES), 1971 to 1974; the National Caries Prevalence Survey, 1979 to 1980; and the National Survey of Oral Health in U.S. Employed Adults and Seniors, 1985 to 1986.

Sinkford (1988) found that, while the prevalence of dental disease was similar in both Black and White children (5 to 17 years), the treatment needs were greater and much more severe in Black children in both primary and permanent dentition. For example, among 5- to 9-year-olds, Black children needed 167.3 restorations per 100 children, compared to 115.9 restorations needed per 100 White children. In addition, Black children needed 14.0 extractions and 10.8 crowns per 100 children, compared to 11.5 extractions and 7.0 crowns per 100 White children. The racial disparities for permanent dentition for children ages 5 to 17 years were even greater.

Child Abuse and Neglect

Reported child abuse and neglect cases have increased steadily since 1976. There was a more than 90 percent increase in reported cases between 1981 and 1986. In 1986, 2.2 million children and adolescents were reportedly abused, neglected, or both (Children's Defense Fund, 1989). This number may be conservative in light of the fact that many cases of abuse and neglect go unreported. Of the total 833,377 primarily substantiated cases of child abuse and neglect cases reported to Child Protective Services nationally in 1990, 203,636 or 24.4 percent were Black children (National Center on Child Abuse and Neglect, 1992).

A disproportionate number of children who are maltreated come from poor families. Children whose family income in 1986 was less than $15,000 experienced substantially more maltreatment compared to those whose families earned $15,000 or more (National Center on Child Abuse and Neglect, 1988). Schorr and Schorr (1988) summarized the situation best: "Economic stress, lack of social support and other protective factors, a fragile, impaired, or immature parent, and sometimes a difficult infant can combine, in the absence of outside help, to create an environment so bad that it prejudices the normal development of the child" (p. 143). Children who are abused or maltreated suffer not only physical harm but also damage to their social, emotional, and cognitive development. As a result, many run away from home, use drugs or alcohol, or get in trouble with the law. A clear pattern can be seen in the connection between a dismal childhood and damage in adolescence and later life. Moreover, abused children are more likely to grow up to be abusive parents themselves.

AIDS

The recent phenomena of drug abuse and the AIDS epidemic are compounding the health risk factors of Black children at a time when the health care system is under-funded and largely unresponsive to them. Blacks and other racial/ethnic minority groups appear more likely to be at risk of AIDS than their White counterparts. Approximately 40 percent of both the AIDS cases and AIDS-related deaths reported during the 1980s have been among Blacks and other racial/ethnic groups, and more than 80 percent of these cases have been among males 13 years or older.

The rate of AIDS per 100,000 Blacks is more than quadruple that of Whites. However, the rates among Black women and children compared with their White counterparts are far greater (U.S. Department of Health and Human Services, 1993a, p. 15). For example, Black women experience more than 15 times the risk of AIDS compared to White women, and Black children represent more than 50 percent of all children with AIDS. In addition, Blacks account for a greater proportion of AIDS cases associated with intravenous drug abuse than other AIDS victims, and higher rates of heterosexual transmission of the HIV virus. Transmission of the virus from mother to infant, therefore, occurs with greater frequency among Blacks (U.S. Department of Health and Human Services, 1991, 1993a).

As of March 1993, the number of AIDS cases among Blacks (88,238 or 30.5%) reflect the astronomical rise in cases in the general population (289,320) (U.S. Department of Health and Human Services, 1993b, p. 11). The numbers of AIDS cases among Black males and females 13 years and over were 68,506 (27.2%) and 17,285 (53.2%), respectively for their subpopulation totals. By comparison, there were 40,136 (15.9%) and 6,617 (20.4%) cases among Hispanic males and females 13 years and over, respectively. Among White males and females 13 years and over, there were 141,082 (55.9%) and 8,258 (25.4%), respectively (U.S. Department of Health and Human Services, 1993b, p. 11).

Somewhat reflective of the condition among Black women, the AIDS cases among Black children under 13 years old (2,447 or 54.6%) were the highest among all racial and ethnic minority groups. Hispanic and White children under 13 years old, on the other hand, represented 1,082 (24.2%) and 907 (20.3%) AIDS cases, respectively (U.S. Department of Health and Human Services, 1993b, p. 11).

As with the reported AIDS cases, AIDS deaths have steadily increased. AIDS deaths for Black males of all ages rose from 6,782 in 1990 to 7,461 in 1991. There was a similar increase for Black females of all ages from 1,805 in 1990 to 2,014 in 1991. By December 1992, the cumulative total of all AIDS deaths among Blacks reached 50,153 or 29.2 percent. Among Hispanics and Whites, AIDS deaths were 28,078 (16.3%) and 92,038 (53.5%), respectively. Cumulative totals as of December 1992 reveal that there were 1,202 (52.6%) AIDS deaths among Black children under 15 years old compared to 548 (24%) among Hispanic children and 513 (22.4%) among White children (U.S. Department of Health and Human Services, 1993a, p. 18).

REDUCING THE VULNERABILITIES OF BLACK CHILDREN

Prescriptive Strategies

Most families rearing children today need more help from sources outside the family than did previous generations. Moreover, most families are living with higher levels of stress because of both external factors (job stability, inflation, etc.) and internal factors (fear of family member succumbing to drug abuse, AIDS, family breakup, etc.). These needs and fears are amplified for high-risk Black children and their families. What is called for is a wide range of social and economic interventions, along with concerted efforts by various sectors of society to improve the health, education, and general welfare of Black children. Specifically, primary care health providers, social service professionals, health educators, housing officials, community groups, and other concerned individuals must work individually and collectively to effect the needed change. In addition, age-appropriate and culturally sensitive health education curricula must be developed to bring about changes in the attitudes and behaviors of Black children. Educational and social support programs could also empower parents in high-risk environments.

Articulating recognition of the enormity of the problem in the publication *Healthy People 2000,* the U.S. Department of Health and Human Services (1991) has outlined three health goals for the nation: (1) to increase the span of healthy life for Americans, (2) to reduce health disparities among Americans, and (3) to achieve access to preventive services for all Americans. The report notes that two sentinel health events are involved, birth and death. "Birth," it proclaims, "frames the potential for a healthy lifetime; death often summarizes how that potential was used" (U.S. Department of Health and Human Services, 1990, p. 43). According to the report, the three goals define the challenge for the year 2000, particularly for health planners, policy makers, and health care providers.

Federal costs for health and education to fund needed programs such as Maternal and Child Health (MCH), the Supplementary Food Program for Women, Infants, and Children (WIC), Head Start, and support for high-risk students for fiscal year 1993 is projected at 1.8 billion dollars (National Commission on Children, 1991). Despite these high national expenditures, however, the costs today of implementing corrective measures are insignificant compared to what they will be tomorrow if lethargy and inaction continue to guide national policy making.

The delivery of health services designed to meet the prenatal and postnatal needs of poor young mothers and their children are, at present, fragmented and ineffective. An increased presence of school-based health clinics, where health education is provided, would be an effective way to encourage adolescents to develop positive and informed attitudes about their health, including values about responsible sexual behavior. Two such health clinics in Chicago's inner-city schools were found to be heavily utilized by Black male and female students (Evans & Evans, 1989).

SUMMARY

Any profile of Black children must consider emotional, psychological, and learning problems, as well as the social and environmental risks to which many of them are subjected. Mental retardation, learning disorders, emotional and behavioral problems, and vision and speech impairments appear to be more prevalent among children living in poverty, often in inner cities, than among children at higher socioeconomic levels.

With reduced funding of the Medicaid program, many health programs for families have now been consolidated into the Maternal and Child Health block grant with the inevitable result of the elimination of a number of services previously covered under Medicaid. Even in cases where services are covered, inadequate funding limits programs in their efforts to serve all eligible clients. For instance, the federal Supplemental Food Program for Women, Infants, and Children (WIC) serves only one-half of eligible applicants. Budget reductions have forced cities and states to cut critically needed services including staff and supplies for public clinics and the school nursing programs (NBCDI, 1990; Children's Defense Fund, 1989). Hospitals that treat uninsured patients face extreme financial difficulties, and many have been forced to close or curtail services to the poor (NBCDI, 1990).

This is the legacy of more than a decade of a conservative administration. The Bush Administration has carried on the legacy of Reaganomics and placed its budgetary priorities on foreign spending and the military rather than on domestic and social programs. In a ranking of national priorities among 142 nations in 1987, the United States ranked 18th in infant mortality (28th in infant mortality if only Black babies are counted), 20th in school-age population per teacher, and 18th in population per physician. But, the United States ranked first in military expenditures, military aid to foreign countries, nuclear reactors, and nuclear tests (Children's Defense Fund, 1989).

At a time when many urban cities with large concentrations of Blacks fare worse in low birth weight births and infant mortality than many developing nations of the Third World, this deplorable state of affairs in the health and welfare of U.S. citizens must and should not continue. According to the Children's Defense Fund (1989), the total number of minority children will have increased by 25.5 percent between 1985 and the year 2000. The proportion of all minority children will have increased from 28.0 percent to 32.7 percent. Specialized programs, such as the ones discussed previously, that address the needs of this emergent population must be developed now.

RECOMMENDATIONS

Based on the issues raised and the prescriptive strategies for change advanced in the foregoing discussion, the following recommendations are made:

- Adequate health care must be provided through programs such as WIC and AFDC to ensure that all children and their families receive medical and preventive health care.
- Quality preschool learning opportunities must be provided for all disad-

vantaged children. This can be done through expansion of the Head Start program to include all eligible children.

- A sound basic education in public school must be afforded all disadvantaged elementary and secondary school students. This can be accomplished through programs such as the Chapter I program.
- Services offered through school programs, such as school-based health clinics, should be integrated with similar services offered by other community agencies, including mental health and social service agencies.
- The system needs to be revamped so that families in severe need are given help during certain life crises. Too often, help comes too late and usually in a punitive form, such as removing children from their homes and placing them in foster care or in the juvenile justice system.
- Families must be empowered, for example, through the provision of counseling or emergency financial subsidies in order to remain functional and intact.

Ultimately, the cost incurred in implementing and operationalizing the programs recommended here, as well as others that have proved to be successful, will be far lower than the price currently being paid for neglected health care, unemployment, and crime. With intensive interventions for populations at highest risk, we can break the cycle of poverty and the related morbidity and mortality associated with Black children in American society. Such change is, indeed, "within our reach."

REFERENCES

Agency for Toxic Substances and Disease Registry. (1988). *The nature and extent of lead poisoning in children in the United States: A report to Congress.* Washington, DC: U.S. Department of Health and Human Services.

Center for the Study of Social Policy. (1992). *Kids count databook.* Washington, DC: Author.

Children's Defense Fund. (1989). *A vision for America's future.* Washington, DC: Author.

Daniel, K., Sedlis, M., Polk, L., Dowuona-Hammond, S., McCants, B., & Matte, T. D. (1990). Childhood lead poisoning, New York City, 1988. *Morbidity and Mortality Weekly Report,* pp. 1–7.

Early childhood vaccination levels among urban children—Connecticut, 1990 and 1991. (1992). *Morbidity and Mortality Weekly Report,* pp. 888–891.

Evans, R. C., & Evans, H. L. (1989). The African American adolescent male and school-based health clinics: A preventive perspective. *The Urban League Review, 12,* 111–117.

Healthy People 2000. (1991). National health promotion and disease prevention objectives. DHHS Publication No. (PHS) 91-50213. Washington, DC: Government Printing Office.

Ince, S. (1991). Baby shots: The immunization controversy. Part 1. *American Baby, 53,* 73–76.

Jones, D. (1992). *A Research Study on Project DAISY—Year 2.* Final Report. Washington, DC: District of Columbia Public Schools.

Measles vaccination levels among selected groups of preschool-aged children—United States. (1991). *Morbidity and Mortality Weekly Report,* January 18, pp. 36–39.

Miller, C. A., Fine, A., Adams-Taylor, S., & Schorr, L. (1986). Monitoring children's health: Key indicators. Washington, DC: American Public Health Association.

National Black Child Development Institute (NBCDI). (1990). The status of African American children. *20th Anniversary Report: 1970–1990.* Washington, DC: Author.

National Center on Child Abuse and Neglect. (1988). Study of National Incidence and Prevalence of Child Abuse and Neglect: 1988, Executive Summary. Washington, DC: Department of Health and Human Services.

National Center on Child Abuse and Neglect. (1992). *National Child Abuse and Neglect Data System. Working Paper No. 1, 1990 Summary Data Component.* Washington, DC: Department of Health and Human Services.

National Commission on Children. (1991). Speaking of kids: A national survey of children and parents. Washington, DC: Author.

Roberts, V. A. (1992). *Emeritus scientists, mathematics and engineers program: Evaluation report.* District of Columbia Public Schools. Washington, DC: Emeritus Foundation.

Schorr, L. B., & Schorr, D. (1988). *Within our reach: Breaking the cycle of disadvantage.* New York: Anchor Press Doubleday.

Schwartz, J., & Otto, D. (1991). Lead and minor hearing impairment. *Archives of Environmental Health, 46,* 300–305.

Senior, A. M. (1991). Profiles of top-scoring African American Students: An analysis of SAT test-takers, *Urban League Review, 15,* 41–51.

Sinkford, J. (1988). Status of dental health in black and white Americans. *Journal of the National Medical Association, 80,* 1127–1128, 1130–1131.

Soewondo, S., Husaini, M., & Pollitt, E. (1989). Effects of iron deficiency on attention and learning processes in preschool children: Bandung, Indonesia. *American Journal of Clinical Nutrition, 50,* 667–673.

Stern, L. (1989). Why your child must be immunized. *Woman's Day* (September 5th), p. 36.

Turner, R. J., Grindstaff, C. F., & Phillips, N. (1990). Social support and outcome in teenage pregnancy. *Journal of Health and Social Behavior, 31,* 43–57.

U.S. Department of Commerce, Bureau of the Census. (1992a). *Statistical Abstract of the United States 1992.* Washington, DC: Government Printing Office.

U.S. Department of Commerce, Bureau of the Census. (1992b). *Current Population Reports,* Poverty in the United States: 1991 (Series P-60, No. 181), Table 5, pp. 10–15.

U.S. Department of Education. (1992). *Digest of Education Statistics 1992.* (NCES Publication No. NCES 92-097). Washington, DC: Government Printing Office.

U.S. Department of Health and Human Services. (1990). *Health status of the disadvantaged: Chartbook 1990.* DHHS Publication No. HRSA HRS-P-DV 90-1). Washington, DC: Government Printing Office.

U.S. Department of Health and Human Services. (1991). *Healthy people: National health promotion and disease prevention objectives.* (DHHS Publication No. PHS 91-50213). Washington, DC: Government Printing Office.

U.S. Department of Health and Human Services. (1992). National Center for Health Statistics, Annual summary of births, marriages, divorces, and deaths: United States, 1991, *Monthly Vital Statistics Report, 40* (13) (September), 22.

U.S. Department of Health and Human Services. (1993a, February). *HIV/AIDS Surveillance Report.* Year-End Edition. Atlanta, GA: Centers for Disease Control and Prevention.

U.S. Department of Health and Human Services. (1993b, May). *HIV/AIDS Surveillance Report.* 1st Quarter Edition. Atlanta, GA: Centers for Disease Control and Prevention.

Youdim, M. B. H., Ben-Shachar, D., & Yehuda, S. (1989). Putative biological mechanisms of the effect of iron deficiency on brain biochemistry and behavior. *American Journal of Clinical Nutrition, 50,* 607–615.

23

Black Health Care Providers and Related Professionals: Issues of Underrepresentation and Change

John Obioma Ukawuilulu and Ivor Lensworth Livingston

INTRODUCTION

Research has consistently shown that African Americans or Blacks (as they will henceforth be called here) have disproportionately higher mortality and morbidity rates than their White counterparts (Report of the Secretary's Task Force on Black and Minority Health, 1985; National Research Council, 1989; CDC, 1990; U.S. Healthy People, 1990). Blacks die in excess of 60,000 annually from preventable illnesses. This disparity in mortality is due in part to the overrepresentation of Blacks in mortality rates associated with cancer, cardiovascular diseases, cirrhosis, diabetes, infant mortality, unintentional injuries, homicide, and, recently, AIDS. Recent statistics show that the gap between Blacks and Whites in terms of their life expectancies has continued to widen (Report of the Secretary's Task Force on Black and Minority Health, 1985).

The vast racial disparities in health that currently exist are a result of several interacting factors and conditions. While this chapter fully acknowledges the overrepresentation of Blacks (and other minorities) in morbidity and mortality statistics, its main thrust is to review and discuss issues relating to the underrepresentation of Blacks in medicine and related medical and other professional occupations and to discuss programs and strategies to improve racial parity in these areas. The basic argument is that there is a correlation between the underrepresentation of Blacks in these medical and other professions and their overrepresentation in morbidity and mortality rates. In short, it is reasoned that if Blacks were proportionately represented in medicine and related science areas, their overall health conditions within the general population would drastically improve (Rice & Winn, 1990).

In elucidating the dominant theme of the underrepresentation of Blacks in medicine and related areas and its consequences, this chapter (1) presents background information and an overview of racial disparities in the preparation for, enrollment in, and matriculation from medical school; (2) discusses the representation of Blacks in medical-related fields and other professions; (3) discusses the rationale for having more racial parity in medical and related professions; and (4) discusses past, present, and future ways of increasing racial parity in these medical and related professions.

PREPARATION, ENROLLMENT, AND MATRICULATION

According to Gunby (1989), although Blacks make up approximately 12 percent of the population, they represent 3 percent of physicians, 3 percent of the dentists, and less than 2 percent of biomedical scientists. In 1989, Blacks represented a mere 6 percent of the total medical school enrollment, 5 percent of medical school graduates, 5 percent of postgraduate trainees, and 2 percent of medical school faculties (Lloyd & Miller, 1989). An even more disturbing picture is provided by statistics on the pool of medical applicants. The disadvantages of Blacks in medical and health-related professions are manifested early in the educational process. According to Woode and Lynch (1992), "The insufficient presence of minorities in medicine manifests itself at all points in the medical education pathway'' (1992). Statistics also show that the percentage of Blacks earning baccalaureate degrees was lower than their share of the U.S. population. Though Blacks comprise more than 12 percent of the U.S. population, in 1989, they received only 5.7 percent of the baccalaureate degrees awarded (see Petersdorf, Turner, Nickens & Ready, 1990).

With regard to the medical education pool, between 1980 and 1988, Blacks comprised about 7.5 percent of medical applicants, an average first-year enrollment of about 7 percent, and total medical school enrollment of about 6 percent (AAMC, 1989). Worse still, the percentage of Black medical school applications declined at about 16.7 percent over the aforementioned period (see Petersdorf, Turner, Nickens & Ready, 1990).

In 1992, 4,000 out of the 37,410 applications received by the nation's 126 medical schools were minority applicants. For nonminority applicants, this represented a 12.3 percent increase over 1991's level. For the minority applicants, there was an increase of 11.9 percent. Out of the 37,410 applicants, about 17,464 students were accepted, while 16,289 students matriculated (AAMC, 1992). For Black female applicants, there was a 12.9 percent increase in the number of applications, a 14.8 percent increase in the number of acceptances, and an 18.0 percent increase in number of new entrants. For Black males, the picture looked mixed. While the number of applicants increased by 5.0 percent, the percent of acceptances decreased by 0.6. However, the percentage of Black male new entrants was up by 6.6. Despite the modest increase, the picture still remained very bleak, especially for Black males.

An analysis of medical school statistics points to some emerging race-gender trends. That is, a gap is developing between the number of female Black medical school applicants and their male counterparts. Also, there are significant differences in three important categories: the applicants, those accepted, and new entrants. The disparity between Black females and Black males was more profound in the percentage of accepted students. While the female students had an increase of 14.8 percent, the percentage of Black males accepted decreased by 0.6 (AAMC, 1992).

Causes of Health and Racial Disparities

Several factors are responsible for the underrepresentation of Blacks in health and health-related professions. These factors include, but are not limited to the following: (1) historical factors (racism and limited number of Black medical schools and schools of public health, (2) poverty, (3) retrenchment of the early 1980s, (4) inadequate or "pipeline" educational preparation, and (5) lack of available and suitable role models.

Historical Factors

There have been and continue to be racial and gender differences in those who attend and graduate from medical school and practice medicine in the United States. Nearly 83 percent of practicing physicians are men. According to Reid-Wallace (1992), full-time faculty at today's medical schools are mainly White males, as are the majority of the students they teach. Also, among medical students enrolled in the 1991–1992 academic year, 38.1 percent were women and 9.6 percent were minorities.

Prior to the landmark civil rights court decisions and the legislation of the 1950s and 1960s, segregation existed in medical schools. Almost all Black physicians were trained either at Howard University School of Medicine or at Meharry Medical College. However, with doors being opened at predominantly White medical schools in the 1960s, other medical schools graduated approximately 15 to 20 Black physicians annually (Shea & Fullilove, 1985). White medical schools began accepting minority students in part because of social outcry, legislative enactments, and support from such agencies as the Office of Minority Affairs of the AAMC. As a result of these and other efforts and realities, Black and other minority enrollment increased, but it peaked in 1974 (Petersdorf, Turner, Nickens & Ready, 1990).

Poverty

Economic factors pose the major obstacle to obtaining medical and health-related professional education. Medical students graduate from medical schools with high debts (mean premed debt is $8,755, and mean medical school debt $45,876) (Nickens & Ready, 1992). These debts must be repaid with interest upon graduation. However, the interest on these loans, coupled with prior financial and other related burdens, especially in the case of Black physicians, can be overwhelming for these graduates. Because many of these medical school graduates are drawn from families that are poor, the economic hardships that come with graduation can be particularly difficult.

The potential financial troubles associated with Black medical school graduates is underscored by the fact that approximately one in three Blacks live below the poverty level and Black unemployment has been twice that of Whites since the 1940s (U.S. Bureau of the Census, 1990). It is from this group that some of the applicants to medical schools are drawn.

The Federal Government's Retrenchment of the 1980s

With the retrenchment of funds by the federal government in the 1980s, it became extremely difficult for Black and other minority students from poor families to enter medical schools and other health-related professions schools. An important report affecting enrollment in medical schools was the Graduate Medical Education National Advisory Committee (GMENAC) Report of 1982. This report acted as a double-edged sword in that, while it noted the surplus of physicians, it also pointed out the underrepresentation problem of Black physicians. However, the debatable issue regarding physician surplus had a debilitating consequence. It contributed, in part, to a withdrawal of federal assistance from both medical schools and students, which adversely affected potential Black students, who disproportionately occupy the lower socioeconomic strata. Similarly, these policies also affected the ability of some medical schools to attract and retain Black medical students (Hanft & White, 1986).

Inadequate Pipeline Preparation

As early as the third grade in school, the disproportionately low representation of minorities in the pool of medical school applicants can be predicted. Statistics show that Black and Hispanic students lag behind their White counterparts in mathematics and reading achievement. This consequently affects the inability of Black college students to take science courses or become premed majors (Simpson & Aronoff, 1988).

A number of studies released during the past decade have documented the inadequate knowledge and performance of U.S. students in science (National Science Board Commission, 1983). Recent information contained in the 1990 Science Report Card (1992) of a national survey of 20,000 students in grades 4, 8, and 12, conducted during the winter and spring of 1990 by the National Assessment of Educational Progress (NAEP), provides additional information in this area: (a) students' lack of preparation in science; (b) their apparent disinclination to enroll in challenging science courses; and (c) the comparatively low achievement of Black and Hispanic students, females, economically disadvantaged students, and non-college-bound students.

Black students have a poor educational background when compared with their White counterparts, which affects how they prepare for, apply to, are accepted by, and matriculate from medical schools. In a related manner, this inadequate educational background also affects their choice of and entry into medical-related and other professions such as science and engineering.

The tragedy is that Blacks and other minorities are eliminated from the educational pipeline even before they reach high school. The National Advisory Committee on Black Higher Education and Black Colleges and Universities (1980), or NACBHE, states that this attrition manifests itself in various forms: (1) general self-selection, (2) being pushed out as a result of discriminatory suspensions and expulsions, and (3) misplacement in special education programs or classes below their ability levels because of standardized test scores. A logical correlate of such educational realities is student drop-out. Although Blacks, like their White counterparts, begin to drop out of school in large numbers around the tenth grade, Blacks (27–29%) tend to have higher high school attrition rates than Whites (15–18%) (Astin, 1982).

These racial and educational realities have important implications for the Black science/mathematics talent pool, which is the reservoir from which medical school and future science profession applicants are pulled. It has been said (Berryman, 1983) that the U.S. science/mathematics pool begins to dwindle after the seventh grade, with the greatest out-migration occurring in grades eleven and twelve. Annually, two in five Black high school graduates enroll in college. Of those Black students enrolling in college, few have an inclination to major in the biological and physical sciences, engineering, and mathematics (Astin, 1982).

With respect to medicine per se, there is no shortage of minority young people interested in careers in medicine. Approximately 5.5 percent of Black college freshmen select medicine as their career choice, compared with 3.2 percent of White freshmen. The unfortunate reality, however, is that Blacks and Hispanics have very low college completion rates and experience difficulty with introductory science courses. Also, although various factors contribute to why Blacks and other minorities drop out of the medical school pipeline, the most salient factor is poor academic preparation prior to college (Petersdorf, 1992).

Lack of Role Models

It is a fallacy to assume that recruitment efforts in themselves are sufficient to attract and keep large numbers of Blacks in medicine, related professions, and the sciences. According to Reid-Wallace (1992), attention must be directed to other important issues such as the barriers (e.g., institutional racism) created by society. These barriers result in too few role models for Black and other minority students to emulate and benefit from. In essence, "We must treat the lack of self-confidence that so often prevents women and minorities from imagining that they too can be physicians" (Reid-Wallace, 1992, p. 380).

Today, greater numbers of Black students attend majority colleges than historically Black colleges and universities or HBCUs. However, HBCUs continue their historical patterns of producing proportionately more than their share of Black scientific and engineering talent (Pearson & Pearson, 1986). A contributing factor to this reality is the vast numbers of academically employed Black scientists, mathematicians, and engineers on the faculties of HBCUs, where they provide visible and dynamic role models for students as teachers, researchers, and administrators. A similar situation exists on the high school level as well (Davis, 1986). On the college level and at majority colleges and universities, the presence of Black faculty members is correlated with the production of Black Ph.D.s.

In the case of medical schools, especially those affiliated with majority White institutions, which currently produce more Black physicians than Black medical schools, the "role model" situation is very dismal. Besides financial conditions and the relatively inadequate premedical school/college preparation mentioned before, the relative lack of available Black role models in medical schools to nurture Black and minority students is a very important contributing factor responsible for their higher failure rate compared with their White counterparts.

According to Pinn-Wiggins (1990), in order to continue making equal access to medical educational and residency training programs available to minorities, there has to be an increase in the numbers (and ranks) of minorities in institutional settings. These minority faculty are not only more receptive and sensitive to the often unique needs of minority students, but they can also serve as important role models as well. Recent evidence shows that only 1.1 percent (185 of 16,819) of those of professional rank were Black, 1.5 percent (228 of 15,267) were Associate Professors, 2.2 percent (514 of 23,387) were Assistant Professors, and 3.6 percent (212 of 5,924) were Instructors (U.S. Medical School Faculty, 1989).

UNDERREPRESENTATION IN OTHER HEALTH-RELATED PROFESSIONS

Table 23.1 shows the percentage distribution of selected Black health professionals in 1983, 1989, 1991, and 1992. It is important to note that for these four years only dieticians (21%, 17.1%, 19.1%, and 21.3%) exceeded their proportionate representation (i.e., approximately 13%) (U.S. Bureau of the Census, 1990) in the U.S. population. Also, only inhalation therapists had the next closest percentages, albeit lower than the desired 13 percent.

There were decreases in health professionals between 1989, 1991, and 1992. The sharpest decrease was in the dentists' category; in 1989 Blacks constituted 4.3 percent of U.S. dentists, but in 1991 Blacks comprised only 1.5 percent of U.S. dentists. Worse, it decreased further in 1992 when Blacks comprised only 1.1 percent of U.S. dentists. A similar trend was also noted in the areas of pharmacy and speech therapy (see Table 23.1). Interestingly, the percentages of Blacks in the biological and life sciences increased between 1989 and 1991, but decreased between 1991 and 1992. The percentage of Blacks in the aforementioned area increased from 2.4 percent in 1983 to 2.9 percent in 1989, and to 5.2 percent in 1991. From 1989 to 1992, there were decreases in the number of Black chemists (see Table 23.1).

Table 23.1

Percentage Distribution of Selected Black Health Professionals (1983, 1989, 1991, and 1992)

Health Professionals	1983	1989	1991	1992
Health Diagnosing				
Physicians	3.2	3.3	3.2	3.3
Dentists	2.4	4.3	1.5	1.1
Health Assessment & Treatment				
Registered Nurses	6.7	7.2	7.1	8.5
Pharmacists	3.8	4.7	3.4	5.6
Dieticians	21.1	17.1	19.1	21.3
Therapists	7.6	6.4	7.2	8.1
Inhalation	6.5	12.5	10.3	8.3
Physical	9.7	4.8	5.8	4.4
Speech	1.5	3.1	1.3	1.7
Physician Assts.	7.7	6.9	8.0	--
Others				
Psychologists	8.6	7.7	7.8	6.2
Biological and Life Scientists	2.4	2.9	5.2	2.8
Chemists, except biochemists	4.3	5.9	5.2	2.8

Source: U.S. Bureau of the Census citing Bureau of Labor Statistics, Employment and Earnings (Based on Current Population Surveys).

Note: Data for 1992 are not fully comparable with data for prior years because of introduction of the occupational classification system used in 1990.

— Percentages for physician assistants are not available for 1992.

It is worth noting that a bias exists in the literature toward addressing racial disparities only in medicine. Most of the research and writings have been concentrated on the underrepresentation of Black physicians. Little or no emphasis has been laid on the other health providers and related professionals. Given the dynamic nature of health and, therefore, the need to assess the role of other Black health professionals and scientists, this restrictive, medical-oriented approach can be counterproductive to reducing the serious racial disparities in this country. Collectively, medicine and all these related professions contribute to the quality and quantity of health care utilization among Blacks and the subsequent benefits derived from these health care and related experiences.

RATIONALE FOR RACIAL PARITY IN MEDICINE AND RELATED AREAS

Many types of health care providers are organized in various ways and provide a broad range of services and care. Also, individuals' health status depends not only on the health services they receive but on a variety of other factors as well (e.g., inherited characteristics, the physical environment, the social environment, occupational experiences, and individual protective behaviors) (Wilkinson, 1992).

Although there is considerable debate concerning the extent to which health services affect health status (Mechanic, 1979), most will argue that health services utilization, while not the only factor, is certainly a salient factor in determining the individual's health status. Therefore, it is argued that the main rationale for increasing Blacks' representation in medicine and related professions is that such representation will, in turn, positively influence the health care utilization practices of Blacks and, ultimately, improve their overall health status. Also, albeit on a more indirect basis, increased representation of Blacks in related science professions can have a profound impact on the health of Blacks. For example, in the case of the biomedical sciences, increased representation can mean a minority voice to argue for the inclusion of more Blacks (and other minorities) in clinical trials, which can provide new and important information about the race-disease-specific efficacy of pharmaceuticals.

The Issues of Accessibility, Availability, and Acceptability

Increasing the number of Black health providers in medicine and related fields will ultimately improve how accessible, available, and acceptable medical care is to the Black community, subsequently leading to better health care utilization among Blacks. It should be pointed out that, whereas affordability of medical care is a necessary condition for subsequent utilization, it is not a sufficient condition. In reality all four of these conditions need to addressed in any effort aimed at improving the health utilization patterns of Blacks.

The degree of access that Blacks have to health care depends on whether there are barriers that limit, among other things, the availability of services. In this respect Holliman (1983) identified three such factors: (1) Blacks are reluctant to obtain early treatment for illnesses because care is provided by non-Black medical personnel (acceptability); (2) doctors are prejudiced against Blacks (acceptability); and (3) access to medical care is reduced because doctors refuse to provide services to poor communities (availability and accessibility). Additional barriers compound the problem of access for Blacks. First, a relatively small number of health care providers are located in the Black community. Second, economic factors, further complicated by distance, contribute to the search for health care being more affordable. Third, even when health services are accessible, Blacks may face discrimination both racial (Rice & Winn, 1990) and economic (i.e., some providers are reluctant to serve Medicaid patients) (U.S. Congress, 1992, p. 9).

The need to increase the number of Black physicians is driven, in part, by the need for more physicians to provide care to the underserved inner cities and rural communities. Traditionally, these communities have a disproportionate number of Black physicians (Hanft & White, 1986; Nickens & Ready, 1992).

Gray (1977) found that Black physicians were practicing in inner-city and ghetto areas of urban centers and were more likely to be primary care specialists with proportionately more Black patients than their White counterparts. When surveyed, approximately 28 percent of matriculants at the four historically Black medical schools planned on locating their practice within inner-city areas compared to 12 percent of matriculants in nonhistorically Black medical schools (Hanft & White, 1986). These and other factors suggest that increasing the number of Black physicians and other health professionals will complement programs aimed at bringing health care to undeserved areas (Association of American Medical Colleges, 1970; Nickens & Ready, 1992).

STRATEGIES TO ACHIEVE RACIAL PARITY IN MEDICINE AND RELATED PROFESSIONS

The United States is and has been a multicultural society. However, as the discussion presented in this chapter indicates, this multicultural diversity is not reflected on a proportional basis, especially for Blacks, in the medical and related professions. Apart from this issue that urgently needs to be addressed, there are the concomitant sociocultural, economic, and technological changes that are occurring in society; Blacks must have the necessary skills and training to achieve any ensuing benefits.

Projections, for example, suggest that the majority work force of the 21st century will consist of Black and other minority workers. In terms of new jobs, it is suggested that ranking of all jobs according to the skills required on a scale of 1 to 6, with 6 being the highest level of skills, indicates that the fastest-growing jobs will require much higher math, language, and reasoning capabilities than current jobs, while slowly growing jobs require less (Workforce 2000,

1987). Blacks have to be adequately trained and prepared to reap the benefits of these changes. Although this chapter is directly concerned with addressing the issue of increased racial parity in the medical and related professions, it is also indirectly concerned with addressing ways of preparing and making Blacks more competitive for these ongoing and projected changes. Ultimately, sustained improvements in the health of Blacks will come when, as a group, they are better educated and more economically self-sufficient.

Past and Present Efforts

Despite the efforts (reported below) that are being made to increase Black representation in health and related fields, the problem of underrepresentation has worsened over the last 16 years. Urgent intervention strategies are needed to address the situation. Several attempts that have been made to help alleviate the problem have in some cases reported successes. What follows is a review of attempts aimed at bringing parity between Blacks and their White counterparts in medicine and related professions.

Organizational Policies and Efforts

In 1970, the Association of American Medical Colleges (AAMC) recognized the problem and enacted policies aimed at establishing parity in the number of Blacks in medicine relative to their proportion in the U.S. population. Also, the 1971 Federal Act that addressed the underrepresentation of minorities and other disadvantaged persons in health fields is an important effort in trying to solve the problem of underrepresentation of Blacks in health professions and related fields. The above legislation provided funds to health professional schools and nonprofit private institutions that provide programs aimed at removing the disparity between the number of Black health providers and their White counterparts. This legislation led to an increase in the identification and recruitment of minorities and other disadvantaged persons for training in health and related fields. It also tracked students at the undergraduate level and provided counseling and financial aid to promising undergraduate students intending to enter the health profession and related fields (Woode & Lynch, 1992).

In 1991, the AAMC again provided leadership in the drive to solve the underrepresentation problem of Black health providers and related professionals. The cornerstone of the new AAMC campaign was to double the number of underrepresented minority matriculants by the beginning of the next decade. This campaign was aptly called Project 3000 by 2000, in recognition of its primary goal of increasing the number of underrepresented minorities entering the first-year class from its then current level of 1,600 to 3,000 by the beginning of the next century (Petersdorf, 1992).

Organizational Programs

Various institutional efforts at colleges and universities have been attempting to improve, among other things, the preparatory skills that Blacks and other minority groups need to successfully apply, enroll, and matriculate for medical and other related professional schools of their choice. Such programs that have demonstrated success, according to George (1991), include the MEDPREP program sponsored by Southern Illinois University, the Minority Affairs Program at the Washington School of Medicine, the summer intervention programs at the Bowman Gray School of Medicine of Wake Forest University, and the Health Careers Enhancement Programs for minorities at the Case Western Reserve University School of Medicine.

Other programs, according to Petersdorf et al. (1990), also demonstrate the importance of utilizing various strategies to be successful in increasing minority application to and matriculation from medical school. Because of space constraints, only mention is made here of three institutions that have educational programs that serve to better prepare and attract minority students to the sciences. These educational institutions are (a) the University of Virginia; (b) Xavier University, a historically Black university located in New Orleans, Louisiana; and (c) Baylor College of Medicine, located in Houston, Texas.

Recommended Approaches

The large disparities in health and health care alluded to in this chapter (and which are elaborated on in other chapters), along with the fast-changing social, economic, and racial composition and technological contexts of American society, all suggest that innovative, long-term, and successful strategies are needed to address the problem of racial and professional parity. Whereas in some cases successful policies and programs from the past should be kept, in other cases new and bold policies, initiatives, and programs must be introduced.

Recruitment Drives

Recruitment drives can be ineffective if not carried out in a comprehensive manner. For example, many colleges engage only in cost-effective programs, concentrating on the immediate applicant pool (premed) students (see Nickens & Ready, 1992). Therefore, innovative and comprehensive recruitment efforts must be launched that, among other things, identify minority applicant pools at the earlier stages of the educational pipeline.

More Articulation Agreements

Nickens and Ready (1992) suggested that schools should develop articulation agreements, continue providing college-level enrichment programs and postbaccalaureate programs, and take steps to make health professional schools hospitable places for minority students.

The Development of Culturally Sensitive Magnet Schools

In terms of long-term efforts, according to Petersdorf (1992), more magnet health sciences high schools should be created with substantial minority enrollments. It is further suggested, however, that such schools be sensitive to, among other things, the cultural background of minority students in attendance.

National Programs to Attract Minorities

Because many health problems of Black and other minority communities are related to the lack of minority health care providers practicing in minority communities, national programs must be increased to attract minorities to practice medicine in inner-city and rural areas. For example, efforts must be made to solidify and improve operations of the National Health Service Corps Program (Hester & Barber, 1990). According to Pinn-Wiggins (1990), "However, the burden of providing access to the health care system for the medically underserved, and too often the medically indigent, should not be that of the minority physician only" (p. 399).

More "Positive" Atmosphere for Medical School and Related Environments

Health professional schools should provide a conducive atmosphere for minority students. There should be a proportionate number of minority faculty persons who will provide role models for the minority students. These schools should also design programs that increase the attractiveness of the health and related professions by emphasizing the positive attributes—glamor, independence, or income—of the profession.

An Africentric Focus

Where applicable, an Africentric curriculum that is scientifically based should be utilized, from elementary school through high school and, most definitely, at the college and university levels as well. Within such curricula, Black historical contributions to the fields of science, medicine, and related areas should be discussed.

More Effective Dissemination of Information Regarding Economic and Related Supports

For example, information concerning the National Institute of General Medical Sciences (NIGMS) minority initiatives should be made more available to qualified Black and other minority applicants. Essentially, the NIGMS is dedicated to increasing the number of scientists who are Black and from other minority groups presently underrepresented in biomedical research. NIGMS has a Minority Opportunities in Research Programs branch that contains two programs designed to increase the number of minority biomedical scientists: the Minority Access to Research Careers (MARC) and the Minority Biomedical Research Support (MBRS). The MARC Program supports research training from the undergraduate level through the postdoctoral level. In fiscal year 1991, the MARC Program had a budget in excess of $13 million. The MBRS Program awards grants to educational institutions with substantial minority enrollments to support research by faculty members, strengthen the institutions' biomedical research capabilities, and provide opportunities for students to work as part of a research team. (For more information see USDHHS, 1992.)

More Aggressive Recruitment of Minority Scientists

Especially in the era of HIV infection and AIDS, more aggressive efforts must be made to recruit Black and other minority physicians and scientists in the biological and life sciences. These areas of most need include clinical research, pharmacology, epidemiology, biostatistics, and public health, to mention only a few. In a related manner, equally aggressive efforts must be directed to include minorities in ongoing research, especially clinical trials, testing the efficacy of emergent drugs and pharmacological therapy.

Greater Representation of Minorities in Specialty Areas

While minorities must continue to seek primary care positions, they should also seek greater representation in the specialty areas (e.g., hematology, pathology, and oncology). Apart from greater participation in these specialty areas, it has been said, for example, that Blacks also need to be in positions that allow them to publish about themselves and their patients (Pinn-Wiggins, 1990), hence the importance of the *Journal of the National Medical Association.*

Innovative Programs to Attract Potential Students, Especially Early in the "Pipeline"

Such programs could include (a) frequent science fairs to attract minority children to science, (b) computer-assisted math and science programs in high school and college, and (c) the return of retired math and science teachers to volunteer their services to those in most need. Such Black or minority retirees would also serve as effective role models for young Black and other minority inner-city kids.

More Lobbying Efforts to Elevate to a National Priority the Issue of Minority Underrepresentation

Apart from existing legislation and policies that address the underrepresentation of Blacks and other minorities in the medical and other related professions, the problem of underrepresentation and its relationship to minority health in general and Black health in particular must be raised to a higher national priority status. It is worth noting that *Healthy People 2000 Objectives,* the federal government's comprehensive projection of Americans' health in the year 2000 (USDHHS, 1991), did not explicitly address the crucial area of underrepresentation and which solutions might remedy the situation. In short, it is argued that the enactment and aggressive enforcement of a national policy addressing racial parity in medicine and related professions will elevate the issue to the visible position it deserves.

CONCLUSION

The underrepresentation crisis is everyone's problem. Although the issues discussed associated with the underrepresentation of Blacks in health and related fields are varied and complex, representation can be achieved only through collective efforts, comprehensive programs, and innovative strategies. Some of these needed efforts, programs, and strategies were discussed in this chapter along with other recommendations to achieve the desirable goal of racial parity in medicine and related areas. If Blacks experience improvements in their life experiences, which occur, in part, through major changes in the status quo, all Americans will stand to benefit. For Blacks, however, the benefits will be more immediate and most profound as they manifest themselves ultimately in lower morbidity and mortality rates.

REFERENCES

American Council on Education. (1986). Fifth Annual Status Report: Minorities in Higher Education. Washington: Office of Minority Concerns.

Association of American Medical Colleges (AAMC). (1970). Report of the Association of American Medical Colleges Task Force to the Inter-Association Committee on expanding educational opportunities in medicine for blacks and other minority students. Washington, DC.

Association of American Medical Colleges. (1983). U.S. medical students, 1950–2000: A comparison factbook for physicians in the making. Washington, DC.

Association of American Medical Colleges. (1985). Minority students in medical education: Facts and figures II. Washington, DC.

Association of American Medical Colleges. (1986a). Datagram: Financial assistance for medical students, 1984–1985. *Journal of Medical Education, 61,* 695–697.

Association of American Medical Colleges. (1989). Minority students in medical education: Facts and figures (Vol. 5). Washington, DC: Author.

Association of American Medical Colleges. (1992). Minority students in medical education: Facts and figures (Vol. 6). Washington, DC: Author.

Astin, A. W. (1982). Minorities in American higher education. San Francisco: Jossey-Bass.

Baratz, J. C., Ficklen, M. S., King, B., & Rosenbaum, P. (1985). Who is going to medical school? A look at the 1984–85 underrepresented minority medical school applicant pool. Princeton: Educational Testing Service.

Berk, M. L., Berstein, A. B., & Taylor, A. K. (1982). Use and availability of medical care in federally designated health manpower shortage areas. U.S. Department of Health and Human Services, National Center for Health Services Research. Washington, DC.

Berryman, S. (1983). *Who will do science?* New York: Rockefeller Foundation.

CDC. (1990). CDC surveillance summaries: Reports on selected racial/ethnic groups: Maternal and child health. *Morbidity and Mortality Weekly Reports, 39.*

Davis, K. (1986). Aging and the health care system: Economic and structural issues. *Daedalus, 115,* 227–246.

George, A. R. (1991). Minority medical education: An association's view. *Journal of the Student National Medical Association, 4,* 33–37.

Gray, L. C. (1977). The geographic and functional distribution of black physicians: Some research and policy considerations. *American Journal of Public Health, 67,* 519–526.

Gunby, P. (1989). Minority physician training: Critical for improving overall health of nation. *Journal of American Medical Association, 261,* 187–189.

Hanft, R. S., Fishman, L. E., & Evans, W. J. (1983). Blacks and the health professions in the 80's: A national crisis and a time for action. Washington, DC: Association of Minority Health Professions Schools.

Hanft, R. S., & White, C. C. (1986). Changing characteristics of minority school matriculants. Washington, DC: Association of Minority Health Professions Schools.

Hanft, R. S., White, C. C., & Fishman, L. E. (1986). Minorities in the health professions: Continuing crises. Washington, DC: Association of Minority Health Professions Schools.

Healthy People 2000. (1990). National health promotion and disease objectives. DHHS Publication No. (PHS) 91-50213. Washington, DC: Government Printing Office.

Hester, R. D., & Barber, J. B. (1990). Health reforms and the black community. *Journal of the National Medical Association, 82,* 291–292.

Holliman, J. S. (1983). Access to health care. In *Securing access to health care: The ethical implications of differences in availability of health services, volume 2.* Washington, DC: President's Commission for the Study of Ethical Problems in Medicine and Biomedical and Behavioral Research.

Keith, S. N., Bell, R. M., Swanson, A. G., & Williams, A. P. (1985). Effects of affirmative action in medical schools: A study of the class of 1975. *New England Journal of Medicine, 313,* 1519–1525.

Lloyd, S. M., & Johnson, D. G. (1982). Practice patterns of black physicians: Results of a survey of Howard University College of Medicine Alumni. *Journal of the National Medical Association, 74,* 129–144.

Lloyd, S. M., and Miller, R. L. (1989). Black student enrollment in U.S. medical schools. *Journal of the American Medical Association, 261,* 272–274.

Mechanic, D. (1979). Correlates of physician utilization: Why do major multivariate studies of physician utilization find trival psychosocial and organizational effects? *Journal of Health and Social Behavior, 20,* 387–396.

Morais, H. M. (1976). *The history of the Afro-American in medicine.* Cornwell Heights, PA: Publishers Agency.

National Advisory Committee on Black Higher Education and Black Colleges and Universities. (1980). Target date, 2000 A.D.: Goals for achieving higher education equity for Black Americans, volume 1. Washington, DC: U.S. Department of Education.

National Center for Educational Statistics. (1992). *The 1990 Science Report Card: NAEP's Assessment of fourth, eight, and twelfth graders.* Office of Educational Research and Improvement. Washington, DC: U.S. Department of Education.

National Research Council. (1989). *A common destiny: Blacks and American society.* Washington, DC: National Academy Press.

National Science Board Commission on Precollege Education in Mathematics, Science, and Technology. (1983). Educating Americans for the 21st century: A report to the American people and the national science board. Washington, DC.

Nickens, H. W., & Ready, T. (1992). The underrepresentation problem: Minorities in the health professions. A paper prepared for the Henry J. Kaiser Family Foundation Funders Forum Preparing Minorities for Health Professions. Washington, DC: AAMC.

Pearson, W., Jr., & Pearson, L. C. (1986). Race and the baccalaureate origins of American scientists. *Journal of the Association of Social and Behavioral Scientists, 32,* 149–164.

Petersdorf, R. G. (1992). Not a choice, an obligation. *Academic Medicine, 67,* 73–79.

Petersdorf, R. G., Turner, K. S., Nickens, H. W., and Ready, T. (1990). Minorities in medicine: Past, present, and future. *Academic Medicine, 65,* 663–670.

Pinn-Wiggins, V. W. (1990). The future of medical practice and its impact on minority physicians. *Journal of the National Medical Association, 82,* 398–401.

Reid-Wallace, C. (1992). Medical schools and America 2000. *Academic Medicine, 67,* 380–381.

Report of the Secretary's Task Force on Black and Minority Health. (1985). Executive Summary, Volume 1. USDHHS, Washington, DC: Government Printing Office.

Rice, M. F., & Winn, M. (1990). Black political health care in America: A political perspective. *Journal of the National Medical Association, 82,* 429–437.

Rice, M. F., & Winn, M. (1990). Black health care in America: A political perspective. *Journal of the National Medical Association, 82,* 429–434.

Sandson, J. I. (1983). A crisis in medical education: The high cost of student financial assistance. *New England Journal of Medicine, 308,* 1286–1289.

Shea, S., & Fullilove, M. T. (1985). Entry of black and minority students into U.S. medical schools: Historical perspective and recent trends. *New England Journal of Medicine, 313,* 933–940.

Simpson, C., & Aronoff, R. (1988). Factors affecting the supply of minority physicians in 2000. *Public Health Reports, 103,* 178–184.

U.S. Bureau of the Census. 1984. Earnings by Occupation and Education. Washington, DC.

U.S. Bureau of the Census. 1990. Population distributions by racial identification. Washington, DC.

U.S. Congress. (1992). Conceptual framework and general methodological issues (pp. 41–50). Office of Technology Assessment, Does health insurance make a difference? Background paper, OTA-BP-H-99. Washington, DC: Government Printing Office.

U.S. Department of Health and Human Services. (1986). Estimates and projections of black and Hispanic physicians, dentists, and pharmacists to 2010 (DHHS Publication No. HRS-P-DV-86-1). Washington, DC: Government Printing Office.

U.S. Department of Health and Human Services. (1990). Seventh Report to the President and Congress on the status of health personnel in the United States (DHHS Publication No. HRS-P-OD-90-1. Washington, DC: Government Printing Office.

U.S. Department of Health and Human Services. (1991). Locating resources for healthy people 2000 health promotion projects. Office of Disease Prevention and Health Promotion, Public Health Service. Washington, DC: Government Printing Office.

U.S. Department of Health and Human Services. (1992). Minority Access to Research Careers Program. Public Health Service, NIH Publication No. 92-3329.

U.S. Medical School Faculty. (1989). The numbers book. Washington, DC: Association of American Medical Colleges.

Wilkinson, R. G. (1992). Income distribution and life expectancy. *British Medical Journal, 304,* 165–166.

Woode, M. K., & Lynch, K. B. (1992). Effective strategies producing black health care providers. In Braithwaite, B. L., & S. E. Taylor (Eds.), *Health Issues in the Black Community.* San Francisco: Jossey-Bass.

Workforce 2000: Work and Workers of the 21st century. Executive Summary. 1987. Indianapolis, IN: Hudson Institute.

V

Legal and Social Policy Issues

24

Politics and Health: The Coming Agenda for a Multiracial and Multicultural Society

Stephanie Kong, B. Waine Kong, and
Singleton B. McAllister

INTRODUCTION

As America heads into the 21st century, the crisis in health care delivery has become increasingly evident to health care providers, managers, politicians, and the general public. After three decades of spending up to 13 percent of the gross national product on health care, many Americans, especially Black Americans, appear to die as often and from the same types of diseases that affected minorities disproportionately in the 1940s and 1950s. What is different today, however, is that heart disease, cancer, and strokes have overtaken infectious diseases as the leading causes of death in minorities as well as in Americans in general (Davies & Felder, 1990).

There is a conflict in American medicine. As a humanistic democratic society, Americans believe that universal access to health care is a basic entitlement of citizenship. However, the cost to implement this basic entitlement may be prohibitive. The health initiatives of the past three decades have emphasized improved access and quantity of available medical services as opposed to effective access, preventive health maintenance, and case management of patients with chronic diseases.

In the health industry, effective access is defined as the ability of patients to receive medically necessary services in a time frame that promotes quality of life and longevity and decreases health risks. Preventive health maintenance is a proactive relationship between the physician and the patient that promotes positive health behaviors and reduces health risks. If health risks are left unabated, they will lead to premature death and disability. Case management involves care planning for the treatment of chronic diseases and catastrophic diseases. Anyone with a chronic disease, such as hypertension or diabetes, must come to terms with the fact that he/she has to alter certain lifestyle parameters until his/her blood pressure or blood glucose is under control. As medical intervention is usually intrusive, physicians must utilize any and all resources to aid the patient in dealing with life-altering diseases.

This chapter examines the interrelationship between politics and health in the context of American society that is both multiracial and multicultural. Focusing specifically on African Americans, it discusses emerging needs and problems, reasons for racial disparities in health, available options, federal and other initiatives, and some selected areas of needed change. The chapter ends with a list of practical recommendations that can serve to improve health care for Americans in general and low-income minorities (e.g., African Americans) in particular.

RACIAL DISPARITIES IN HEALTH AND RELATED CARE

A crisis in health care for minorities exists today: far too many minority people continue to suffer and die from preventable diseases and conditions. It is important to note that patients who do not have health insurance are less likely to be given routine diagnostic tests, less likely to have some surgical procedures performed, and more likely to die during a hospital stay than patients who are insured. African-American men, on average, do not live long enough to collect the benefits from the Social Security program they may have contributed to for 30 years (Balfe & Bieber, 1986; Tallon, 1989).

Even with everything else held equal, African Americans would have less access to health care. After comparing the morbidity and mortality of a group of African-American and White physicians for over thirty years, Dr. John Thomas of Meharry Medical College concluded that the rate of death among African-American physicians mimics that of low-income African Americans. This does not necessarily mean that higher socioeconomic status does not correlate with improved health status and longevity. Unique issues associated with being an African-American physician may be present. However, African Americans, regardless of socioeconomic status, have more heart disease but less coronary bypass surgery and angioplasty and transplants, more renal failure but less kidney transplantation (Thorpe, Siegal & Dailey, 1989; Walker, 1992).

AREAS IN NEED OF CHANGE

Racial disparities in health can be corrected, in part, by the systematic monitoring of patients' quality of life and by implementing culturally sensitive community-based risk-reduction programs (e.g., smoking cessation, exercise, dietary improvements, and early detection of diseases), which can help to prevent or control health risk factors in high-risk minority communities. The top ten causes of death can be significantly reduced by behavior life-style changes. Preventive health practices could eliminate up to 45 percent of deaths from cardiovascular diseases, 23 percent of deaths from cancer, and more than 50 percent of the disabling complications of diabetes (USDHHS, 1990).

Health planners need to design systems that consider the unique access problems that impede the effective delivery of health for all segments of our society, especially those Americans who are socially and economically disenfranchised. Special care and planning must also be directed to those patients who have "age" as a complicating factor. Flexibility is another desirable characteristic that should be incorporated into the system to provide a range of necessary and sufficient health care for all citizens. Without consideration of these components, any national reform will fall short of the commitment to provide needed health care to a multiracial, multicultural population.

Although most doctors and lay citizens believe that the political realm of social inequities in health is not a part of their responsibility, all segments of the population in fact need to participate actively in planning for the future of health care. Any segment of the population that does not participate will most likely be disadvantaged and suffer related consequences.

The estimated costs of supporting the American health care system exceed $800 billion. Expenditures for African Americans' health care exceed $50 billion per year. In one way or the other, health care is being addressed by religious, private, and voluntary organizations, government agencies, and commercial and industrial enterprises as well as individuals (Johnsson, 1992). Even with 34 million Americans without medical coverage, a massive infusion of money is probably not what is needed to assure adequate health care for all citizens.

On a per capita basis, the United States already spends more than any other country on health care. What is needed is reform that assures effective access for all citizens, cost control, and improved quality of life. While health care reform will require a high degree of cooperation between consumers, doctors, insurance companies, health maintenance organizations (HMOs), business leaders, and government officials to remove the barriers to health care for minorities, complete cooperation is not likely. There are too many competing interests to expect unified solutions. As much as health planners try, it is impossible to design and advocate a system that does not threaten the interests of some segment of the health care system. At the same time, the costs of medical care cannot continue to accelerate indefinitely. Because the health care industry will have to do more for less, the intractable and chronic health problems of minorities pose a very real challenge to society.

SELECTED AREAS OF CONCERN

Public Law 101–527, a 1990 act designed to improve the health of individuals of minority groups who are from disadvantaged backgrounds, provides a good summary of important areas of concern relating to minority health affairs. A selection of these areas follows.

- Racial and ethnic minorities are disproportionately represented among individuals from disadvantaged backgrounds.
- The health status of individuals from disadvantaged backgrounds, including racial and ethnic minorities, in the United States is significantly lower than the health status of the general population of the United States.
- Minorities suffer disproportionately high rates of cancer, stroke, heart disease, diabetes, substance abuse, acquired immune deficiency syndrome (AIDS), and other diseases and disorders.
- The incidence of infant mortality among minorities is almost double that for the general population.
- Blacks, Hispanics, and Native Americans constitute approximately 12 percent, 7.9 percent, and 0.01 percent, respectively, of the population of the United States.
- Blacks, Hispanics, and Native Americans in the United States constitute approximately 3 percent, 4 percent, and less than 0.01 percent, respectively, of physicians and 2.7 percent, 1.7 percent, and less than 0.01 percent, respectively, of nurses.
- The number of individuals in the health profession who are from disadvantaged backgrounds should be increased for the purpose of improving the access of other such individuals to health services.
- Minority health professionals have historically tended to practice in low-income areas and to serve minorities.
- Minority health professionals have historically tended to engage in general proactive medicine and specialties providing primary care.
- Access to health care can be substantially improved by increasing the number of minority health professionals.

Minorities have not benefitted equitably from the dramatic improvements in medical procedures, technology, knowledge about disease processes, and preventive health over the last century. While there has been an increase in life expectancy, the health and death gap between minorities and White Americans continue to be wide across the entire life span (USDHHS, 1990).

African Americans, particularly men, have increased mortality in 13 of the 15 leading causes of death. According to the U.S. Department of Health and Human Services, life expectancy for African Americans is 6.2 years less than for Whites. The average White female in the United States lives 14 years longer than the average African-American male (USDHHS, 1990).

EXPLANATIONS FOR RACIAL DISPARITIES IN HEALTH

The health status of African Americans and other disadvantaged groups will continue to lag as long as disparities in education, jobs, living conditions, and opportunities persist. It can be said that health is a function of the social, economic, and physical environments interacting with one's genetic endowments. Health is always more than simply a medical issue. Although various explanations can be offered as to why racial disparities in the prevalence of certain diseases exist, four models discussed by Thomas (1992) will suffice at this point.

The Genetic Model

This model works on the hypothesis that the distribution of certain genes explains racial disparities in health. The theory downplays the environment's influence and indicates that the best thing one can inherit is advantageous genes, because the environment asserts a very limited influence on one's life expectancy. People's health status, then, is a function of their predispositions. However, biological determinism has severe limitations. There is no hard evidence to show that racial differences in health status have a genetic basis. Health is a dynamic concept that interacts with physiological and social factors.

The Behavioral Model

This model holds that health outcomes are the result of an individual's lifestyle—habits, customs, how one "chooses" to live. High-risk behaviors include cigarette smoking, high-fat diets, lack of exercise, unsafe sex, refusal to take advantage of available health care and health information, ignoring symptoms, and solving conflicts with violence. Flaws include a lack of understanding of the historical roots of these behaviors and its potential for blaming the victim. Nonetheless, when the behavioral model is properly applied, a thorough understanding of it will be helpful in planning for community health interventions. Real savings in health care will only be realized through the promotion of preventive health that involves individual life-styles as well as environmental and social factors as they impact on preventive measures.

The Socioeconomic Model

This model holds that differences in health status are economically based. Low incomes generate less "healthy" life-styles. The compromises that one makes when economically disadvantaged produce poor health outcomes. The stresses and frustrations of daily living increase high-risk behaviors and promote imprudent choices. When one is in pain, quick fixes are very appealing. A person just trying to get enough calories to survive will not have the luxury of choosing what he or she eats. Low-paying jobs place these workers in the most unsanitary and accident-prone circumstances. A concentration of poor minorities produces an over-large demand on community resources, resulting in overcrowded and inadequately supported clinics and substandard, ill-equipped hospitals. These factors result in higher mortality, inadequate housing, and overburdened social services that can deny minorities access to health care.

The Social Status Model

This model holds that disparities in health status are a result of the social stratification of American society that encourages continuing discrimination against minorities. The class structure produces inequities for oppressed groups in every facet of life. Health status is but one area. Less access to education also affects health beliefs and health-seeking behaviors by promoting "home remedies" and a stigma associated with seeking help.

The long-term solution to health disparities between minorities and White Americans can and should be addressed by the sociopolitical process. The 1992 national elections brought universal access to health care to center stage. Now that there is a Democratic president and a Democratic majority in the Senate and House of Representatives, Americans will have a chance to assess various Democratic proposals.

SOME AVAILABLE OPTIONS

Most health planners now embrace some form of managed care as the wave of the future. This trend does not minimize the fact that powerful interest groups who stand to benefit or lose by changes in the existing health care system are articulate and formidable. Any change in the financing, organizing, and delivering of health care goods and services will be both resisted by some and promoted by others who stand to gain.

The reported success of managed care in the management of patients with less-expensive services and reducing costs is encouraging (Smith, 1991). Also, most forms of managed care and prepayment plans have achieved lower costs for total health care (Hoy, Curtis & Rice, 1991). According to Kronenfeld (1993), "Managed care is a term used in the last 5 or so years that describes attempts to control use of services, to require prechecking with the insurance company before certain procedures or surgeries are done, and to help an individual co-ordinate care. HMOs (health maintenance organizations), PPOs (preferred provider organizations), and IPAs (independent practice associations) are all examples of managed care in today's health care environment" (p. 7).

It is much cheaper to help a patient to stop smoking than to pay for oncology services later. Citizens can be taught to take care of most of their health problems and also become realistic about what medicine can and cannot do for them. A common cold will last for 7 days if a doctor is involved and a week without medical care. Managed care is the least likely to disrupt business as usual and most likely to reduce waste. Managed care can also cap costs to employers. Most of the savings, however, come from reduced need for hospital and physician services (Robinson, 1991). It is inconceivable, then, that this concept of managed care will be omitted from any plan adopted by the Clinton Administration.

Although there are several options to explore, currently reform-minded politicians are looking at the following 6 options:

1. The "Pay or Play" option requires all employers to provide coverage for their employees. If employers choose not to insure their employees, they will have to pay a surcharge into a special government-controlled fund. A governmental agency or a managed care organization would, in turn, supply coverage (Springer & Lundberg, 1992).

2. The "Tax Credits" option gives employers tax credits to enable low-income citizens to buy coverage. Health insurers back "small-group reform" that would make it easier for small businesses to obtain insurance coverage for their employees. Twenty states already have some form of this plan (Sullivan, 1992).

3. The "Expanded Medicaid" option would cover people who are unattractive to insurance companies and who are too poor to buy insurance even with tax credits. This plan would expand the Medicaid program to provide health care to the unemployed and eligible low-wage earners. The disincentive in this system is that the burden is shifted to taxpayers to cover people who insurance companies will not cover. Taxpayers are not likely to think kindly about any system that raises taxes. In addition, because of the low level of reimbursement through the Medicaid program, these patients often do not receive the best care. Other key features include federal statutory authority to preempt state-mandated benefits and not to allow insurance companies to cancel high-cost members. Insurance would be available to all employees of a group regardless of preexisting medical conditions (Tallon, 1989).

4. The "Single Payer" option is the Canadian or national health insurance system that covers everyone. The plan is resisted by most physicians, who would go on salary; hospitals, which would be more controlled; and insurance companies, which might become superfluous. It is, however, a good solution for patients who are presently shut out of the private insurance system. This system also addresses the fear of many workers that they will lose their coverage on becoming unemployed. The single-payer model also assumes a much diminished role for insurance companies. Most single-payer plans allow individuals to choose among contracted providers.

The single payer system has universality, portability, accessibility, comprehensiveness, and public administration. If the United States were to adopt the Canadian system, the monies presently allocated to private insurance, Medicare, Medicaid, and grants to states would be redirected to fund this single-payer, publicly financed insurance plan. The single-payer system eliminates cost shifting from privately to publicly funded programs, facilitates data collection and public health research (especially outcome data), and allows one agency to negotiate all health care contracts, provider fees, and the orderly introduction of technology. Given the resistance of the present providers and the universal distrust that government can run something so large and complicated, it will not be easy to adopt a single-payer system in the United States in the near future, especially as the plan is being characterized as "socialized medicine" (Russell, 1989).

5. The "Hospital Based" option would maximize the situation that an abundance of hospitals and employees are available to take care of the health needs of their communities. This plan would expand the hospitals' role in primary care. Segments of a community would be allocated to hospitals for their care. While the hospitals would prefer this option, hospitals are perceived to be "dinosaurs" and stuck with systems that are unresponsive. If the government cannot manage health care, hospitals are not likely to do better.

6. The "Enthoven" Plan (Clinton, 1992), which is also called "managed competition," is most likely to be adopted by the Clinton Administration. It would establish a competitive health care system that rewards the most efficient health agencies and providers with the most customers, thereby creating an economic incentive for effective use of health care resources. The plan would include a private-sector system, employer-based coverage, controlled costs for insurance, and community standards to determine quantity and quality of care. Consumers would be able to shop for coverage by comparing price and quality. Small businesses could obtain affordable coverage through purchasing cooperatives.

At the heart of the managed competition system is a change in the tax treatment of employer-provided health benefits. Currently, employer-provided benefits are tax free, regardless of cost. Under managed competition, the tax break would be limited to the cost of the lowest-priced comprehensive plan offered in a given area. This is intended to put the breaks on medical inflation. The down side of this plan is that another layer of administration will be added along with increasing costs.

HEALTH REFORM AND THE STATES

According to the Constitution, the responsibility for health and welfare rightfully belongs with the states. The preemption clause, however, gives the federal government the right and responsibility to intervene in this issue, provided the states are not excluded. While most states will begin reform slowly and will readily relinquish control and costs to the federal government, several states are becoming impatient with the "promises" of the federal government for the past 20 years and have gone ahead with their own plans.

Minnesota is setting up a state-subsidized insurance program to help families who work but have no insurance. The money to fund this program comes from a 2 percent tax on the income of doctors, hospitals, and other health providers.

Florida has guaranteed basic health care to all its 2.5 million uninsured citizens by 1995. Governor Chiles believes this can be accomplished if existing allocations are managed better. A new law gives employees until the end of 1994 to offer medical coverage to their workers.

Vermont narrowed its options to two proposals to provide universal health care. One would be based on a single-payer plan similar to the Canadian system; the other would be a multi-payer plan more like the German model. Their intention is to implement one plan by 1995. Vermont's sweeping reform package also calls for centralized health planning and for global budgeting, which means that the state will have to decide in advance on how much it will spend on health care annually. Under this plan, insurance companies must accept everyone who applies, although rates can be adjusted for preexisting medical conditions.

Oregon will pay only for top-priority medical procedures. Based on priority rankings of 709 procedures, the Oregon Medical program, as proposed, would no longer pay for anything below item 587 and excludes payment for the common cold, hemorrhoid removal, and life support for babies born prematurely. While rationing services, Oregon will be able to cover an additional 120,000 people with Medicaid benefits.

A STEP IN THE RIGHT DIRECTION

In recognition of the relatively short life span and the burden of chronic illness among minorities, the Office of Minority Programs (OMP) formed a fact-finding team headed by the presidents of Meharry Medical College and Xavier University. The charge to the team was to recommend ways to significantly increase the participation of minorities in all phases of biomedical research and to reduce the burden of illness among minorities through targeted research (Minority Programs Fact Finding Team Recommendations, 1992).

Within the four groups identified as "minorities" by the OMP (African Americans, Hispanic Americans, American Indians, and Asian Americans), the six major health problems were heart disease, stroke and hypertension, homicide and preventable accidents, cancers, infant mortality and perinatal morbidity, cirrhosis and liver failure, and diabetes.

The fact-finding team recognized the interrelationship among health, social, and economic well-being and recommended that the National Institutes of Health (NIH) do the following:

- Provide clear goals and adequate funding for research to extend healthy life and to reduce the burden of illness among minority populations to equal that of the general population by the year 2000. Research programs should be focused in three areas: life-span issues, chronic diseases, and infectious diseases.

- Undertake additional longitudinal data-collection studies among the many diverse groups referred to as minority in order to better determine what factors affect their health status and needs. More should be done to increase the participation of minorities in clinical trials and epidemiological studies.

- Develop new and varied research methods and procedures to address successfully the health needs of minorities.

- Sanction OMP to ensure that programs meet overall guidelines, to ensure the general and timely dissemination of research results among the minority communities, and to encourage collaboration between major research institutions and minority institutions.
- Improve the scientific literacy of all children in the United States, with particular emphasis on convincing more minority children to choose science as careers.
- Support the training and professional development of science teachers, especially minority teachers.
- Increase the recruitment and retention of minority science students at the pre-college and college entrance levels.
- Help to increase the transfer of talented minority students who have demonstrated scientific knowledge and skills from associate or technician programs at 2-year institutions to baccalaureate programs in the biomedical and life sciences at 4-year institutions.
- Support the training of undergraduate minority students in the biomedical sciences.
- Use the NIH-sponsored Predoctoral Fellowship Program and its various institutional training grants to support the transition of undergraduate minority research trainees to graduate and investigator training.
- Fund an array of programs that will support the professional development of minority biomedical scientists.
- Expand programs at institutions with a significant minority presence as a method of promoting "centers of excellence" for the training of minority science students and the conduct of state-of-the-art faculty research.
- Continue its historic progress along the path that leads to the achievement of the twin goals of the NIH minority health initiative—to improve the health of minorities and to increase the participation of minorities in all phases of biomedical research.

Federal Minority Health Initiative

Partly as a response to these recommendations, NIH, under the leadership of former Secretary of Health and Human Resources Dr. Louis Sullivan and NIH Director Dr. Bernadine Healy, increased funding for programs aimed at minorities under the "Minority Health Initiative" (Palca, 1992). The components of the health-promotion program include $20 million to support the following:

1. behavioral intervention trials on perinatal research nutrition and low-birth-weight infants
2. behavioral interventions aimed at ages 10–24 with emphasis on violence and sexual behavior

3. minority participation in health screening and adherence to medical regimens
4. research on factors affecting severity and progression of chronic diseases and relieving impairment
5. modification of behaviors that adversely affect health

The allocations for the training initiatives will provide research training, support for students receiving master's degrees to move to institutions that grant doctorates in biological sciences, support middle and high school life-science programs, and evaluate its success in recruiting, motivating, and training minority students.

This encouraging initiative takes several steps in the right direction. At this moment in history, there is probably more sensitivity to minority health issues than at any previous time. There is every indication that the new Democratic administration will be more responsive to minority needs in general. The appointees are, by reputation, genuinely committed to equal participation of minorities in a pluralistic society.

IMPLICATIONS OF PRESENT AND FUTURE VIEWS

Contemporary health philosophy has moved to an emphasis on the individual life-style rather than on associated social and political conditions. Focusing on issues over which the individual has control ("blaming the victim") is much more palatable to politicians than focusing on issues that require the expenditure of large sums of scarce resources. As a result, doctors are exhorted to get people to change their life-styles and not to focus on issues of access. The epidemiologists have provided much ammunition (most of it believable) for politicians and social planners to convince the public that change in the wider social sphere is not where the focus should be. The implications of this view, some of which are mentioned below, can be far-reaching for minority groups in general and African Americans in particular.

- In a society where African Americans and other minorities may be seen by some as inferior and deviant from the White norm, ill-health is perceived as just another example of how undisciplined and shortsighted minorities are.
- Ethnicity is increasingly invoked to explain epidemiological differences. The impact of other factors such as class and wealth are often not considered when ethnic comparisons are made. In focusing on African Americans as "culturally distinct," we also focus on the subculture as deviant, deficient, and resistant to change.
- The complex problem of becoming "ill" and the inequities in seeking help from the health care system and benefiting from medical care are often considered to be the result of peoples' beliefs, experiences and expectations rather than a wider crisis.

Indifference to diversity does not ensure equal access. If difference and diversity are not considered and we carry on as business as usual, minorities will receive less favorable treatment. The height of racism is "treating everyone the same." Understanding and sensitivity to the needs of "individuals" are needed to meet unique needs. The haste of some to characterize the behavior of a patient as ignorant, hostile, or uncooperative may result from the insensitivity and lack of understanding of health care providers.

Minority physicians see a disproportionate number of patients who have no insurance or who are inadequately covered by Medicaid and Medicare. For sub-specialty care, minority patients are primarily sent to White specialists, White hospitals, and White diagnostic and treatment centers primarily because there are very few privately owned minority hospitals, HMOs, Independent Practice Associations (IPAs), Preferred Provider Organizations (PPOs), or other health care institutions.

Minorities are underrepresented in most health and allied health professions as well as in upper-level health policy and managerial positions in major health-related facilities and organizations such as boards, commissions, hospitals, academic health centers, HMO's, nursing homes, and public health departments. As a result, cultural factors and the cultural acceptability of such services may also serve as a major barrier to health care for minorities. Often, health services and programs are developed and implemented for minorities without the benefit of input or participation from the minority communities.

On the other hand, programs that may be culturally sensitive to the values, beliefs, and social structures of minorities are not considered by White administrators. In addition, racial and cultural differences (e.g., language and lifestyle) between provider and patient can impede access to health services. Minority patients may experience better medical outcomes if their providers are from the same cultural background as well as being able to communicate better and have a more positive influence on many of the factors that affect health outcome (Protor & Rosen, 1982).

The health care system fails if patients are made to believe they are always causing problems or deviant if they are single parents, homosexual, do not speak "correct English," overly modest about revealing their bodies (even their faces) to nurses and physicians, or wear odd-looking clothes and "dreadlocks." Moreover, it may be necessary to have someone else (sometimes a child) interpret and explain a sensitive health problem. Without sensitivity or insight about patients' cultures, certain inappropriate actions may ensue. For example, Muslims may be served bacon and eggs and Rastafarians (a religious sect initially hailing from Jamaica) may be served pork chops. Also, visiting times are inflexible and do not account for transportation and work schedules.

Currently, rather than identifying and meeting the needs of each individual in a justified response and providing appropriate services to a multiracial society, the institutional response is to see the needs of minorities as "abnormal" or "special." This attitude automatically generates resistance.

RECOMMENDATIONS FOR IMPROVING HEALTH CARE

Efforts to improve health care seem to be experiencing a "bandwagon effect." A good example is the more than 300 health care bills introduced as of April 1992 in the 102nd Congress (Mizrahi, 1992). Based on the previous discussion in this chapter, the following recommendations are offered to improve the current system of health care:

1. Employers should be required either to offer employer-based health insurance or to pay a payroll tax. All Americans not currently covered by employer-based health insurance would be covered by a single unified federal health plan that combines Medicare, Medicaid, and state-mandated benefits.

2. Insurance companies must be prohibited from excluding individuals for preexisting conditions and waiting periods.

3. The federal government should promote competition by privatizing the consolidated federal health plan.

4. All programs approved by the national standard benefit criteria should be required to have utilization management and quality assurance protocols.

5. Provider payment should mandate physicians and hospitals to accept a standard payment for services and eliminate cost shifting.

6. Medical liability should be reformed by mandating arbitration, placing restrictions on contingency fees, requiring that expert witnesses be certified, and elimination of joint liability.

7. Incentives must be provided for the redistribution of physician specialties by providing grants to medical students who select primary care as their specialty; scholarships and low interest loans for medical students in underserved areas with forgiveness of loans after 5 years of service in underserved areas; tax breaks for physicians who serve in underserved areas; federal grants for primary care residency programs; and tax credits for corporations who donate to primary care residency programs.

8. It is mandatory that federal programs as well as other health insurance carriers provide substantial support for culturally relevant preventive health programs in minority communities. These programs should promote healthy life-styles and educate African Americans and other minority citizens about effectively interfacing with the health care system.

9. Physicians who meet objective professional standards should not be excluded from managed-care organizations that contract with the federal government.

10. Programs should encourage the availability of private long-term care as now in existence that is associated with accidental death and dismem-

berment insurance. Also, the federal government should offer tax credits for the purchase of long-term care coverage and provide subsidies to low-income African-American and other minority beneficiaries, enabling them to purchase private long-term care insurance.

It is reasoned that this 10-point program is straightforward, fair, and attainable, benefits the economy, does not overburden taxpayers, and, most important improves health care for all Americans.

SUMMARY

Intense, well-targeted, community-based, and culturally appropriate outreach and education programs are necessary to reach and educate minorities and enhance their access to health services. It is essential that health professionals, religious leaders, elected officials, and other community leaders become involved in promoting healthy life-styles and behaviors to bring about improvements in health care to their communities.

Racism is subtly incorporated into most services from mainstream institutions. As a result, health planners and providers need to recognize minority perspectives or racism as major issues on the general agenda of health services. A comprehensive approach to overcome racism in health care is essential to avoid ineffective solutions. The elimination of discrimination in health care employment would increase sensitivity to minority patients. The more White physicians and staff become accustomed to relating to minorities as equals and superiors, the more positive attitudes and sensitivity will increase.

Minorities in the United States are victims of the existing health care system—lacking access to appropriate, affordable, and quality health services. In spite of the economic progress of some minorities, a substantial portion remain disproportionately poor, experience significantly higher rates of chronic diseases and mortality, and are substantially more likely to be uninsured. General improvement in the health care system and increased access will not substantially alter this reality. Special focus is needed to meet these minority and race-related health and other needs. Minorities in general and African Americans in particular are more likely to respond to culturally sensitive, intimate, and personal interventions that cannot be planned without substantial input and participation from members of these groups.

REFERENCES

Balfe, B. E., & Bieber, G. (1986). A health policy agenda for the American people: The issues and their development. *Journal of the American Medical Association, 256,* 1021–1026.

Clinton, B. (1992). The Clinton Health Care Plan. *New England Journal of Medicine, 327,* 804–807.

Davies, N. E., & Felder, L. H. (1990). Applying brakes to the runaway American health care system. *Journal of the American Medical Association, 263,* 73–76.

Hoy, E. W., Curtis, R. E., & Rice, T. (1991). Change and growth in managed care. *Health Affairs, 10,* 18–36.

Johnsson, J. (1992). State health reform: Five trends that will transform hospitals. *Hospitals* (October 5), 2638.

Kronenfeld, J. J. (1993). *Controversial issues in health care policy.* Newbury Park, London: Sage Publications.

Minority Programs Fact Finding Team Recommendations. (1992). Presented to the National Institutes of Health Associate Director for Minority Programs (February).

Mizrahi, T. (1992). Toward a national health care system: Progress and problems. *Health and Social Work, 17,* 167–171.

Palca, J. (1992). NIH spells out plans for a $45 million initiative. *Science, 256* (April), 24.

Protor, E., & Rosen, A. (1982). Expectations and preferences for counsellor race and their relation to intermediate treatment outcomes. *Journal of Counseling Psychology, 28,* 40–46.

Public Law 101–527. (1990). 101st Congress, November 6th, (H.R. 5702), 104 Stat. 2311.

Robinson, J. C. (1991). HMO market penetration and hospital cost inflation in California. *Journal of the American Medical Association, 20,* 2719–2723.

Russell, L. (1989). Proposed: A comprehensive health care system for the poor. *Brookings Review, 7,* 13–20.

Smith, L. (1991). A cure for what ails medical care. *Fortune, 1* (July), 44–49.

Springer, M., & Lundberg, G. D. (Eds.). (1992). *Caring for the uninsured and underinsured.* Chicago, IL: American Medical Association.

Sullivan, L. S. (1992). The Bush administration's health care plan. *New England Journal of Medicine, 327,* 804–807.

Tallon, J. R. (1989). A health policy agenda proposal including the poor. *Journal of the American Medical Association, 261,* 1044.

Thomas, V. G. (1992). Explaining health disparities between African-American and white populations: Where do we go from here? *Journal of the National Medical Association, 84,* 837–840.

Thorpe, K. E., Siegal, J. E., and Dailey, T. (1989). Including the poor: The fiscal impacts of Medicaid expansion. *Journal of the American Medical Association, 261,* 1003–1007.

U.S. Department of Health and Human Services. (1990). *Vital Statistics of the United States 1988.* Mortality (Part B) volume 11. USDHHS Publication No. (PHS) 90–1102. Washington, DC: Government Printing Office.

Walker, B. (1992). Health policies and the black community. In R. Brathwaite and S. E. Taylor (Eds.), *Health issues in the black community* (pp. 315–320). San Francisco: Jossey-Bass Publishers.

25

Barriers to Health Services Utilization and African Americans

Woodrow Jones, Jr., and Antonio A. Rene

INTRODUCTION

Health beliefs and behaviors are determined by a number of factors, including the availability, accessibility, and quality of the health care delivery system. In addition to these factors, race has been shown to be particularly relevant to how health care is delivered in America. Although it admittedly has been difficult to separate the influence of related variables, such as socioeconomic class and acculturation, the fact remains that African Americans face barriers to the attainment of adequate health services.

Despite the recent advances in the reduction of mortality and morbidity, there are still disparities between African Americans and White Americans on every measure of illness and death (Blendon, Aiken, Freeman & Corey, 1989). These disparities have become a consistent reality for each new cohort and do not seem to be diminished by governmental efforts toward health promotion and prevention. As with other federal programs, health promotion and prevention programs suffer from vague statutory guidance, inept administration, poor coordination, and unanticipated consequences (Blum, 1974).

The condition of an individual's health is, in part, beyond the control of governmental policies. If we accept the view of health as involving the interaction of heredity, environment, and behavior, we can quickly surmise that government policies or individual behavioral changes can not eradicate genetic factors. In such cases, all an individual can do is take preventive measures to reduce the risk of the onset of disease.

Environmental determinants, including such diverse elements as clean air, water pollution, housing, and crime, directly impact the health conditions of populations. These determinants are directly influenced by public and private decisions about the production of resources, as well as by governmental policies to reduce the effects of the environment on health. Policies directed toward air and water pollution, housing, poverty, welfare, and families all contribute to an environment that is either supportive or repressive of health activities and can influence the individual's feeling of well-being.

Health behaviors are important in reducing the risk of many illnesses. Yet, environmental and social constraints work to limit the individual's ability to develop beneficial health practices. Poor housing, poverty, crime, and unemployment create an environment in which health care is not a high priority (McCulloch, 1989). Furthermore, lacking control over their environment prevents many African Americans from exercising health practices that would prolong life and allow them a greater sense of well-being (Rodin, Timko & Harris, 1985).

Health services reflect the matrix of social, economic, and political factors that segment American society. Cultural diversification can serve only to exacerbate these differences when patients interact with medical practitioners whose orientation toward the health care system is totally incongruous (Romano, 1990). It is at this critical point that race and ethnicity directly influence the interaction and subsequent experiences between patients and health care providers.

This chapter examines explanations of differences in utilization behavior and the pattern of utilization in the African American community. The thesis presented here is that specific problems faced by African Americans prevent them from developing the health behaviors necessary for a healthy life-style. Problems of access continue to undermine their ability to utilize health services in a society that claims to have the best health care system in the world.

EXPLAINING DIFFERENCES IN UTILIZATION BEHAVIORS

Three major factors explain the health utilization behaviors of African Americans: institutional racism, economic inequality, and access barriers. Institutional racism focuses on the discriminatory practice of the health care delivery system. Economic inequality has a direct bearing on the amount and quality of health care one can purchase. The final explanation focuses on the barriers to access to health services. Each of these explanations has a common thread, that race is a factor in the distribution of health care services in this country.

Institutional Racism

Institutional racism has been an important part of the explanation of why African Americans underutilize medical services (Gayles, 1972). Discrimination in the provision of medical services stems from the historical relationship between African Americans and dominant medical institutions in the South. During the slavery period, slaves received good primary care because of their property value (Rice, 1985–1986). In the post-Reconstruction era, many medical institutions excluded African Americans from receiving primary care. Following World War II, many urban institutions provided special wards or supported separate facilities for African Americans. Until recently, African Americans in urban settings received poor health care as a result of poverty, unemployment, biases in public health facilities, and the lack of African-American physicians and administrators.

The history of the integration of health care is at best a sporadic and inconsistent pattern of federally mandated integration. The covert racism that exists in many institutions today is manifested in a number of ways, most often in the adoption, administration, and implementation of policies toward the poor. Many rules and regulations governing the present health care system discriminate in the quality of care provided the poor. The poor are most likely to experience long waits, to be unable to shop for services, and to receive inadequate care. Thus, as the incidence of poverty among African Americans is high, they are more likely to be victims of the health care system.

Overt racism is evident in the observable practices of institutions that deliver health care. The admission practices of institutions, bed assignments, and the assignment of physicians have historically discouraged African Americans from seeking health care from non-institutional sources. When these sources are not available, long periods of travel become necessary for the acquisition of services, especially in rural areas. Invariably, the delivery of primary care for African Americans usually takes place in the emergency rooms and outpatient wards of public hospitals (Cockerham, 1992).

Covert or overt, racism has not been eradicated by federal and state civil rights laws. African Americans who are poor still do not have priority in the delivery of health services. Therefore, their utilization behaviors tend to decline in direct correlation with perceived racism in health service institutions. Present policies do not eradicate discrimination in health institutions; instead, they encourage delay in seeking health care until the patient's condition has deteriorated and has become concomitantly more expensive.

Economic Inequality

The economic conditions in which most African Americans find themselves directly affect their health care. Our present employer-based health insurance system excludes many African Americans because of high unemployment rates. Households without adequate funding tend to be composed of members who are in a poor state of health. Being below the poverty line is an important criterion for attaining public assistance. For those who compose the working poor, there is no public alternative when employers do not provide insurance.

The uneven distribution of resources is reflected by a number of indicators from census reports. With an African-American unemployment rate approximately twice that of Whites and with nearly 37.4 percent of African-American families having no employed member, there is little hope for adequate health care. In 1990, 37 percent of the African-American population had incomes of less than $15,000; in 1970, a little under 33 percent were at that level. In 1990, 31.9 percent of African American families were below the poverty line, in comparison with 11 percent of the White families (U.S. Bureau of the Census, 1990). Alarmingly, 44 percent of all African-American children were living in households below the poverty line in 1990 (U.S. Bureau of the Census, 1991). Further, in female-headed households, 69 percent of the children were below the poverty line.

Despite the gross disparities, some segments of the African American population have experienced significant changes, most notably African-American families where both spouses work. Such families earned a median income of $21,899 in 1990, which was 59 percent of the median income of White families (U.S. Bureau of the Census, 1991). In the case of African-American husband-absent householders, the median income decreased to $12,537 or 61 percent of the median income of similar White families (U.S. Bureau of the Census, 1991).

Lacking resources necessary to obtain adequate health insurance, African-American families have a lower utilization rate than Whites. African Americans are more likely to seek care from nonprofit clinics or public free clinics where the demands for health services are high because of the increasing number of homeless persons. As an alternative, many individuals seek home remedies or practice folk medicine. Most often, families delay seeking care until conditions worsen and become life-threatening. This problem is further compounded by increasing suburbanization and the growing poverty in rural communities. In both contexts, African Americans are the victims of an economic system that dictates their ability to receive health services and the quality of their health.

Access Barriers

When financing is available, the use of health services can be viewed as an individual choice. Much attention has been focused on the determinants of health service utilization and how these determinants act as potential barriers to access (Aday, Andersen & Fleming, 1980). Most studies of utilization have tended to focus on these barriers and to lead to policies that might augment the delivery of services. Yet, effective health service access and utilization require additional forms of assistance that are informational, psychological, and organizational (Crandall & Duncan, 1981). Accordingly, the models used to explain health care barriers for African Americans can best be described as a set of attitudinal and situational factors. Attitudinal factors include attitudes that might serve as determinants of health behaviors (Hulka & Wheat, 1985). For example, perceived health status, perceived racism, and perceived social stress might limit patients' seeking services when illnesses occur.

Among attitudinal barriers are beliefs about health and health behaviors, including fears about medical care, physicians, and diseases. These beliefs stem from the socialization and religious experiences of African Americans. Studies indicate that African Americans' feelings of apathy are generated by a sense of loss of control in medical settings. Having little sense of competency or control of events in hospitals and in physicians' offices, many African Americans develop a sense of fear and do not seek further medical services (Windle, 1980).

Situational barriers include cultural and financial conditions that might prevent health service access (Andersen & Neuman, 1973). Each situational factor partially explains why patients might underutilize services or fail to comply with treatment. Many of these factors are linked to economic inequality and the environment as interpretations of underutilization (Bice, Eichhorn & Fox, 1972). For example, situational factors include geographic accessibility, that is, the "fiction of space," which is a function of the time and physical distance that must be traversed to acquire care. Rural settings are the extreme in the division of physical distance and time (Kennedy, 1979). African-American rural patients tend to view a physician visit in terms of hours of travel. Conversely, inner-city patients tend to regard the physician visit in terms of "freeway minutes."

A final set of situational factors is composed of the socio-organizational dimension of the service provider. These attributes include the organizational perceptions and treatment of the patients (Gillum, 1979). The doctor-patient relationship, as viewed through the eyes of the patient, is critical for follow-up treatment. All aspects of this relationship can be influenced by such factors as sex, age, fee structure, specialization, and organization of the practice. When the patient perceives these factors as obstacles, then utilization behaviors decrease.

In sum, three factors—institutional racism, economic inequality, and access barriers—prevent the reduction of present inequities in health services delivered to African Americans. Unfortunately many of these inequities are a direct result of the failure of governmental policies to adequately plan and deliver health services. This failure is manifested in utilization patterns derived from national surveys and mortality studies.

HEALTH UTILIZATION BEHAVIORS

One of the major health problems faced by African Americans is unmet health needs resulting from inadequate health service access and utilization. The explanations discussed in the previous section suggest that the general economic, social, and political climate in which the African-American community exists is not conducive to the acquisition of health services or for good health.

One key variable in the study of utilization is the subjective health assessment of African Americans. The difficulties inherent in the study of subjective health assessment, as a measure of health status, are widely recognized (Fiedler, 1981). Implicit in the use of these assessments is the assumption of an accepted normative standard of health. However, objective health and subjective health assessments can be very different, as the latter tend to reflect the norms of a relevant reference group and to change according to psychological states. Even though subjective health assessments must be considered as global interpretations

Table 25.1
Perceived Health Self-Assessment by Race, United States, 1991

	Excellent	Very Good	Good	Fair	Poor
White	39.6	28.9	22.0	6.8	2.7
Black	31.3	25.8	29.1	10.0	3.8
All Persons	38.5	28.5	23.0	7.2	2.8

Source: U.S. Department of Health and Human Services. (1992). Current Estimates from the National Health Interview Survey, 1991. *Vital and Health Statistics,* Series 10, No. 184. (PHS) 93-1512. Washington, DC: Government Printing Office.

rather than specific reflections of objective health, they do provide a useful measure of the health service needs and health perceptions of a population.

In the National Health Interview Survey of 1991, subjective health assessment was measured by asking respondents to assess their health status on a 4-point scale, from "poor" to "excellent." Overall, most respondents in the national survey of households view their health as excellent. Whites are more likely to view their health as excellent than are African Americans. The percentage distribution varies as the health status categories change from "good" to "poor." A higher percentage of African Americans are more likely to view their health as "good," "fair," or "poor" (see Table 25.1). These differences, especially where African Americans report lower levels of "excellent" health and higher levels of "poor" health, may be due to some extent to the higher unemployment and lower education of African Americans compared with their White counterparts.

The health service utilization behaviors of African Americans have not reduced the apparent needs indicated by their self-assessment of their health status. Utilization behaviors are measured by both physician and hospital utilization and are divided into the two dimensions of contact and volume (Strand & Jones, 1985). Contact measures the achievement of entry into the system, and volume measures the utilization after entry.

The health service utilization behavior of African Americans are presented in Table 25.2. Overall, 78.5 percent of Americans have had contact with a physician in the last year, and 6.5 percent were admitted to a hospital during the preceding year. In both cases, there are contact differences associated with race, volume of contacts, and interval since the last contact. The length of time since the last

Table 25.2
Hospital and Physician Contact by Race for All Causes, and Excluding Deliveries, United States, 1991

	African American	White	Total
Hospital Contact	6.2	6.7	6.5
Hospital Volume			
1 episode	5.1	5.2	5.1
2 episodes	.8	1.0	.9
3 or more	.3	.4	.4
Physician Contact	77.6	79.0	78.5
Contact Interval			
> 1 year < 2 yrs.	11.4	9.6	9.9
> 2 yrs. - < 5 yrs.	7.8	8.1	8.1
> 5 yrs.	3.2	3.4	3.5

Source: U.S. Department of Health and Human Services. (1992). Current Estimates from the National Health Interview Survey, 1991. *Vital health statistics,* Series 10. No. 184 (PHS) 93-1512. Washington, DC: Government Printing Office.

visit is an indicator of the frequency of utilization. African Americans are more likely than any others to delay seeking care for a period between 1 to 2 years. However, they were less likely to delay care beyond 2 years, in comparison with others.

An explanation may be in the tendency of the poor to delay seeking care until conditions worsen and also the tendency to seek primary care in emergency rooms. The findings on race and hospital contact, however, are not generally supportive of racial differences. African Americans who have health insurance or Medicaid or Medicare are slightly less likely to use hospital services (Weaver & Inui, 1975). In a related manner, because of changing and emerging demographic trends, it is important to determine the impact of homelessness on these estimates of utilization.

CONCLUSION

The growing numbers of uninsured and underinsured have created a national concern for health care reform. African Americans represent a large proportion of the population that cannot afford adequate health. Compounding their lack of insurance are the inequities inherent in the health services available to African Americans. Institutional racism, economic inequality, and access barriers prevent an inadequate health care system from being responsive to their needs.

Although these findings are based on national surveys of households, their implications are useful in evaluating substantive policy issues concerning the health care needs of African Americans and in assessing the need for future research in this area. The limited utilization of health services by African Americans can be improved by national health insurance reform. The very fact that utilization among this group is low further suggests that cultural and racial differences may act as a barrier to the perception of health status and the utilization of health services even when those services are subsidized.

Finally, adequate health care begins with health perceptions. It is important to begin to study the perceptions of health and illness from the viewpoint of African Americans. In-depth analysis of the cultural dimensions of health perceptions and behaviors would help in understanding the uniqueness of the health care experiences of these Americans. A health policy that promotes access and socialization to the health care system could reduce the present underutilization of health services and the problems of the uninsured.

REFERENCES

Aday, L., Andersen, R., & Fleming, G. V. (1980). *Health care in the U.S.: Equitable for whom?* Beverly Hills, CA: Sage.

Andersen, R. M., & Neuman, J. (1973). Societal and individual determinants of medical care utilization in the United States. *Milbank Fund Quarterly, 51*, 95–124.

Blendon, R. J., Aiken, L. H., Freeman, H. E., & Corey, C. (1989). Access to medical care for black and white Americans. *Journal of the American Medical Association, 261*, 278–281.

Blum, H. L. (1974). *Planning for Health.* New York: Human Sciences Press.

Bice, T. W., Eichhorn, R. L., & Fox, P. D. (1972). Socioeconomic status and the use of physicians' services: A reconsideration. *Medical Care, 10*, 261–271.

Cockerham, W. C. (1992). *Medical sociology* (5th ed.). Englewood Cliffs, NJ: Prentice-Hall.

Crandall, L. A., & Duncan, P. R. (1981). Attitudinal and situational factors in the use of physician services by low income persons. *Journal of Health and Social Behavior, 22*, 22–64.

Fiedler, J. L. (1981). A review of the literature on access and utilization of medical care with special emphasis on rural primary care. *Social Science and Medicine, 15C*, 129–137.

Gayles, J. N. (1972). Health brutality and the black life cycle. *Black Scholar, 5*, 2–9.

Gillum, R. F. (1979). Determinants of dropout rates among hypertensive patients in an urban clinic. *Journal of Community Health, 5*, 94–100.

Hulka, B. S., & Wheat, J. R. (1985). Patterns of utilization: The patient perspective. *Medical Care, 23*, 438–460.

Kennedy, V. C. (1979). Rural access to regular sources of medical care, *Journal of Community Health, 4*, 199–203.

McCulloch, P. C. (1989). The ecological model: A framework of operationalizing prevention. *Journal of Primary Prevention, 11*, 30–45.

Rice, M. F. (1985–86). On assessing black health status. *Urban League Review, 9*, 6–
12.

Rodin, J., Timko, C., & Harris, S. (1985). The construct of control: Biological and
psychological correlates. *Annual Review of Gerontology and Geriatrics, 5*, 3–55.

Romano, J. (1990). Basic orientation and education of the medical student. *Journal of
the American Medical Association, 143*, 411.

Strand, P. J., & Jones, W., Jr. (1985). *Indochinese refugees in America: Problems of
adaptation and assimilation.* Durham, NC: Duke University Press.

U.S. Bureau of the Census. (1991). *Current Population Reports,* Series P-60, No. 174,
and unpublished data.

U.S. Bureau of the Census. (1990). *Current Population Reports,* Series P-60, No. 175,
and unpublished data.

U.S. Department of Human Services. (1992). Current Estimates from the National Health
Interview Survey, 1991. *Vital and Health Statistics,* Series 10, No. 184. DHHS
No. (PHS) 03-1512, Washington, DC: Government Printing Office.

Windle, C. (1980). Correlates of community mental health centers' underservice to non-
whites. *Journal of Community Psychology, 8*, 140–146

Weaver, J. L., & Inui, L. T. (1975). Information about health care providers among
low-income minorities. *Inquiry, 12*, 330–343.

26

Improving the Health Status of African Americans: Empowerment as Health Education Intervention

Collins O. Airhihenbuwa and Agatha G. Lowe

INTRODUCTION

It is well documented that African Americans have poorer health and excess premature deaths compared with White Americans. It is also known that most of these deaths are preventable. The main argument presented in this paper is that the health status of African Americans can be improved through empowerment as health education intervention.

Health education has been defined as "any combination of learning experiences designed to facilitate voluntary adaptations of behavior conducive to health" (Green, Kreuter, Deeds & Partridge, 1980, p. 7). The primary focus of health education is health promotion and disease prevention associated with individuals, families, and communities. Although it is reasoned that health educators have a crucial role to play in improving the health status of African Americans, they alone cannot be responsible for health promotion, but must combine efforts with other health professionals, government sectors, and communities so that societal goals for health are realized.

In developing health education interventions one of three basic approaches are employed. The first, the "Preventive Model," focuses on the individual decision-making process for the purpose of adopting positive health behavior to prevent diseases at the primary level (i.e., prevent disease at the asymptomatic phase so that it does not lead to an impairment), secondary level (i.e., prevent impairment from leading to disability), and tertiary level (i.e., prevent disability from leading to dependency). The second is the "Radical-Political Model," which focuses on changing social, environmental, and political structure to tackle the problem of ill health at its root. Third, the "Empowerment Model" focuses on facilitating choices for the individual and community by supplementing knowledge acquisition with value clarification and practice in decision making through nontraditional teaching methods (Tones, Tilford & Robinson, 1991). It has been argued that the Preventive Model has a tendency to blame the victim while the Radical-Political Model may bias consciousness-raising efforts toward the interests of the health educators rather than that of the community. The Empowerment Model incorporates elements of the Preventive and Radical-Political models and will be discussed relative to its application to the African-American population. There is a need to focus on preventive health practices by empowering African Americans to capitalize fully on the opportunities available to them so that they can make a difference in their own health outcomes.

In this chapter the aims are as follows: (a) to compare selected disparities between the health status of African Americans and that of Whites, (b) to suggest some of the factors that have contributed to these disparities, and (c) to recommend how African Americans might be empowered to promote their own health.

DISPARITIES IN HEALTH STATUS BETWEEN AFRICAN AMERICANS AND WHITES

Although this chapter focuses on empowerment as a health education strategy among African Americans, it is important to present an overview of some data on health status even though these data are on health care delivery and their inadequacies. The information that follows is designed to illustrate the importance of disease prevention and health promotion as a way of alleviating the deteriorating health conditions among African Americans.

Disparities in the health status of the African-American and White populations have been and continue to be realities in the United States. Blacks of both sexes and in all age groups are more likely than Whites to be ill or to die prematurely. The 1989 mortality data for Black men showed a continued reduction in life expectancy and no change for both sexes, in sharp contrast to the extension of life by 0.4 years for Whites of both sexes (Health Trends, 1992). The age-specific excess deaths for Blacks compared with Whites in 1991 ranged from 64 percent for persons aged 15–25 to 11 percent for persons 65 years and older (Fingerhut & Makuc, 1992).

A Black baby is more than twice as likely as a White infant to die before the first birthday (Edelman, 1989). In 1989, the infant mortality rate for Whites was 8.2 per thousand live births compared to 17.7 for Blacks (Health Trends, 1992). The gap is even wider (8.1 for Whites and 18.6 for Blacks) when the mother's race is used to classify infant mortality rate. The percent of low-birth-weight births among Black mothers is almost three times that of Whites. The 1989 rate of 13.3 percent (compared to 5.7 percent for Whites) has been increasing annually from the 12.7 percent in 1980 (USDHHS, 1991). Effective use of preventive services can significantly improve maternal and child health.

Some researchers argue that poor health is the result of low socioeconomic status rather than ethnicity. Though low economic status is linked with poor health status, as will be later discussed, one must also appreciate other factors, such as structural discrimination and institutional racism, that favor the disproportionate representation of African Americans in low-income groups, which ultimately results in poor health status. Focusing on individual income fails to address the social context and environment in which a disproportionate number of African Americans find themselves (Auslander, Haire-Joshu, Houston & Fisher, 1992). Even when income levels are the same in the two population groups, many other factors, such as total assets, housing, prior socioeconomic status, and social mobility, influence health status (Kumanyika & Golden, 1991).

The goal of the public health system in the United States should, therefore, be directed toward achieving social equity in the health status of all Americans. In the discussion that follows, an examination is made of some of the reasons that the gap in health services between the races continues to persist. Issues relating to health institutions and health personnel will be addressed first.

HEALTH INSTITUTIONS

An examination of the availability of health care resources to the population reveals that the condition has worsened for African Americans since the 1985 Secretary's Task Force Report on the Status of Black and Minority Health (Hale, 1992). Indeed, in a 1988 response issued by the Commission on Minority Participation in Education and American Life, the investigators concluded that America was "moving backward" in its efforts to secure equity for minority citizens (Jacob, 1989).

The reductions in federal financing programs slowed the decentralization of health care resources through block grants and attenuated the increasing accessibility of minorities and the disadvantaged to health care services. For example, the Health Education-Risk Reduction (HERR) Grants Program was cut by 25 percent as a consequence of the 1980s block grant policy (Kreuter, 1992).

Even when services are available they may not be as accessible to Blacks as to Whites, as the Black family is often faced with different barriers that complicate accessibility to health services. Some of the barriers include physicians' refusal to attend to patients who are indigent (Davidson, 1982) and patients who are Black (Charatz-Litt, 1992). Other barriers include limited accessibility to medical facilities, long waiting time at the office, inconvenient office hours, racial discrimination, and absence of privacy within public and private clinics and emergency rooms (Davidson, 1982).

HEALTH AND RELATED PERSONNEL

The underrepresentation of Black professionals in the health care delivery system has complicated the problem of accessibility (Airhihenbuwa, 1989). Although Blacks constitute 12.1 percent of the U.S. population and 13.6 percent of the population aged 20–29, they received only 5.3 percent of the medical degrees in 1989 (Petersdorf, Turner, Nickens & Ready, 1990). Similarly, a recent survey showed that African Americans accounted for only 5.8 percent of the total number of doctorates awarded in health education between 1980 and 1988 (Airhihenbuwa, Olsen, St. Pierre & Wang, 1989). Of the total number of graduates from schools of public health in the 1981/82 academic year, only 2.5 percent were Black (Airhihenbuwa et al., 1989). When Blacks expressed a preference in their health care providers, it was a desire to be attended to by a Black health care provider (Protor & Rosen, 1981) and comfort in the knowledge of Black counselors' presence on the counseling staff (Miles & McDavis, 1982).

An increase in the number of Black health professionals could definitely improve accessibility and, subsequently, the quality of health care delivery to Black clients. Even if health care recipients are not treated by Black personnel, the knowledge of the presence of Black staff in a particular health care facility helps to alleviate some of the apprehension Black clients may have about the service they will receive (Airhihenbuwa, 1989). Seemingly, the presence of Black faculty in health education and other public health academic departments should directly or indirectly enhance the recruitment and, more important, the retention of Blacks in these programs (Airhihenbuwa et al., 1989).

A COMBINATION OF ISSUES

Structural discrimination and institutional racism are also synergistically responsible, in large part, for the persistent disparity of services available and accessible to Blacks as opposed to Whites. This has been demonstrated in the way the policies and practices of the White medical community negatively impact the health of Blacks (Charatz-Litt, 1992) as well as in the history of racism as an established characteristic of the health care delivery system (Muller, 1985). These discriminatory practices are often exacerbated by limited resources in time and money to access health care.

Investigators have documented the continual disproportionate decrease in income levels among Blacks compared with Whites (Horton & Smith, 1990; Auslander et al., 1992). Based on constant dollars, 30 percent more Blacks than Whites had an annual income of less than $5,000 in 1987 than in 1970 (Horton & Smith, 1990). Today, approximately 34 percent of African Americans are below the poverty level compared to 11 percent of Whites (Auslander et al., 1992).

Opportunity costs, or the synergy of time and money required to access available health services, is a major barrier for economically disadvantaged health consumers (Airhihenbuwa, 1992). Because their daily activities are not always quantifiable in dollars, their time is often less valued by the health care professionals.

Services that are available, accessible, and affordable must also be acceptable to the clients. Racism has separated Blacks and Whites to the extent that White health care professionals are often unaware of the Black experience (i.e., suffering, discrimination) and the effect it has on Black people. This ignorance may prevent professionals from understanding both the cultural appropriateness of their clients' behaviors and the adaptive qualities of such behaviors. White professionals may, therefore, discount the value of, or incorrectly label the behavior of a Black client as abnormal. Conversely, ignorance of the Black life-style may also contribute to the health care workers' tendency to attribute certain behaviors to racial differences when such behavior should be ascribed to personal malfunctioning and/or psychopathology.

As the majority of Black clients receive care from White professionals, cultural differences are often encountered. Many Blacks are suspicious of White health care institutions because of past abusive usage of Blacks for medical experimentation and demonstration (Savitt, 1982; Jones, 1982; Pernick, 1985).

Investigators analyzed the 10 leading causes of death in 1976 and reported that 50 percent of them were due to unhealthy behavior or life-style, 20 percent to environmental factors, 20 percent to human ecological factors, and only 10 percent to inadequacies in health care (Healthy People, 1979). Thus, 90 percent of our total health is determined by factors over which doctors have little or no control. By focusing on these factors—life-styles, social conditions, and physical environment—health educators have been successful at improving the health of the population (Airhihenbuwa, 1989).

The latest studies on health promotion have shown that improved self-esteem, building skills, and providing support are the three most important factors that lead to positive health behavior change (Keeling, 1992). These factors are often identified as the key ingredients in successful programs designed to empower people, groups, and communities. Strategies for promoting these factors are explored within the context of the African-American family and community.

HEALTH EDUCATION INTERVENTIONS

Secretary Sullivan (1989) of Health and Human Services has pointed out that one answer to the disproportionately high rates of infant deaths and deaths from chronic degenerative conditions among Blacks is an increased emphasis on health education and preventive care. This call for health education and preventive strategies is appropriate and timely. However, one must be cautious not to develop health promotion and disease prevention programs under the assumption that individuals have total control over factors that influence their health. There is a tendency to believe that, given the right information and perhaps the right circumstances, individuals would be willing and able to change their health conditions.

Indeed, largely as a result of health promotion programs, many Americans now engage in a variety of risk-reduction activities; as a result, some Americans have experienced improvement in, for example, lipid profiles, protection against hypertension, and decrease in obesity, as well as healthier cardiovascular systems (Sprafka, Burke, Folsom & Hahn 1989). However, there are serious limitations in placing so much of the responsibility for health promotion and disease pre-vention on the individual (Becker, 1986; Lamarine, 1989). Becker (1986) be-lieves the focus on the individual "enables us to ignore the more difficult, but at least equally important problem of the social environment, which both creates some lifestyles and inhibits the initiation of others" (p. 19).

The assumption that information will assist in changing behavior presumes that the information is correct. Yet, the content of some programs can be mis-leading or so confusing that the individual has difficulty sorting out the facts. Lamarine (1989) states that the scientific data base of many of the recommended programs are not clearly established, and there is thus much misinformation. For health education programs designed for African-American communities, the situation is even worse, particularly when cultural influences of health behavior such as food selection practices are ignored.

The ability to manipulate one's environment is achieved by acquiring the skills to critically review information and by raising one's level of consciousness through support from and sharing with friends and families in order to make appropriate decisions regarding health-enhancing activities. The decision-making task is a serious challenge because most of the preventable diseases require lifelong changes and because failure to act does not always result in immediate illness. Consequently, individuals whose daily survival is a struggle may perceive limited benefit in adopting lifelong changes such as abstaining from eating certain foods, engaging in unprotected sexual intercourse, smoking, or alcohol abuse. To gain the benefit of accentuating the connectedness between one's livelihood and positive health practices, African Americans must be empowered to develop the skills and support that are necessary to make those positive health decisions.

What Is Empowerment?

Empowerment is defined here as "a process of helping people to assert control over the factors which affect their health" (Gibson, 1991, p. 369). The complex and multidimensional empowerment model combines ideas from social reform, behavior change, social action, social support, and life-stage theories, perceptions of self-efficacy, and organizational and community-development theories (Freire, 1989; Kieffer, 1984). It recognizes that people have competencies that can be developed if the opportunities are provided and insists that people be involved in plans that affect their lives (Rappaport, 1981; Fahlberg, Poulin, Girdano & Dusek, 1991). Envisioned as a process, empowerment is positive in that it focuses on the strengths, rights, and abilities of people, organizations, and communities and has also been used synonymously with indices of its presence such as coping skills, mutual support, community organization, support systems, neighborhood participation, personal efficacy, competence, self-esteem, and self-sufficiency (Rappaport, 1981, 1984; Kieffer, 1984; Gibson, 1991). Each of these synonyms are based on extensive theoretical frameworks that are beyond the scope of this chapter.

The objective changes resulting from empowerment are various because they reflect the varied needs of individuals, groups, organizations, and communities and the contexts where empowerment occurs. They may comprise groups of empowered institutions and individuals or single groups of people living in, for example, housing units. In the following section, the discussion focuses on how African Americans can be empowered within the context of health promotion and disease prevention.

The Empowerment of African Americans

Despite the barriers, Blacks of all socioeconomic levels have begun to empower themselves and are making changes in the problems that affect their health. For example, programs targeting the prevention of the human immunodeficiency viral infections include the SISTERLOVE Women's AIDS Prevention Project of Atlanta and Blacks Educating Blacks about Sexual Health Issues (BEBASHI) of Philadelphia. The National Black Women's Health Project in Atlanta focuses on health and other social issues relating to Blacks. In recognition of the pivotal role Black women play in the family, these and other organizations seek to empower women to assume responsibility for their family's and ultimately their community's health, and the women are responding. In Atlanta, for example, some women are saying no to drugs and unsafe sex and are encouraging members of their families, friends, and neighbors to do the same (Lowe, 1992). In effect, Blacks are recognizing that they are not a top priority in the government's agenda for health care and therefore are helping themselves.

Gilkes (1983) interviewed individuals who had been successful in community-development programs to determine the patterns and processes involved in the transition from powerlessness to political involvement. The sample comprised 23 Black female professionals who were committed to the empowerment of the Black community through affecting changes in the quality of life of individuals and groups, as well as influencing changes in the social structure. Personal and community empowerment were accomplished through focusing their educational and career choices and by using strategies to maintain their ties and commitment to the community. The acquisition of knowledge and skills and the support they received from others were key ingredients in helping them to achieve their goals. In another study, a group composed primarily of African-American women in a housing project in Harlem used assistance from local politicians, nonprofit groups, and organizations to run a series of successful housing cooperatives in apartment buildings that had been abandoned as unprofitable by the landlords (Saegert, 1989).

Kieffer (1984) described the process of empowerment as a developmental one, comparable to the stages of infancy through adulthood, that represents the transition from a feeling of powerlessness to one of feeling more powerful, whether or not this has been accompanied by the acquisition of actual power. African-American women exemplified other aspects of empowerment described by Kieffer (1984) in that they had "a strong sense of pride and determination, a deeply felt rootedness in the community, a commitment to self reliance, and feelings of attachment within a caring community" (p. 18). The threat to their sense of personal and family integrity triggered the empowering response. Kieffer argued that these threats to integrity, rather than "consciousness raising," or deliberate educational efforts, motivate people to become involved in projects.

Bandura (1977) demonstrated that personal expectations of one's ability to influence events in life (self-efficacy) will determine whether an individual will initiate behavior to deal with the situation, how much effort will be expended, and how long the effort will be sustained in the face of obstacles and aversive experiences. Those persons who believe they have the skills to cope with situations will be less likely to avoid them than others who do not see themselves as having the skills. This being the case, skill development among Blacks is pivotal to their empowerment.

Techniques used to facilitate the transition from powerlessness to empowerment have embraced consciousness raising, training members in social competence, encouraging and accepting the client's definition of the problem, identifying and building upon existing strengths, analyzing how powerlessness is affecting the situation, identifying and using sources of power in the client's situation, teaching specific skills, mobilizing resources, and looking out for the welfare of the clients (Gutierrez, 1990). The ideal modality recommended for promoting empowerment is the small group, because it facilitates the use of techniques such as consciousness raising, engaging in mutual aid, knowledge and skill development, modeling behaviors, and problem solving. Individuals in these groups can evaluate their effectiveness in influencing others and can receive support in learning and practicing new skills.

Interpersonal skills reflect the ability to influence others and to work to change institutions and social structures in order to attain personal and collective goals (Saegert, 1989; Gutierrez, 1990; Ozer & Bandura, 1990). This is true whether the goal is empowering individuals or empowering institutions. Groups also provide support through the change process, a format for obtaining concrete assistance, and a potential power base for future action (Gutierrez, 1990). The outcomes of empowerment include changes at individual, interpersonal, institutional, and community levels.

Individual psychological changes associated with empowerment include a sense of personal power, a positive and potent self-esteem, increasing self-efficacy, developing group consciousness, and an understanding of political and social realities that influence life circumstances or situations, reducing self-blame, and assuming personal responsibility for change (Kieffer, 1984; Gutierrez, 1990). For African Americans, support, either within community groups or in the larger society, is essential in promoting changes at individual and group levels. Overall, such experiences do benefit society, as African Americans who are empowered will have a greater sense of political efficacy, a greater desire for control over their environment, more civic mindedness, and a general belief that success results from internal rather than external factors. The outcome will, in time, result in a positive contribution to the improved health status of African Americans.

CONCLUSION AND RECOMMENDATIONS

African Americans in different parts of the country are assuming responsibility for finding solutions to the health and social problems that affect them and their families, in spite of the structural and psychological barriers that consign a disproportionate number of them to the lower socioeconomic strata of society. The greatest contribution the government can make is to remove the barriers that frustrate the efforts of grass-roots organizations to facilitate the empowerment of the Black family, which remains one of the strongest institutions in the Black community. The Black family must become a collaborator before programs can effectively meet the needs of the Black population (Airhihenbuwa, 1989). Collectively and separately, family members must receive the required skills and support and develop the self-esteem necessary to lead to positive health behavior change. However, families are not always knowledgeable about the necessary skills and support that lead to self-efficacy and empowerment. Therefore, it is recommended that health educators, working with others in public health and social and economic development, particularly those of African descent (students as well as professionals), must begin by working with the community to identify and help address the needs of the community, as prioritized by the community.

It is also recommended that preventive health initiatives can be introduced simultaneously or after the community's prioritized needs have been addressed. An example has been demonstrated by the Black Students Leadership Network, which combines community service with political activism. This has resulted in empowering, for example, Blacks in housing projects to have control over forces and decisions in the environment (e.g., influencing the decisions of town councils and community agencies regarding services provided in the community) that affect the destiny of their families and communities (Collison, 1992). Additionally, health and other social issues can be triangulated into those that are positive and should be encouraged for increased self-esteem, those unique but indifferent to health that should be left untouched, and those that are negative and should be changed. (For more on a model for health promotion in the African-American community that addresses these issues, see Airhihenbuwa, 1992.)

Health promotion programs have been effective in helping individuals to decrease their risks of disease, such as cancer, cardiovascular problems, and hypertension. However, targeting individuals for most health reduction efforts, without considering the effect of the various environments, may be counterproductive, because few have control over most environmental factors that influence them. The sociopolitical and environmental forces that influence health behavior must be manipulated within the context of the culture, utilizing source expertise who can also serve as positive role models to influence behavior change (Airhihenbuwa et al., 1992). Finally, to promote preventive activities, Black and White health professionals need to become advocates of the people for whom the options of choice are rapidly decreasing. They need to focus on environmental and social issues that rob people of hope and dignity and contribute to poverty and crime. These and other outcomes, if left unaddressed, can become additional risk factors to the health of African Americans.

NOTE

Direct all correspondence to Dr. C. O. Airhihenbuwa, Associate Professor of Health Education, Pennsylvania State University, One White Building, University Park, PA 16802.

REFERENCES

Airhihenbuwa, C. O. (1989). Health education for African Americans: A neglected task. *Health Education, 20,* 9–14.

Airhihenbuwa, C. O. (1992). Health promotion and disease prevention strategies for African-Americans. In R. L. Braithwaite & S. E. Taylor (Eds.). *Health issues in the black community* (pp. 267–280). San Francisco: Jossey-Bass.

Airhihenbuwa, C. O., DiClemente, R. J., Wingood, G. M., & Lowe, A. (1992). HIV/ AIDS education and prevention among African-Americans: A focus on culture. *AIDS Education and Prevention, 4,* 267–276.

Airhihenbuwa, C. O., Olsen, L. K., St. Pierre, R. W., & Wang, M. Q. (1989). Race and gender: An analysis of the granting of doctoral degrees in health education programs. *Health Education, 20,* 4–7.

Auslander, W. F., Haire-Joshu, D., Houston, C. A., & Fisher, E. B. (1992). Community organization to reduce the risk of non-insulin-dependent diabetes among low-income African-American women. *Ethnicity and Disease, 2,* 176–184.

Bandura, A. (1977). Self-efficacy: Toward a unifying theory of behavioral change. *Psychological Review, 84,* 191–215.

Becker, M. H. (1986). The tyranny of health promotion. *Public Health Review, 14,* 15–25.

Charatz-Litt, C. (1992). A chronicle of racism: The effects of the white medical community on black health. *Journal of the National Medical Association, 84,* 717–725.

Collison, M. N. K. (1992). Network of black students hopes to create a new generation of civil rights leaders. *Chronicle of Higher Education* (September 30), A28–A29.

Davidson, J. M. (1982). Physician participation in Medicaid: Background and issues. *Journal of Health Politics and Policy Law, 6,* 703.

Edelman, M. R. (1989). *Black children in America.* In J. Dewart (Ed.), *The state of Black America 1989* (pp. 63–76). New York: National Urban League, Inc.

Fahlberg, L. L., Poulin, A. L., Girdano, D. A., & Dusek, D. E. (1991). Empowerment as an emerging approach in health education. *Journal of Health Education, 22,* 185–193.

Fingerhut, L. A., & Makuc, D. M. (1992). News from NCHS. *American Journal of Public Health, 82,* 1168–1170.

Freire, P. (1989). *Education for Critical Consciousness.* New York: Continuum Publishing Company.

Gibson, C. H. (1991). A concept analysis of empowerment. *Journal of Advanced Nursing, 16,* 354–361.

Gilkes, C. T. (1983). Going up for the oppressed: The career mobility of black women community workers. *Journal of Social Issues, 39,* 115–139.

Green, L. W., Kreuter, M. W., Deeds, S. G., & Partridge, K. B. (1980). *Health Education Planning: A Diagnostic Approach.* Palo Alto, CA: Mayfield Publishing Company.

Gutierrez, L. M. (1990). Working with women of color: An empowerment perspective. *Social Work, 35,* 149–153.

Hale, C. B. (1992). A demographic profile of African Americans. In R. L. Braithwaite & S. E. Taylor (Eds.) *Health issues in the black community* (pp. 6–19). San Francisco: Jossey-Bass.

Health Trends. (1992). New vital statistics confirm worsening of black health. *Ethnicity and Disease, 2,* 192–193.

Healthy People, the Surgeon General's report on health promotion and disease prevention. (1979). U.S. Department of Health, Education and Welfare, DHEW (PHS) No. 79-55071A. Washington, DC: Government Printing Office.

Horton, E. P., & Smith, J. C. (1990). (Eds.). Statistical record of black Americans. Detroit, MI: Gale Research, Inc.

Jacob, J. E. (1989). Black America, 1988: An overview. In J. Dewart (Ed.), *The state of Black America 1989* (pp. 1–7). New York: National Urban League, Inc.

Jones, J. (1982). *Bad Blood: The Tuskegee syphilis experiment—A tragedy of race and medicine.* New York: Free Press.

Keeling, R. (1992). Taking the next steps in HIV prevention in young adults. Paper presented at the VI International Conference on AIDS Education, The second decade of HIV: Paths to pursue, (April).

Kieffer, C. H. (1984). Citizen empowerment: A developmental perspective. In J. Rappaport, C. Swift, & R. Hess (Eds.), *Studies in empowerment: Steps toward understanding and action* (pp. 9–36). New York: Haworth Press.

Kreuter, M. W. (1992). PATCH: Its origin, basic concepts and links to contemporary public health policy. *Journal of Health Education, 23,* 135–139.

Kumanyika, S. K., & Golden, P. M. (1991). Cross-sectional differences in health status in U.S. racial/ethnic minority groups: Potential influence of temporal changes, disease, and life-style transitions. *Ethnicity and Disease, 1,* 50–59.

Lamarine, R. J. (1989). First do no harm. *Health Education, 20,* 22–24.

Lowe, A. G. (1992). The effects of an HIV/AIDS prevention program on the knowledge, attitudes, behavior, beliefs and empowerment of African-American women. Doctoral dissertation. University Park, Pennsylvania: Pennsylvania State University.

Miles, G. B., & McDavis, R. J. (1982). Effects of four orientation approaches on disadvantaged Black freshmen students' attitudes toward the counseling center. *Journal of College Student Personnel, 23,* 413–418.

Muller, C. (1985). A window of the past: The position of the client in twentieth century public health thought and practice. *American Journal of Public Health, 75,* 470–476.

Ozer, E. M., & Bandura, A. (1990). Mechanisms governing empowerment effects: A self-efficacy analysis. *Journal of Personality and Social Psychology, 58,* 472–486.

Pernick, M. S. (1985). *A calculus of suffering.* New York: Columbia University Press.

Petersdorf, R. G., Turner, K. S., Nickens, H. W., & Ready, T. (1990). Minorities and medicine: Past, present, and future. *Academic Medicine, 65,* 663–670.

Protor, E., & Rosen, A. (1981). Expectations and preferences for counselor's race and their relation to intermediate treatment outcomes. *Journal of Counseling Psychology, 28,* 40–46.

Rappaport, J. (1981). In praise of paradox: A social policy of empowerment over prevention. *American Journal of Community Psychology, 9,* 1–25.

Rappaport, J. (1984). Studies in empowerment: Introduction to the issue. In J. Rappaport, C. Swift, & R. Hess (Eds.), *Studies in empowerment: Steps toward understanding and action* (pp. 1–7). New York: Haworth Press.

Saegert, S. (1989). Unlikely leaders, extreme circumstances: Older black women building community households. *American Journal of Community Psychology, 17,* 295–316.

Savitt, T. L. (1982). The use of blacks for medical experimentation and demonstration in the old south. *Journal of Southern History, 48,* 331–335.

Sprafka, J. M., Burke, G. L., Folsom, A. R., & Hahn, L. P. (1989). Hypercholesteremia prevalence, awareness and treatment in blacks and whites: The Minnesota Heart Survey. *Preventive Medicine, 18,* 423–432.

Sullivan, L. W. (1989). Shattuck lecture—The health care priorities of the Bush administration. *New England Journal of Medicine, 321,* 125–128.

Tones, K., Tilford, S., & Robinson, Y. K. (1991). *Health education: Effectiveness and efficiency* (pp. 1–16). London: Chapman and Hall.

USDHHS. (1991). *Health United States and Prevention Profile.* Public Health Service, Centers for Disease Control, National Center for Health Statistics Pub. No. (PHS) 91-1232. Hyattsville, MD.

27

Improving the Health of the Black Community: Outlook for the Future

Ivor Lensworth Livingston and J. Jacques Carter

> Of all the forms of inequality, injustice in health is the most shocking and the most inhuman.
>
> Martin Luther King, Jr.

The 1990 census estimated that African Americans, or Blacks, as they will be called here, make up 12.3 percent of the United States population, by that being the nation's largest minority group. It is projected that the Black population will grow to an estimated 16.9 percent of the nation's population in 2050 (O'Hare, 1987). Blacks as a group are disproportionately poorer and experience a greater incidence of morbidity and mortality from chronic diseases and other health conditions than their White counterparts. As the nation approaches the 21st century, it is troubling that the moral, social, legislative, and economic consciences of America have not been sufficiently touched to eradicate these racial and class-related health injustices.

The previous 26 chapters in this volume provided a comprehensive and detailed view on various health problems and concerns of Blacks living in the United States. This chapter is mainly concerned with providing some closure as to the outlook for the health of the Black community, now and as we approach the 21st century. Although this chapter will, at times, reiterate and supplement some of the racial disparities in health alluded to before, this information is presented under a guiding framework for action. It is the belief of these authors that, while many agree that change is needed on both the macro and micro levels to achieve and sustain racial parity in health, no framework exists to show both the inter-relationship between these interdependent levels and where and how needed changes/interventions can be achieved. This chapter introduces a conceptual model that provides a framework for individual, social, and political action. This model (see Figure 27.1), which provides an interactionist view on health and encompasses the trio of the [E]nvironment, [I]ndividual, and [O]rganization, is called the E-I-O Model.

THE E-I-O MODEL

Any effort to intervene to improve the overall health conditions of Blacks is very difficult, not insurmountable. However, because of the multifaceted nature of health, interventional efforts, for example, by health educators, scientists, and politicians are more likely to succeed if they are guided by a theoretical framework. The E-I-O model of health provides such a framework for action, and the subsequent discussion about intervention and change to achieve racial parity in health is presented under the E-I-O model's three main parameters: the environment, the individual, and the organization.

The E-I-O model is derived, in part, from the Health Field Concept (or HFC). It was primarily modified to make it consistent with an interactionist perspective on health as well as certain emergent views of health. An example of the latter is the view that, although health is multifaceted in nature, a salient factor that contributes to good health is the personal action of individuals. Good health lies ultimately within individuals, and they are ultimately responsible for its outcome.

Originally, the HFC was used to formulate strategies for improving the health of Canadians. The utility of the HFC in addressing emergent public health concerns of contemporary society has been expressed in the past (Terris, 1984). (For more background information on the HFC, see LaLonde, 1974.)

The E-I-O model consists of three broad domains: (1) the environment (i.e., events external to the person's body and over which he/she has little or no control), (2) the individual (i.e., a person's biologic makeup, his/her skills/resources and lifestyle activities), and (3) the organization (i.e., the organized structures in society responsible for directing/influencing the daily activities and health of individuals). Various subdivisions of each of the major parameters of the E-I-O model are seen in Table 27.1.

The desirable qualities individuals[I] must have for good health under skills/resources and life-style are indicated with a plus (+) and the undesirable qualities with a minus (−). A major feature of the E-I-O model is the complementary position of the major parameters and, hence, their implied and real importance. The E-I-O model demonstrates the functional importance among the three domains by means of the arrows indicating reciprocal relationships. The domain of the environment[E], because of the significant influence of the wider society, subsumes the other two domains. An additional characteristic (which is also a strength) of the E-I-O model is its illustration of ways interaction can occur within as well as among the three dominant domains. This characteristic is very important, especially when there is a need to intervene to address a health-related issue.

Using the E-I-O model as a guide, this chapter presents discussions about

Figure 27.1
An Interactionist View of Health: The E-I-O Model

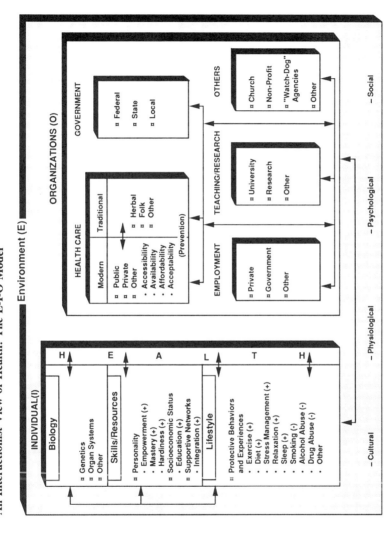

Source: This model was developed specifically for this chapter by Ivor Lensworth Livingston, Ph.D., M.P.H.

Note: Bi-directional arrows indicate the reciprocal relationships between the various sections of the model.

(+) Desirable qualities/experiences

(−) Undesirable qualities/experiences

racial disparities in health and about how improvements can be made. Because of space limitations and the vast disparities in health and related conditions that exist between Blacks and Whites, only a selection of topics can be included.

THE ENVIRONMENT: A MOSAIC OF AREAS FOR IMPROVEMENT

The *Oxford English Dictionary* defines environment as "the conditions under which any person lives." As the "umbrella" domain in the E-I-O model, the environment is external to the individual, yet it influences health in many ways through a mosaic of subdomains, for example, the cultural, physiological, psychological, and social. For Blacks living in the United States, the sociostructural and sociopolitical realities of poverty, institutional racism, and environmental racism underscore the importance of the environment as a focal point for needed interventional activities and change.

Poverty as an Impediment to Health

Currently, the poverty level for Blacks is 32.7 percent, versus 11.3 for Whites (U.S. Bureau of the Census, 1992). The existing realities of institutional racism and the accompanying legacy of poverty underscore the need for collective action and change in the status quo.

Some legislative enactments have had a positive influence on Black behavior and poverty experiences. These include, for example, the Civil Rights Act of 1964; Medicaid and Medicare legislation of 1965; and Title VI of the Civil Rights Act, which prohibited racial discrimination in any institution receiving federal funds. All of these laws combined to create a "Civil Rights Era" in health care for Blacks (Sidel & Sidel, 1984; Shea & Fullilove, 1985). The passage of Medicare (Title XVIII) and Medicaid (Title XIX) legislation was intended to open the health system to Blacks, the handicapped, the indigent, and the elderly poor (Cobb, 1981). In spite of these legislative and other accomplishments, however, Blacks remain disproportionately poor and unhealthy.

Low-income people have death rates that are twice the rates for people with incomes above the poverty level (Amler & Dull, 1987). Poverty reduces a person's opportunities for long life by increasing the chances of, for example, infant death, chronic disease, and traumatic death (Healthy People 2000, 1990).

No single indicator of health status makes the connection between poverty and poor health clearer than does infant mortality. It has been said (Institute of Medicine, 1985) that poor pregnancy outcomes, including prematurity, low birth weight, birth defects, and infant death, are associated with low income, low educational level, low occupational status, and other indicators of social and economic disadvantage. Therefore, because Black babies are twice as likely as White babies to die before their first birthday, the poverty-health relationship for Blacks is especially significant and in need of urgent improvement.

Because Blacks are disproportionately poor, race (i.e., being Black) is increasingly viewed as a proxy of ill health. Therefore, given the relationship between low socioeconomic status (SES) or poverty and health for Blacks, it is evident that for any meaningful improvements to occur, major interventional efforts are needed at the "macro" or structural levels of American society. If successful, these interventions should produce greater equality in living standards and general economic well-being for Blacks as a group.

Infrastructure Decline and Environmental Hazards

From a structural point of view, major interventions are needed from federal, state, and local governments to address (e.g., through revitalization projects) the decaying infrastructure of inner cities (see chapter 21). Help is needed (e.g., through more effective governmental regulation and community "grass-roots" actions) to reduce the amount of environmental hazards that currently exist and are increasing.

More than 57 percent of Blacks live in central cities, which is viewed as the highest concentration of any racial and ethnic group (Bullard, 1992). Urban decay includes, but is not limited to, densely congested neighborhoods, unsanitary and dilapidated housing, crime-ridden and drug-infested communities, inadequate and/or unwilling police presence, high unemployment and ill-staffed, deteriorating schools. From a physical point of view, the decay of inner cities also means increasing exposure to pollution and environmental hazards for their residents.

Pollution and Environmental Hazards

Modernization has brought with it different types of pollution and environmental hazards. Pollutants include exhaust fumes from motor vehicles, natural and artificial chemical emissions from factories, chemical fertilizers, herbicides, and pesticides used in agriculture, and other industrial wastes (Doll, 1992). A major environmental hazard affecting Blacks is lead poisoning. Estimates suggest that one American child in six has toxic amounts of lead in his or her blood and that 400,000 infants are born each year with undesirable toxic lead levels. Lead is ingested by children who eat paint peelings from lead-based paint on walls. The incidence of Black children with blood levels greater than 15 ug/dL of blood is 55 percent. It is important to note that lead toxicity begins at blood levels as low as 10 to 15 ug/dL (Walker, Goodwin & Warren, 1992).

Toxic pollution hazards, because of their negative impact on Blacks and other minorities, need to be eliminated through the collective interaction of Black community residents (e.g., grass-roots organizations) as well as by the variety of organizations (e.g., church, nonprofit, and watchdog agencies) suggested in the E-I-O model seen in Figure 27.1. A disproportionate number of uncontrolled toxic waste sites are located in Black and Hispanic communities (Commission for Racial Injustice, 1987). Also, large commercial hazardous waste landfills and disposal facilities are more likely to be found in rural communities in the southern Black Belt (General Accounting Office, 1983; see also discussion in Chapter 21).

With Blacks disproportionately represented in the inner cities and poor communities of America, they are at greater risk of severe health dysfunctions. Intervention through organizational involvement is needed to address issues of environmental racism and environmental equity (see Mohai & Bryant, 1992).

The interacting parts of the E-I-O model, as seen in Figure 27.1, provide the means by which, for example, racial parity concerning environmental pollution can be achieved. Not only should Black community residents[I] become informed and empowered to protect their local communities[E], but they should receive and/or acquire assistance through various organizations[O], such as teaching/research universities (through research), government (through legislation and regulation), and others like nonprofit and watchdog agencies (through surveillance and lobbying strategies). Figure 27.1 displays the interactions within and among these major parameters of the E-I-O model.

THE INDIVIDUAL: IMPROVEMENTS THROUGH PREVENTION, RESPONSIBILITY, AND EMPOWERMENT

As a contemporary writer has noted, "Men as a rule find it easier to rely on healers than to attempt the more difficult task of living wisely" (David, 1993, p. 32). Health resides within the individual; therefore, improvements in Black health will, to a large extent, be influenced by Blacks' biology, skills/resources, and life-style. For example, in the case of biology, Blacks should be provided with genetic counseling, when needed, about sickle cell anemia, identifying carriers of the sickle cell trait (see chapter 9).

In terms of skills/resources, Blacks should be educated about the *positive* value (see Figure 27.1 for the + signs) of such qualities as mastery (+) (Pearlin, Lieberman, Menaghan & Mullan, 1981), hardiness (+) (Kobasa, 1979) empowerment (+) (Braithwaite & Lythcott, 1989; Livingston, 1993), and being socially integrated in groups (+) (Livingston, Levine & Moore, 1991). Research has demonstrated a positive relationship between these qualities and health. Because of the overriding and direct importance of life-style activities on health in general and the health of Blacks in particular, a more detailed discussion follows around this individual[I] domain of the E-I-O model.

Life-style Activities

The astronomical costs of treating preventable diseases only strengthen the case for prevention. For example, smoking-related illness costs our health care system more than $65 billion annually to treat; the yearly cost of treating alcohol and drug abuse is at least $16 billion; and the lifetime costs of caring for a person with AIDS now exceed $100,000 (Fineberg, 1993).

Approximately 85 percent of human illness is attributed to life-style activities. Because of the importance of this relationship, more empirical and population-based studies are needed to assess both interracial and intraracial differences in life-style, adjusting for potentially confounding covariates such as socioeconomic status (SES).

Health Habits Survey

An important national survey conducted in 1990 assessed the health habits of Americans 18 years and older (Piani and Schoenborn, 1993). Specifically, the study measured the prevalence of selected health promotion and disease prevention knowledge practices (stratifying for race and gender). Selected results of this survey are presented in Table 27.1. The results reported in this study can, along with other information presented, serve as a basis for action/intervention within the context of the E-I-O model. Relevant sections of the report are included in sections that immediately follow.

Blacks must be educated to become more aware of the relationship between health promotion, risk factors, and well-being. However, for many Blacks this education, which should come from designated organizations[O], will amount to nothing short of "resocialization," especially for those Blacks with low incomes and low educational attainments (see chapters 16 and 26).

Because the behavior of Black people (like any other group) is so entwined in the social, cultural, and psychological experiences of the wider society[E], any request to change or alter these behaviors is tantamount to a request to abandon parts of one's own culture or way of life. This issue is compounded by the reality that the positive replacement "values" may not seem attractive at first and, unfortunately, will not instantaneously translate into "good" or "better" health for Blacks; hence, the proposed changes may meet skepticism and a reluctance to be "changed." Also, given the sociopolitical realities of poverty[E], in addition to a lack of, for example, mastery (+) and empowerment (+), the likelihood that Blacks will accept a different value system becomes even more remote. These issues underscore the need for sociostructural changes in society[E], as well as innovative and culturally sensitive health promotion/education strategies by organizations[O] to educate Blacks about the need to adopt more beneficial and health-oriented life-styles.

Nutrition, obesity, and exercise. Through effective health education intervention, Blacks can become empowered to exercise (+) and eat healthful, low-fat diets (+), which reduces the risk of obesity and related disease such as coronary heart disease (see chapter 2) and cancer (see chapter 6). Also, obesity and sedentary lifestyles appear as risk factors for a variety of health dysfunctions, for example, hypertension and diabetes, both of which are risk factors for heart disease (see chapter 18). It is interesting to note (see Table 27.1) that Black females (46.8%) walked less for exercise than did White females (49.5%); both Black males (34.0%) and females (21.3%) reported less physical activity than White males (38.3%) and females (28.9%) when asked about being physically

Table 27.1

Percentage of Persons 18 Years and Over on Selected Health Promotion and Disease Prevention Activities by Race and Gender, United States, 1990

| Selected Activities | Race | | | |
| | Black | | White | |
	Male	Female	Male	Female
General Health Habits:				
• Eats breakfast	47.0	46.7	55.6	59.8
• 20% > body wt.	31.1	40.4	29.7	24.0
• Pap smear exam. in past year	——	54.3	——	49.7
• Breast exam in past year	——	55.3	——	53.1
• Blood pressure ck. in past year	84.7	92.6	82.9	90.6
• Told had high pressure two or more times	20.0	22.3	15.1	16.7
• Told had high blood pressure & taking meds.	70.1	73.8	66.9	71.3
• Ever had blood cholesterol ck.	35.4	47.4	52.4	56.8
• Moderate stress in past 2 weeks	44.5	50.7	55.8	61.5
• Stress has some effects on health	32.0	43.8	34.4	46.8
• Walked for exercise in past 2 weeks	42.8	46.8	40.8	49.5
• Know the value of exercise (3x week, 20 mins/session)	3.1	4.5	5.2	5.4

Table 27.1—Continued

Selected Activities	Race			
	Black		White	
	Male	Female	Male	Female
• > physically active than others like self	34.0	21.3	38.2	28.9
• Currently smoke	32.5	21.2	28.0	23.4
• Currently smoke & knowledge about smoke & heart disease	81.8	87.3	89.0	91.0
• Know about risk of smoking & heart disease	85.5	86.4	92.2	92.5
• Had at least 1 drink (beer, wine or liquor) in past year	62.7	33.3	73.6	53.6
• Seen dentist within past year	46.0	56.4	60.8	67.2
• Had mammogram within past 3 years (35+ years old)	____	44.9	____	51.5
• Had at least 1 working smoke detector in house	71.2	71.1	79.6	79.7
• Wear seat belts most of time when riding in car	56.4	59.7	62.6	72.5
• Ever heard of radon	52.7	46.7	78.8	70.3

Source: A. Piani and C. Schoenborn (1993). Health promotion and disease prevention: United States, 1990. NCHS, *Vital and Health Statistics,* Series 10, No. 85, DHHS Publication No. (PHS) 93-1513. Hyattsville, MD.

active relative to others like themselves. Regarding hypertension status, Blacks were more hypertensive than Whites and currently taking their hypertension medication (see Chapter 4). Interestingly enough, however, given that cholesterol is a prime risk factor for heart disease, both Black males (35.4%) and females (47.4%), compared with their White male (52.4%) and female (56.8%) counterparts, reported a lower prevalence of ever having a blood cholesterol check. It must be noted that the racial comparisons made between these percentage distributions reflect substantive as opposed to statistical differences.

For Black females, however, obesity-related conditions may be a result of life-style activities as well as race-related predispositions (The NHLBI Growth and Health Study Research Group, 1992). However, other studies (e.g., Burke et al., 1992) reported that total (caloric) intake was higher in Black women, while physical activity and fitness levels were significantly higher in White women. Also, White women were more likely to diet and more likely than Black women to perceive obesity as harmful. As seen in Table 27.1, Blacks reported being more obese than Whites, which was particularly significant for Black females (40.4%) compared with White females (24.0%). Changes in life-style behaviors regarding nutrition and exercise should contribute to an improvement in morbidity and mortality rates associated with these and other dysfunctions in Blacks.

Smoking. Because of the relationship between cigarette smoking and health, smoking (−) needs to be seriously addressed among Blacks. A higher percentage of Blacks are currently smokers and a smaller percentage have quit smoking, compared with Whites (U.S. Bureau of the Census, 1991) (see chapter 14). Smoking and the use and abuse of illicit substances among pregnant women are thought to be a major factor in low-birth-weight babies (i.e., less than 2,500 grams), a strong predictor of infant mortality (Petitti & Coleman, 1990) (see chapter 15). As seen in Table 27.1, while Black males (32.5%) currently smoked more than White males (28.0%), as a group fewer Blacks reported knowing about the risk of heart disease associated with cigarette smoking.

Alcohol consumption. The relationship between alcohol consumption (−) and health dysfunctions has been reported in the past (Livingston, 1985). Black men had a cirrhosis death rate that in 1988 was 1.7 times greater than that of White men, while Black women had a rate that was 1.9 times that of White women. Also, age-adjusted incidence rates for cancer of the esophagus and oral cavity/ pharynx among Black men were 16.1 and 21.5, respectively. These rates contrasted with rates of 5.3 and 14.9 among comparable White men (NCHS, 1991). Other health outcomes related to the abuse of alcohol and other drugs include homicide (Gary, 1986), excessive mortality (Whitfield, Davis & Barker, 1986), and HIV infection and AIDS (Massachusetts Department of Public Health, 1992). Table 27.1, however, shows that Blacks, as a group, reported a lower prevalence than Whites when asked if they had had at least one drink in the past year. The manner in which the question was asked could, however, be responsible for the results.

HIV infection and AIDS. AIDS is disproportionately experienced by Blacks. Whereas only 12 percent of the U.S. population are Black, 28 percent of AIDS patients are Black (CDC, 1991). Organizational input is required to modify the perception Blacks have of HIV/AIDS (Livingston, 1990) as well as sexual practices of Black youth and adolescents. Inner-city Black adolescents, however, are particularly at risk. It has been reported that sexually transmitted diseases are two to three times more common in inner-city populations, and the adolescent pregnancy rate is nearly twice as high among Blacks as among Whites. Also, the high prevalence of intravenous drug use in the inner city increases the risk of HIV infection for Black adolescents (Jemmott, Jemmott, & Fong, 1992) (see chapter 11).

Other life-style practices. Despite improvements in oral health in the U.S. population in the past several decades, there is still considerable evidence of unnecessary oral disease (National Institute of Dental Research, 1989). Approximately 44.5 percent of Blacks, compared with 59.3 percent of Whites, had a dental visit in the past 12 months (Bloom, Gift & Jack, 1992). These racial disparities are reflected in Table 27.1 as fewer Blacks (males = 46%; females = 56.4%) than Whites (males = 60.8%; females = 67.2%) reported seeing a dentist within the past year. Major interventions are needed in this area.

As seen in Table 27.1, fewer Black females (44.9%) than White females (51.5%) reported having had a mammogram within the last three years. Asked about injury-control activities (i.e., having a working smoke detector in the house and wearing seat belts when riding in a car), more Whites than Blacks responded affirmatively. In ever having heard about radon, fewer Blacks than Whites responded affirmatively.

ORGANIZATIONS: INPUT, INTERVENTION, AND IMPROVEMENT

Health care in the United States has been described as follows: "In a significant measure what we [i.e., Americans] have is not a health care system but a disease care system. We have created a medical-care complex that is pretty darn good at diagnosing disease, managing disease, and sometimes curing disease—but not nearly so good at preventing disease. And sometimes it is only too good at creating disease" (David, 1993, pp. 31–32). As can be seen in the E-I-O model (Figure 27.1), organizations[O], although subsumed by the environment[E], have pivotal roles in influencing the health of individuals[I]. The influence of organizations on Black health can be assessed in terms of what they do (e.g., educating, treating, researching, regulating) or what they fail to do. What follows are some issues and activities that are important for organizations as they interface with Blacks and around which important interventional efforts can be directed to improve the health status of Blacks.

Parity in Access to Wider Societal Resources

It is increasingly agreed that racial disparities in the quality of health among Americans mainly result from differences in both need and access. Blacks are more likely to require care but are less likely to receive (quality) health care services (Orentlicher, 1990). In attempting to find meaningful solutions to improve the health of Blacks, policymakers must have the courage to pursue difficult, yet long-term and sustainable solutions (e.g., meaningfully addressing institutional racism) rather than short-term solutions, which are likely to result in short-lived improvements at best.

Health Care: A Right or a Privilege?

According to Cockerham (1992) health care is more "an opportunity rather than a commodity, it should be available as a right to all Americans, regardless of living conditions or financial status" (p. 262). However, historical lessons learned from the United Kingdom suggest that if increased access to health care is not accompanied by fundamental changes in the institutional structure of society (e.g., reducing poverty), the health of poor people does not dramatically improve (Wilkinson, 1986).

Access to Health Care and Related Factors

Any comprehensive organizational[O] effort aimed at improving utilization of health services by Blacks must address the accompanying interrelated issues of affordability, availability, and acceptability of health care (see health care organizations in the E-I-O model in Figure 27.1).

Affordability of Health Care

Insurance coverage affects whether or not persons (i.e., Blacks) gain access to care and the manner in which that care is delivered. "Most basically, individuals completely lacking health insurance may delay or forego care that has the potential to dramatically improve their health and functioning and even prevent premature death" (U.S. Congress, Office of Technology Assessment, 1992, p. 43). Studies have reported that the uninsured have a higher relative probability of in-hospital death than the insured. Of specific importance, however, is the report that the probability of in-hospital death was greater for Blacks than for Whites (Johnson, 1991).

Availability of Health Care

Historically, many White physicians would not accept Blacks as patients. This fact, coupled with the dearth of Black physicians, has contributed to a situation in which many Blacks have no identified physician and/or no regular source of care except hospital clinics or emergency rooms (McDavid, 1990). Various factors affect the relative lack of available health care facilities and personnel for Blacks. It was reported (Airhihenbuwa, 1989) that in a national profile on medical access the ratio of Black families to White families who needed medical care but did not obtain it was approximately 2:1.

Acceptability of health care

Organizational intervention is needed to improve the perception Blacks have of medical care and the quality of services rendered to them as a group. Although several factors may contribute to how acceptable the health care services are to Blacks, a salient issue has been racial compatibility between provider and patient (Protor & Rosen, 1982). This being the case, how Blacks utilize health care services may be significantly improved if there is a visible representation of Black (and other minority) health care providers in these health care facilities.

Areas for Organizational Input and Intervention

Because of their visibility and direct relationship to the morbidity and mortality of Blacks, the following selected areas need more aggressive organizational interventions.

Heart disease and *stroke* together account for 30 percent of the excess deaths among Blacks, with Blacks having a stroke mortality rate that is 66 percent higher than that of Whites (Kim, 1989). Therefore, because 30 percent of excess deaths among Blacks can be attributed to heart disease and stroke, the area of cardiovascular (see chapters 1 and 2) and cerebrovascular (see chapter 3) diseases (and their related areas) must be targeted for exploratory, etiologic, and race-specific research.

Excessive *delays in seeking medical care* (e.g., thrombolytic therapy) for myocardial infarction may contribute to the higher mortality rates from CHD reported for Blacks (Maynard, Fischer & Passamani, 1987) despite the fact that coronary artery disease is actually more severe in Whites (Simmons et al., 1988). Inner-city Blacks experience, on average, delays up to three times as long as those reported for White patients (Cooper et al., 1986). Interventions in this area can, for example, be spearheaded by the National Medical Association, along with other black-related medical organizations, by more aggressively educating Blacks about these CHD-related issues (e.g., early warning signs of impending heart attacks and preventive risk factors), especially directed at Blacks who are at greatest risk (i.e., low SES, obesity, smoking, and a sedentary life-style).

In terms of *cancer*, evidence is now accumulating that the causes of increased cancer morbidity and mortality in Blacks are related more to poverty and lack of education than to any inherent racial characteristics (Baquet, Horm, Gibbs & Greenwald, 1991). Again, organizations such as outreach hospital programs, health auxiliaries of black churches, and counsellors at inner-city schools (see Livingston, 1993) can educate Blacks (both youth and adults) about, for example, dietary risk factors associated with cancer.

In terms of *HIV/AIDS,* the federal government and black community organizations must work together to educate at-risk (e.g., sexually active and IV-drug using) segments of the Black population about the etiology of AIDS and how "risky" behaviors (e.g., unprotected sex) place them at risk of being infected with HIV. Also, modern health care organizations and the federal government must keep an "open mind" and, where feasible, collaborate with other groups and organizations (e.g., traditional health care workers, Third World Organizations) who may have important information regarding possible cures for AIDS.

As the *underutilization of Blacks in research* means that Blacks and Hispanics are less likely to participate in surveys and clinical studies, there is little information about risk groups within these minority populations (Anderson, Mullner & Cornelius, 1987). In almost any area of clinical or psychosocial research, there is a need to know if Blacks are affected differently than Whites and, if so, to know why. For example, it is important to know for which diseases, such as breast cancer, Blacks may be at no greater risk than Whites (Schatzkin, Palmer, Rosenberg et al., 1987).

Racial disparities in medical treatment mean that Blacks are less likely to have angiographic studies done or to have coronary-artery bypass surgery performed (Strogatz, 1980). Even after adjusting for age, sex, payor, income, and primary and secondary diagnoses, Whites still undergo more coronary-artery bypass grafting (CABG) procedures (Wenneker & Epstein, 1989). A recent national study found that for patients insured by Medicare, race is strongly associated with CABG rates (Goldberg et al., 1992).

Racial status has also been found to correlate with the likelihood that a patient with kidney disease will receive long-term hemodialysis or a kidney transplant (Kjellstrand & Logan, 1987). Also, discriminatory and other practices regarding end-stage renal disease (ESRD) have been reported in the past (Livingston & Ackah, 1992).

CONCLUSION

Improving the health status of Blacks, although difficult, is not an insurmountable task. Sustained success, however, will require action that leads to bold, innovative, comprehensive, and culturally sensitive directives. As discussed in this chapter and as illustrated in the E-I-O model, the outlook for positive improvements in the health of Blacks can only come through a mutually agreed-upon framework for collective action involving active participation at the environmental[E], individual[I], and organizational[O] levels. The interrelationship among these three areas is aptly illustrated in Figure 27.1.

While organizations involving the federal government, the health care sector, education, and private concerns will and should play their respective roles, a positive and sustaining outlook on health, especially for Blacks at risk, will be ultimately achieved only through Black self-help, motivation and, most important, empowerment (Braithwaite & Lythcott, 1989). In short, Blacks have to become more responsible for their health, not only at the individual level but also at the other interfacing levels involving organizations and the environment.

Blacks have to become re-energized and demand more control over their health and welfare. Apart from becoming empowered to engage in protective lifestyle behaviors (e.g., increasing their levels of exercise; eating less cholesterol-laden foods; controlling excess body weight; consuming less alcohol; having annual, or more frequent as needed, physical examinations; and learning how to control stress) Blacks must collectively demand, for example, through the legislative process and lobbying efforts, that equal rights for all means just that, and nothing less. A re-energized Black community that demands more for itself and its members can achieve the following: (a) needed support to clean up and rebuild inner-city communities; (b) curtailment of toxic dumping in minority communities; (c) creation of jobs and low-interest loans for entrepreneurial activity that stimulates economic growth and prosperity; (d) inner-city communities that are safe and relatively crime-free; (e) rebuilding of inner-city schools, libraries, and recreational parks as places for Black children to study, play, and explore and extend their God-given potential; and (f) the strict enforcement (or introduction if needed) of federal, state, and local ordinances restricting the sale of alcohol, especially in poorer sections of Black communities. In short, there needs to be a cultural, spiritual, psychological, and economic revitalization within the Black community that will, in turn, contribute to racial parity in health.

In closing, inaction and/or failure to improve the health conditions of Blacks living in America will have disastrous moral, political, physical, and social consequences. In terms of cardiovascular and cerebrovascular diseases, the number one and three killers, respectively, of all Americans, Richard Gillum stated in chapter 1 that Blacks continue to experience excess mortality compared to Whites for diseases of the heart, hypertension, and stroke. In terms of cancer, the number two killer of all Americans, Ki Moon Bang stated in chapter 6 that the overall trends in cancer incidence and mortality have been increasing among Blacks, and it is estimated that Blacks have approximately a 30 percent cancer-related mortality compared with their White counterparts. Eugene Tull and colleagues, in chapter 7, documented the serious current and projected problems of diabetes mellitus and its complications in the Black population. And, in a related manner in chapter 10, Stephen McLeod and Maurice Rabb focused on the infrequently addressed racial problems in ophthalmology, where they highlighted among various issues the real problem of diabetic retinopathy among Blacks.

The remaining chapters in this book, whether they were addressing the issue of AIDS, intentional or unintentional injuries, drug use and dependency, infant mortality, stress, mental health, nutrition, homelessness, Black elderly, environmental health and declining infrastructures, growth and development of Black children, politics and health, health care utilization, and the need for empowerment through health education, all further underscore the magnitude and urgent need to achieve racial parity in health. If substantial and sustained changes are not achieved, it is safe to say that the ensuing consequences will, with time, bring unprecedented misery and upheaval the likes of which this nation has never known. The time to act is now, because yesterday was too late!

REFERENCES

Airhihenbuwa, C.O. (1989). Health education for African Americans: A neglected task. *Health Education, 20,* 9–14.

Amler, R. W., & Dull, H. B. (1987). *Closing the gap: The burden of unnecessary illness.* New York: Oxford University Press.

Anderson, R., Mullner, R. M., & Cornelius, L. J. (1987). Black-white differences in health status: Methods or substance? *Milbank Quarterly, 65,* 72–99.

Baquet, C. R., Horm, J. W., Gibbs, T., & Greenwald, P. (1991). Socioeconomic factors and cancer incidence among blacks and whites. *Journal of the National Cancer Institute, 83,* 551–557.

Bloom, B., Gift, H. C., & Jack, S. S. (1992). Dental services and oral health: United States, 1989. National Center for Health Statistics. *Vital Health Statistics, 10,* 15–17.

Braithwaite, R. L., & Lythcott, N. (1989). Community empowerment as a strategy for health promotion for black and other minority populations. *Journal of the American Medical Association, 261,* 282–283.

Bullard, R. D. (1992). Urban infrastructure: Social, environmental, and health risks to African Americans. In B. J. Tidwell (Ed.). *The state of Black America.* New York: The Urban League, Inc.

Burke, G. L., Savage, P. J., Manolio, T. A., Sprafka, J. M., Wagenknecht, L. E., Sidney, S., Perkins, C. C., Liu, K., & Jacobs, D. R. (1992). Correlates of obesity in young black and white women. The CARDIA study. *American Journal of Public Health, 82,* 1621–1625.

Centers for Disease Control (CDC). (1991). HIV/AIDS surveillance report, June 1–8. Atlanta, GA: Center for Infectious Diseases, CDC.

Cobb, W. M. (1981). The black American in medicine. *Journal of The National Medical Association, 78,* 1185–1244.

Cockerham, W. C. (1992). *Medical sociology* (5th ed.). Englewood Cliffs, NJ: Prentice-Hall.

Commission for Racial Justice. (1987). Waste and race in the United States: A national report on the racial and socioeconomic characteristics of communities with hazardous waste sites. New York: United Church of Christ.

Cooper, R. S., Simmons, B., Castaner, A., Prasad, R., Franklin, C., & Ferlinz, J. (1986). Survival rates and prehospital delay during myocardial infarction among black persons. *America Journal of Cardiology, 57,* 208–211.

David, R. (1993). The demand side of the health care crisis. *Harvard Magazine, 95,* 31–32.

Dever, G. E. A. (1984). Epidemiology and health policy (pp. 25–46). *Epidemiology in health services management.* Rockville, MD: Aspen Systems Corporation.

Doll, R. (1992). Health and the environment in the 1990s. *American Journal of Public Health, 82,* 933–943.

Fineberg, H. V. (1993). The power of prevention. *Harvard School of Public Health 1991–1992 Annual Report*. Boston, MA: Harvard School of Public Health.

Gary, L. E. (1986). Drinking, homicide and the black male. *Journal of Black Studies, 80,* 397–410.

General Accounting Office. (1983). Siting of hazardous waste landfills and their correlation with racial and economic status of surrounding communities. Washington, DC: General Accounting Office.

Goldberg, K. C., Hartz, A. J., Jacobsen, S. J., Krakauer, H., & Rimm, A. A. (1992). Racial and community factors influencing coronary artery bypass graft surgery rates for all 1986 Medicare patients. *Journal of the American Medical Association, 267,* 1473–1477.

Healthy People 2000. (1990). *National health promotion and disease prevention objectives*. DHHS Publication No. (PHS) 91-50213. Washington, DC: Government Printing Office.

Institute of Medicine. (1985). *Preventing low birthweight*. Washington, DC: National Academy Press.

Jemmott, J. B., Jemmott, L. S., & Fong, G. T. (1992). Reductions in HIV risk-associated sexual behaviors among black male adolescents: Effects of an AIDS prevention intervention. *American Journal of Public Health, 82,* 372–377.

Johnson, C. (1991). Challenge for the minority physician: Gaining quality health care for the underserved. *Journal of the National Medical Association, 83,* 563–568.

Kim, T. F. (1989). Research seeks to reduce toll of hypertension, other cardiovascular disease in black population. *Journal of the American Medical Association, 261,* 195.

Kjellstrand, C. M., & Logan, G. M. (1987). Racial, sexual, and age inequalities in chronic dialysis. *Nephronology, 45,* 257–263.

Kobasa, S. C. (1979). Stressful life events, personality, and health: An inquiry into hardiness. *Journal of Personality and Social Psychology, 37,* 1–11.

Lalonde, M. (1974). *A new perspective on the health of Canadians*. Ottawa: Canadian Department of Health and Welfare.

Livingston, I. L. (1985). Alcohol consumption and hypertension: A review with suggested implications. *Journal of the National Medical Association, 77,* 129–135.

Livingston, I. L. (1990). Perceived control, knowledge and fear of AIDS among college students: An exploratory study. *Journal of Health and Social Policy, 2,* 47–65.

Livingston, I. L., Levine, D. M., & Moore, R. (1991). Social integration and black intraracial blood pressure variation. *Ethnicity and Disease, 1,* 135–149.

Livingston, I. L., & Ackah, S. (1992). Hypertension, end-stage renal disease and rehabilitation: A look at black Americans. *The Western Journal of Black Studies, 16,* 103–112.

Livingston, I. L. (1993). Stress, hypertension and young black Americans: The importance of counseling. *Journal of Multicultural Counseling, 21,* 132–142.

Massachusetts Department of Public Health. (1992). Disparities in health status among racial and ethnic groups in Massachusetts, April.

Maynard, C., Fisher, L. D., & Passamani, E. R. (1987). Survival of black persons compared with white persons in the Coronary Artery Surgery Study (CASS). *American Journal of Cardiology, 60,* 513–518.

McDavid, L. M. (1990). An overlooked resource: The black patient (pp. 67–70). Conference Proceedings: Primary care research: An agenda for the 1990s. Agency for Health Care Primary Research (AHCPR), September.

Mohai, P., & Bryant, B. (1992). Race, poverty, and the environment. *EPA Journal, 18,* 6–8.

National Center for Health Statistics. (1991). Vital statistics of the United States, 1988, Volume II, mortality part A. Public Health Service. Washington, DC: Government Printing Office.

National Institute of Dental Research. (1989). Oral health of United States children. The National Survey of Dental Caries in U.S. Children: 1986-1987. Epidemiology and Oral Disease Prevention Program. NIDR/NIH 89-2247. Bethesda, MD.

O'Hare, W. P. (1987). Black demographic trends in the 1980s. *Milbank Quarterly, 65* (supp.), 35–55.

Orentlicher, D. (1990). Black-white disparities in health care. *Connecticut Medicine, 54,* 625–628.

Pearlin, L. T., Lieberman, M. A., Menaghan, E. G., & Mullan, J. T. (1981). The stress process. *Journal of Health and Social Behavior, 22,* 337–356.

Petitti, B. D., & Coleman, C. (1990). Cocaine and the risk of low birthweight. *American Journal of Public Health, 80,* 25–32.

Piani, A., & Schoenborn, C. (1993). Health promotion and disease prevention: United States, 1990. NCHS, *Vital and Health Statistics,* Series 10, No. 85, DHHS Publication No. (PHS) 93-1513. Hyattsville, MD.

Protor, E., & Rosen, A. (1982). Expectations and preferences for counselor race and their relation to intermediate treatment outcomes. *Journal of Counseling Psychology, 28,* 40–46.

Schatzkin, A., Palmer, J. R., Rosenberg, L., et al. (1987). Risk factors for breast cancer in black women. *Journal of the National Cancer Institute, 78,* 213–217.

Shea, S., & Fullilove, M. T. (1985). Entry of black and other minority students in U.S. medical schools: Historical perspectives and recent trends. *New England Journal of Medicine, 313,* 933–940.

Sidel, V. W., & Sidel, R. (Eds.). (1984). *Reforming medicine: Lessons of the last quarter century.* New York, NY: Pantheon Books.

Simmons, B. E., Castaner, A., Campo, A., Ferlinz, J., Mar, M., & Cooper, R. (1988). Coronary artery disease in blacks of lower socioeconomic status: Angiographic findings from the Cook County Hospital registry. *American Heart Journal, 116,* 90–97.

Strogatz, D. S. (1980). Use of medical care for chest pain: Differences for blacks and whites. *American Journal of Public Health, 80,* 290–294.

Terris, M. (1984). Newer perspectives on the health of Canadians: Beyond the Lalonde report. *Journal of Health Policy, 5,* 327–337.

The National Heart, Lung, & Blood Institute Growth and Health Study Research Group. (1992). Obesity and cardiovascular disease risk factors in black and white girls: The NHLBI growth and health study. *American Journal of Public Health, 82,* 1613–1620.

Thomas, S. B. (1922). Health status of the black community in the 21st century: A futuristic perspective for health education. *Journal of Health Education, 23,* 7–13.

U.S. Bureau of the Census. (1992). *Current Population Reports, Poverty in the United States: 1991.* Series P-60, No. 181. Washington, DC: Government Printing Office.

U.S. Bureau of the Census. (1991). *Statistical Abstract of the United States* (111th Edition). Washington, DC: Government Printing Office.

U.S. Congress, Office of Technology Assessment. (1992). Does health insurance make a difference? Background paper, OTA-BP-H-99. Washington, DC: Government Printing Office.

Walker, B., Goodwin, N. J., & Warren, R. C. (1992). Violence: A challenge to the public health community. *Journal of the National Medical Association, 84,* 490–496.

Wenneker, M. B., & Epstein, A. M. (1989). Racial inequalities in the use of procedures for patients with ischemic heart disease in Massachusetts. *Journal of the American Medical Association, 261,* 253–257.

Whitfield, C. L., Davis, J. E., & Barker, L. R. (1986). Alcoholism. In L. R. Barker, J. R. Burton, & P. D. Zieve (Eds.), *Principles of ambulatory medicine* (2nd ed.). Baltimore: Williams and Wilkins.

Wilkinson, R. G. (1986). *Class and health.* London: Travistock.

Index

Abel, G. G., 131
Abu-Bakare, A., 101
Access to care. *See* Health care; Health care utilization
Acquired immune deficiency syndrome (AIDS): and access to health care, 165; and age- and race-related mortality, 158; and AZT, 162; and behavioral research, 166; and bisexuality, 157–158; and the Black community, 157–158, 337–338, 409; and clinical research, 163; and collective efforts to control, 166; and contaminated blood products, 159; and costs of treatment, 404; and distribution of cases, 158; and economic consequences, 157; epidemiology of, 157–158; and future imperatives, 165–166; gender-specific manifestations, 159; and health care system and institutional racism, 165; and HIV infection, 161–162; and HIV-related renal disease, 162; and homosexuality, 157–158; and insurance, 157; and issues in therapy, 162–163; and mortality-specific deaths, 159; origins of, 164–165; pediatric cases of, 159; and perinatal transmission, 159; and poverty, 157; prevalence of, 338;

prevention of, 162, 165–166; and race and racial differences in mortality, 338, 344; and racist attitudes, 165; and sexually transmitted diseases, 157, 165–166; signs and symptoms of, 161–162; and survival times, 162; and women, 159
Acton, R. T., 97, 100
Acute myocardial infarction (AMI), 5
Adair, R., 258, 261–264
Adams-Campbell, L. L., 271, 274
Addiction, and treatment and rehabilitation, 210–211. *See also* Alcoholism; Chemical dependency; Illicit drug use and abuse
Adebimpe, V. R., 259–260
African Americans: and activism around health issues, 326; and central cities, 315; and empowerment, 393–395; families of, 315; and home ownership, 318; and housing discrimination, 316–317; and lending institutions, 316–317; and location of waste sites, 319–323. *See also* Blacks
Agency for Toxic Substances and Disease Registry, 333, 335
Ahmed, F., 218, 222–225, 230
Aid to Families with Dependent Children (AFDC), 334, 340

About the Editor and Contributors

IVOR LENSWORTH LIVINGSTON, Ph.D., M.P.H., is a Graduate Associate Professor of Medical Sociology/Social Epidemiology and Social Psychology, and Director of Undergraduate Studies, Department of Sociology and Anthropology, and Adjunct Associate Professor, Department of Community Health and Family Practice, School of Medicine, Howard University. He was educated at Howard University, Harvard University, and Johns Hopkins University. He is an affiliated member of the Resource Persons Network, Office of Minority Health Resource Center, U.S. Department of Health and Human Services. He also advises many organizations on a variety of issues, including hypertension, stress, mental health, and HIV/AIDS. His main research interests include the social epidemiology of cardiovascular and immunological diseases in African Americans and people of color in the Third World. Dr. Livingston is the author of *The ABC's of Stress Management*, and he has been published in many national and international journals including the *Journal of the National Medical Association, National Journal of Sociology, Ethnicity and Disease, Stress and Medicine, Health Promotion International,* and *Social Science and Medicine.*

LAWRENCE Y. AGODOA, M.D., is Director, Minority Health Program and End-Stage Renal Disease Program, Division of Kidney, Urologic, and Hematologic Diseases, National Institute of Diabetes and Digestive and Kidney Diseases, National Institutes of Health, Bethesda, Maryland.

FEROZ AHMED, Ph.D., is a professor in the School of Social Work, Howard University. His areas of interest are demography and health and social behavior. For the past several years, he has been working on infant mortality among African Americans, particularly in the District of Columbia.

COLLINS O. AIRHIHENBUWA, M.P.H., Ph.D., is an associate professor of health education and an affiliate faculty member of the Black Studies Program at Pennsylvania State University. His research focuses on the influence of cultural identity on health determinants and health outcomes among Africans and African Americans in order to develop culturally appropriate health promotion strategies.

OMOWALE AMULERU-MARSHALL, Ph.D., M.P.H., is currently the Southern Regional Director for the Center for Health and Development, a Boston-based organization dedicated to the health and development of African and African-descended people. He is the founding director of the Cork Institute on Black Alcohol and Other Drug Abuse. He has lectured across the United States and abroad on a variety of topics, most recently on the prevention and treatment of chemical slavery among African Americans.

KI MOON BANG, Ph.D., M.P.H., is currently serving as Chief of Respiratory Disease Surveillance, the National Institute for Occupational Safety and Health (NIOSH), Centers for Disease Control in Morgantown, West Virginia. He is also a faculty member in the Department of Community Health and Family Practice, Howard University College of Medicine. His specialty areas are cancer and pulmonary epidemiology.

GREGG BARAK, Ph.D., is a professor and Chairman of the Department of Sociology, Anthropology, and Criminology at Eastern Michigan University. Among his numerous publications are those that specifically address the ''Black experience.''

DEBORAH E. BLOCKER, D.Sc., M.P.H., R.D., is an assistant professor in nutrition and the Food Science Program at Hunter College, City College of New York. Her current research interests include folic-acid metabolism, specifically looking at the neurological effects of folic deficiencies in neurologic functioning, and folic-acid and vitamin B_{12} deficiency in diabetic peripheral neuropathy.

LEE R. BONE, R.N., M.P.H., is an instructor in the Department of Health Policy and Management, Division of Behavioral Sciences and Health Education and Health Services Research and Development Center, School of Hygiene and Public Health, Johns Hopkins University. Her research interests include the design, planning, implementation, and evaluation of community-based educational and behavioral interventions/programs that address public health problems affecting vulnerable populations, health promotion, and disease prevention in chronic illnesses (e.g., high blood pressure and diabetes).

CHRISTINE M. BRANCHE-DORSEY, Ph.D., M.S.P.H., is an epidemiologist, Epidemiology Branch, National Center for Injury Prevention and Control, Centers for Disease Control and Prevention. Her research interests include descriptive and analytic studies on unintentional injuries, but mainly drowning and sports-recreation injuries.

ROBERT D. BULLARD, Ph.D., is a professor of sociology at the University of California, Riverside. He has worked on and conducted research in the areas of urban land use, housing, community development, industrial facility siting and environment quality.

J. JACQUES CARTER, M.D., M.P.H., is an instructor in medicine, Harvard Medical School, and Attending Physician, Department of Medicine, Division of General Internal Medicine, New England Deaconess Hospital, Boston. His current research interests include (1) medical education with special emphasis on primary care, (2) public health planning and management, and (3) health care delivery systems.

TERENCE L. CHORBA, M.D., M.P.H., is a medical epidemiologist, National Center for Injury Prevention and Control, Centers for Disease Control and Prevention. His research interests include developing vehicular injury control programs at CDC in conjunction with the National Highway Traffic Safety Administration.

ALEXANDER E. CROSBY, M.D., M.P.H., is a medical epidemiologist, Centers for Disease Control and Prevention, National Center for Injury Prevention and Control, Epidemiology Branch. His work consists of conducting descriptive and analytic research and providing community technical assistance in the areas of suicide, child abuse and neglect, interpersonal violence among adolescents, and assaultive injuries among minorities.

CHARLES CURRY, M.D., is a professor and Director of the Division of Cardiovascular Diseases, College of Medicine, Howard University. He is an acknowledged expert on the problem of cardiovascular disease and hypertension in African Americans. He is on the Board of Directors of the American College of Cardiology and International Society for Hypertension in Blacks.

BRENDA T. FENTON, M.Sc., is currently a doctoral student in the Department of Epidemiology and Public Health at the Yale School of Medicine. Her research interests include anxiety disorders in the African American population.

GARY H. FRIDAY, M.D., is Associate Director of Clinical Development at Astra U.S.A., Westborough, Massachusetts and assistant professor of neurology at the Medical College of Pennsylvania. His current research interests include neuroepidemiology, risk factors for stroke, and clinical trials of new treatments in the area of central nervous system diseases.

RICHARD F. GILLUM, M.D., is a special assistant to the Associate Director for Cardiovascular Epidemiology at the National Center for Health Statistics. He has been recognized for his various scholarly contributions, especially in the area of the epidemiology of cardiovascular diseases.

WAYNE L. GREAVES, M.D., is an associate professor of medicine and the Hospital Epidemiologist at Howard University Hospital. He has published and lectured on infectious diseases and epidemiology both nationally and internationally. His research has focused on hospital-acquired infections, sexually transmitted diseases, and the problem of AIDS in minority communities.

ARLENE I. GREENSPAN, M.P.H., Dr.P.H., P.T., is an Epidemic Intelligence Service Officer, Epidemiology Branch, National Center for Injury Prevention and Control, Centers for Disease Control and Prevention, U.S. Public Health Service. Her current research includes descriptive and analytic studies related to unintentional injuries, focusing on unintentional firearm injuries, motor-vehicle injuries, and head injuries.

GERALD GROVES, M.D., M.P.H., Dr.P.H., is an assistant professor of psychiatry at the University of Pennsylvania Medical School and a Veterans Administration Research Fellow in Substance Abuse. He is currently engaged in research on the elimination of cocaine from hair in recently abstinent crack addicts and on HTLV-I/II infection in chronic intravenous opioid addicts.

MARCELLA HAMMETT, M.P.H., is an epidemiologist presently at the National Center for Disease Control and Prevention, National Center for Injury Prevention and Control, where she has worked on numerous projects focusing on violence as a public health problem. Currently, she is developing a project that will describe patterns of homicide victimization among African American females, while also attempting to develop a grass-roots violence-prevention program in conjunction with local organizations in Atlanta.

DARNELL F. HAWKINS, Ph.D., is a professor, Department of African American Studies and Sociology, Faculty Affiliate, Criminal Justice Department, University of Illinois at Chicago. His areas of specialization include criminology/ deviance, sociology of law, race and ethnic relations, applied sociology and public analysis, and survey research methodology.

MARTHA N. HILL, Ph.D., R.N., is an associate professor, Johns Hopkins University School of Nursing, and adjunct associate professor, Johns Hopkins University School of Medicine, Division of Internal Medicine. She has an extensive background in all aspects of high blood pressure (HBP) control. Her activities range from establishing and managing community-based HBP detection and control programs and nurse-run clinics through writing and speaking about patient and professional education to promote HBP control.

CAMILLE A. JONES, M.D., M.P.H, is Director, Epidemiology Program, Division of Kidney, Urologic, and Hematologic Diseases, National Institute of Diabetes and Digestive and Kidney Diseases, National Institutes of Health, Bethesda, Maryland. Her research interests include the areas of racial differences in the epidemiology of end-stage renal disease, interstitial cystitis, and definition of population values for measures of renal function (creatinine, microalbuminuria).

DIONNE J. JONES, M.S.W., Ph.D., is a senior research associate/editor, the *Urban League Review,* Research Department, National Urban League, Washington, D.C. Her areas of expertise include research and evaluation and the analysis of sociocultural problems associated with high-risk and other students.

WOODROW JONES, Jr., Ph.D., M.P.H., is a professor of political science and Associate Dean of Liberal Arts at Texas A&M University. His areas of specialization include health policy, Black health care, and environmental health policy. He has published numerous articles and books on the issues of health care in Black America.

B. WAINE KONG, Ph.D., is the executive director of the Association of Black Cardiologists, Inc. He is also president of Medical Organization Management (MOM), Inc., a national consulting/management firm with headquarters in Miami, Florida. His research interests include quality-of-life monitoring in the treatment of chronic diseases and the survival of minority physicians in the current health care climate.

STEPHANIE KONG, M.D., is Vice President of Medical Affairs, Physicians Corporation of America, a national HMO with headquarters in Miami, Florida. She has been most influential in pioneering concepts to empower minority physicians to compete effectively in job and related areas.

DAVID M. LEVINE, M.D., Sc.D., M.P.H., is a professor and Director of Internal Medicine, Department of Medicine, School of Medicine, School of Hygiene and Public Health, Johns Hopkins University. His areas of concentration/expertise include preventive health behavior and risk reduction; long-term management and control of public-health chronic disease problems (e.g., hypertension); health manpower; and health services research, organization provision, quality, and costs of health care.

AGATHA G. LOWE, R.N., Ph.D., is a Visiting Associate Community Health Educator with the Chicago Cluster Group responsible for developing a Primary Health Care Curriculum for inner-city school children. She has been involved with the development and implementation of international health projects for Project HOPE.

MOHAMMED H. MAKAME, M.D., M.P.H., is a post-doctoral fellow at the W.H.O. Collaborating Center for Diabetes Registries, Research and Training, University of Pittsburgh. He is also a practicing diabetologist at the Mnazimmoja Referral Hospital, Zanzibar, Tanzania. His current research interests include the evaluation of factors associated with the development of diabetes in African-heritage populations and the development of diabetes intervention programs for African countries.

RON C. MANUEL, Ph.D., is an associate professor of sociology, Department of Sociology and Anthropology, Howard University. He teaches courses in the sociology of aging and statistics. His current research focuses on identifying the social psychological interactants with personal health behaviors influencing health and longevity.

SINGLETON B. McALLISTER, J.D., is a senior legislative counsel with the national law firm of Shaw, Pittman, Potts, and Throwbridge of Washington, D.C., which is legal counsel to the National Association of Black Cardiologists, National Medical Association, and National Association for Sickle Cell Disease. She previously served as senior counsel to the U.S. House of Representatives Committee on the Budget; Special Assistant to the late Congressman Mickey Leland; Legislative Director to Congressman William H. Gray, III; and aide to former Congressman Parren J. Mitchell (then Chairman of the House Small Business Committee). She also served as Vice President of the organization of Women and Government Relations.

STEPHEN DALE McLEOD, M.D., is a fellow at the Doheny Eye Institute of the University of Southern California in Los Angeles. His ophthalmologic research and clinical emphasis is on diseases of the cornea and the anterior segment.

KERMIT B. NASH, M.S.W., Ph.D., is a professor of social work at the University of North Carolina, Chapel Hill. He is also the principal investigator of the Psychosocial Research Division and of a grant on the impact of mutual support and self-help on adults with sickle cell disease at the Duke-UNC Comprehensive Sickle Cell Center. His major areas of specialization include health, mental health, chronic conditions, and groups.

MAURICE F. RABB, M.D., is a professor of ophthalmology, Department of Ophthalmology, University of Illinois at Chicago; Chief, Division of Ophthalmology, Mercy Hospital and Medical Center, Chicago, Illinois; Chief of Medical Retina Service, Illinois Masonic Medical Center, Chicago, Illinois; and Medical Director, National Society to Prevent Blindness.

ANTONIO A. RENE, Ph.D., is an assistant professor of epidemiology at Tulane University School of Public Health. His research interests include environmental assessment, environmental attitudes, and the social epidemiology of diseases that affect African Americans.

VERONICA A. ROBERTS, Ph.D., is Director of Chapter 1 Evaluation Unit, Research and Evaluation Branch, District of Columbia Public Schools. Her areas of expertise include research in learning and cognition, employing a variety of developmental theories.

JEFFREY M. ROSEMAN, M.D., Ph.D., M.P.H., is an associate professor of epidemiology at the School of Public Health, University of Alabama at Birmingham (UAB). He is currently director of the Jefferson County Juvenile Diabetes Registry and of the UAB Center for Risk Assessment and Diabetes Prevention. He is an investigator in a 10-year longitudinal study of gestational diabetes in African Americans.

JULIE C. RUSSELL, Ph.D., M.P.H., is an epidemiologist, National Center for Injury Prevention and Control, Centers for Disease Control and Prevention, U.S. Public Health Service. Currently, her research focuses on behavioral risk factors, injuries to adolescents, and surveillance methods related to motor-vehicle injuries.

JOSEPH TELFAIR, Dr.P.H., M.S.W., M.P.H., is an assistant professor, Department of Maternal and Child Health, School of Public Health, University of North Carolina, Chapel Hill. His areas of specialization include public health sociology; health education; evaluation research; and health issues of children, families, people of color and the poor.

EUGENE S. TULL, M.P.H., Dr.P.H., is an assistant professor of epidemiology at the Graduate School of Public Health and the W.H.O. Collaborating Center for Diabetes Registries, Research and Training, University of Pittsburgh. His research interests include the evaluation of the factors associated with Type 1 diabetes mortality in African Americans, assessment of environmental and genetic factors associated with Type 1 diabetes frequency in African-heritage populations, and the development of intervention programs to change life-style risk factors for diabetes and other chronic diseases.

JOHN OBIOMA UKAWUILULU, Ph.D., is a research associate/project director in the Department of Psychology, George Washington University. He is also a research associate and adjunct assistant professor at the Howard University Research and Training Center and the Department of Sociology/Anthropology, Howard University. His current research interests include age-related trends of health practices and the sociological analysis of minority individuals with disabilities.

DAVID R. WILLIAMS, M.P.H., Ph.D., is an associate professor, Department of Sociology; an associate research scientist, Survey Research Center, Institute for Social Research; and a faculty associate, African American Mental Health Research Center, at the University of Michigan. He specializes in the study of socioeconomic and race differences in health status. His publications have dealt with variations in mental and physical health by race and poverty, social support and health, and religion and mental health.